THREE
SECONDS
UNTIL MIDNIGHT

S. HATFILL, R. COULLAHAN, & J. WALSH

Cover design by Ivica Jandrijevic
Interior layout and design by www.writingnights.org
Book preparation by Chad Robertson

ISBN: 978-170-0120298
LIBRARY OF CONGRESS CATALOGING-IN-PUBLICATION DATA:
NAMES: Hatfill, Steven; Coullahan, Robert; Walsh Jr. John., authors
TITLE: Three Seconds Until Midnight / S. Hatfill, R. Coullahan, & J. Walsh
DESCRIPTION: Independently Published, 2019
IDENTIFIERS: ISBN 978-170-0120298 (Perfect bound) |
SUBJECTS: | Non-Fiction | Emergency and Disaster planning | Global pandemic |
Public Health |
CLASSIFICATION: Pending
LC record pending

Printed in the United States of America.
Printed on acid-free paper.

24   23   22   21   20   19   18   17   8   7   6   5   4   3   2   1

Dedicated to the Memory of William C. Patrick III
Soldier, Scientist, and Patriot

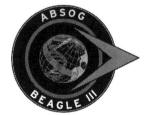

The single biggest threat to man's continued dominance on the planet is the virus.

—Dr Joshua Lederberg
1958 Nobel Prize in Physiology or Medicine.

CONTENTS

TABLE OF FIGURES

FOREWORD

THIS VOLUME IS CO-AUTHORED by 3 highly qualified authors, each of whom has extensive experience in disaster planning and epidemic response. It starts with the basic problem of emerging RNA viruses and then uses the 1918 influenza pandemic as a case study while incidentally covering many other aspects of the problems of disaster medicine and pandemic infections.

RNA viruses are the most variable of viruses and influenza is particularly problematic for reasons described in this book. The first half of the book deals with specifics such as the problem of a highly variable agent that is spread by the respiratory and contact routes, with the history of a pandemic that infected much of the world carrying a 1-10% case fatality rate.

In 1918, influenza penetrated every continent except Antarctica, wreaking havoc even in tropical Africa (unharvested manioc) and the Arctic (Eskimos unable to fish and hunt). In the absence of control, prophylaxis or treatment, the most developed areas suffered even more. The 1918 influenza, even with the less rapid transportation of the time, was causing epidemic disease in Europe within 3 months. Today, with airplane travel, the agent would be widely disseminated within days. The 1918 disease was fulminant with death occurring as soon as 24-48 hours. The same would hold today without an organization of control strategies, development of vaccines, or effective antivirals.

This book attacks the problem of control without vaccines or antiviral drugs. Vaccines would require 3-9 months to develop for a new strain of influenza even though we understand how to make influenza vaccines. Even assuming a vaccine could be rapidly available, it would still require testing and distribution. We have one good antiviral, oseltamivir; it is available in limited amounts, must be given within 24-48 hours of onset to be effective, and resistant strains of the organism arise readily. Thus, physical barriers would be the primary defense even today.

The book examines the need for home quarantine and protection of hospital contacts because of the relatively small amounts of vaccine and antivirals that are now available. Hospital care and home care would be quickly overwhelmed because of the number of patients and a lack of realistic instructions concerning personal protection, sufficient N95 respirators and expertise in using this basic mode of aerosol protection, and lack of sufficient numbers of protective gloves. The book then goes on to examine our shortfalls just for the U.S.

In the medical field there will be shortages of hospital beds, critical care facilities, clinics, physicians, nurses, drugs (and not just anti-influenza drugs), etc.

Many other effects must be planned for and remedied. First, there is the impact on electric power and petrol which will then lead to shortages of transportation which in turn will result in food shortages. The authors go on to examine the complexity of today's cities, megacities, and regional problems. There is attention to the role of the internet and its impact on disinformation and on control.

These and other problems are all treated well. The approach is comprehensive, beginning with an explication of the historical approaches, a discussion of the modern problem, and going on to outline the future solutions. The development of megacities, complex megaregions, globalization, and just-in-time inventories are only some of the complications not fully addressed in today's planning.

The conclusion is that none of the current approaches is funded or up to the needs of today. The sources of this problem are multiple. One is the involvement of non-medical planners such as politicians or DHS. Another is the lack of follow through or sustained effort. These approaches are also hampered by a simple lack of adequate technology. All the current efforts are piece meal and do not adequately take into account dealing with highly transmissible diseases.

The next lethal pandemic could well come from an RNA virus, perhaps with critical mutations. There are already known strains of avian influenza with high human mortality rates; they lack only increased transmissibility to become as dangerous as the 1918 influenza. I believe that it is only a matter of time until the next pandemic influenza strain or other RNA virus, results in a pandemic disease of high lethality.

This book throughout, and particularly in the last chapters, covers preparation for such a virus with modern and imaginative methods. It begins with surveillance for the earliest emergence using modern DNA-based technology operating in areas suspected to be incubators for emerging viruses. It goes on to disease surveillance in populations and modern methods of response from individual patient containment and care to the disposal of corpses. It partially relies on some methods and equipment developed by the DoD and modified for civilian use. Possibly current public health practitioners will resist the intrusion of military solutions, but they only need examine case studies of recent outbreaks of influenza (Mexico, 1999, spread of epidemic before acknowledged) and Ebola (extensive resources deployed in West Africa for its control and medical care of staff-infections while caring for evacuated patients in modern U.S. hospitals).

A partial antidote for this lies in the concept of a "fusion center" which would serve to coordinate several facets of surveillance, dispatch "ground truth" verification teams on short notice, and have experienced teams available to deal with incipient epidemics.

One of the most interesting approaches is the concept of trains equipped for dealing with highly infectious, lethal viruses. The history of medical-care trains dates to the 1850's and they were most recently used in WW2 by the French. The proposed trains would provide housing and support for the medical crew, cars for the safe care of infected patients, provision for water, food preparation, ambulances for transport of patients to the train, etc. These trains would provide a surge capacity to many areas. In addition, they would allow treatment to be brought to areas such as inner cities with inadequate facilities. They provide none of the rapidity of aeromedical resources, but have a dimension of capacity and ground mobility useful in providing patient care in the numbers needed at sites.

Throughout, the authors emphasize rapid responses, adequate numbers for response, and personnel trained for hazardous infection work with multidisciplinary talents. They also point out that this can only be achieved with trained, dedicated personnel and not with a roster of people to call for epidemiological and patient care responses. The book does not attempt to cover control of the zoonotic aspect of diseases.

C.J. Peters MD (COL) Ret.
Former Chief; Medical Division and Disease Assessment Division, USAMRIID.
Former Head; Special Pathogens Branch, Center for Disease Control and Prevention
Director; Biodefense UTMB Center for Biodefense and Emerging Infectious Diseases
Author; (1998), *Virus Hunter: Thirty Years of Battling Hot Viruses Around the World.*

PREFACE

THIS BOOK IS A STORY ABOUT both the past and the future and it deals with an extremely serious respiratory disease called Influenza. While many equate Influenza or the "flu" with the "common cold," it is important to realize that these are two very different infectious disorders. The "common cold" is caused by over 100 different viruses that attack the lining of the nose and throat and while miserable, it rarely causes serious complications. In contrast, some Influenza viruses can cause serious and sometimes fatal lung infections with the potential to cause devastatingly lethal global pandemics (infections that spread to multiple countries).

In March of 1918, a dangerous strain of the Influenza virus suddenly appeared in a small rural area of Kansas. The strain became pandemic and by late June in Europe, it transformed itself into a rampant pulmonary disease with catastrophic lung damage. Many victims turned purple from respiratory failure and died within a day from the onset of their symptoms. This new lethal variant quickly spread around the world and it went on to become one of the three deadliest plagues ever recorded in human history. More individuals died of Influenza in the first 11-months of the 1918 Influenza outbreak than during the 4-years of the Medieval "Black Death" caused by the Bubonic Plague in the 1300's.

From 1996 until 2014 the United States has spent a conservative $79 billion towards a National Biological Defense.[1] Yet in 2014, the Government demonstrated that it could not properly implement a simple syndromic surveillance system at five U.S. airports to screen for possible Ebola cases from West Africa. This event prompted us to examine 18-years of recorded GAO (Government Accountability Office) reports and testimony to determine the current state of U.S. preparedness for another lethal 1918-type Influenza pandemic. What we found was billions of wasted dollars, the purchase of defective equipment, out-of-date pandemic supplies, conflicting national guidelines, and the massive stockpiling of poorly chosen antiviral drugs with a questionable effectiveness in a pandemic. These stockpiled drugs remain a major feature of the US Government's 2015 (updated 2017) Influenza Pandemic Response Plan. They are to be used as a stopgap measure until a new protective Influenza vaccine can be manufactured and disseminated to the American population.

In this respect, a very limited supply of any new vaccine may not be ready for 1-3 months after the start of a serious Influenza outbreak and there are only 81-million doses of the stockpiled antiviral drugs. In addition, the federal plan unrealistically shifts the most severe problems of a pandemic response to the local authorities of our towns and cities. Unfortunately, most local authorities demonstrate an inconsistent planning for how they would manage a very conservative 1918-type scenario involving 91,473,620 infected Americans with a projected national total of 1,903,000 Influenza deaths caused by a 1918-type Influenza strain.

Our study determined that the U.S. does not currently have a public health workforce sufficient to manage this type of event. Our hospitals do not have the "surge" medical personnel necessary to take care of overwhelming mass casualties and no significant dedicated national pandemic training programs are underway. Even if sufficient drugs and vaccines were present, we do not have consistently reliable plans for how to distribute these through the local communities in time to make a difference. With only limited initial antiviral drugs and vaccine supplies, we lack a logical well-thought out plan for deciding who in society is to be prioritized for treatment.

While highly touted by the Government, the current National Pandemic Influenza Plan will at best, only ensure that U.S. politicians, the military, and the "essential" personnel of the Federal and State bureaucracies have first access to the limited drugs and the initial doses of vaccine. This will be followed weeks later, by the vaccination of healthcare workers and emergency services personnel. By this time, the peak of the epidemic may have already passed.

In 2015, the U.S. Director of National Intelligence clearly expressed the effect of such a pandemic when he stated, "If a highly pathogenic avian influenza virus, like H7N9, were to become easily transmissible among humans, the outcome could be far more disruptive than the great influenza pandemic of 1918. It could lead to global economic losses, the unseating of governments, and the disturbance of geopolitical alliances."[2]

There is a consensus among scientists that another 1918-event will eventually happen again. As we will explain further, based on the current understanding of emerging infectious diseases, there are some disturbing signs that this may happen sooner rather than later.

As a nation we are still unprepared.

NOTES FOR THE PREFACE

[1] Tara Kirk Sell and Matthew Watson. Federal Agency Biodefense Funding, FY2013-FY2014 Biosecur Bioterror. 2013 September; 11(3): 196–216. doi: 10.1089/bsp.2013.0047

[2] Clapper, J. (2015). Statement for the Record, Worldwide Threat Assessment of the US Intelligence Community, Senate Armed Services Committee.

PROLOGUE

FOLLOWING THE END OF THE SECOND WORLD WAR, a group of physicists from the Manhattan atomic bomb project began to publish a journal they called "The Bulletin of the Atomic Scientists". The first publication of the journal occurred in 1947 and its cover depicted an artist's rendition of a fictional "Doomsday Clock". The clock represented the scientists' perceived risk for a catastrophic global nuclear war. The time of "Doomsday" was designated to be at 12:00 AM and the clock's hands were set at 7-minutes to midnight.

Since 1947, the "Doomsday Clock" has been set forward and backward every few years. Following the first test explosion of the fission/fusion thermonuclear Hydrogen Bomb in 1953, the countdown clock was set ahead to 2-minutes until midnight. In 2007, the clock was set further ahead to include the projected effects of an ever-expanding world population. For several years the lock's minute hand had been set back to 3-minutes before Midnight, but with the problems in the Mideast and North Korea, the clock was again reset to 2-minutes.

In all practicality, if the nuclear scientists responsible for the Doomsday Clock were knowledgeable in the biology of infectious diseases, the countdown might have been set to three-seconds until Midnight. The reasons for this are complex and yet still easy to understand. Basically, they involve an ever-expanding human population living under historically unprecedented high densities with an over-dependence on complex systems for the supply of food and other services to any nation's major urban areas.

From 1918 to 1960, the total number of people living on Earth has increased from 1.8 billion to 3 billion. By 2011 this figure had reached 7 billion and it is projected to rise to 8 billion by 2028 and to 9.8 billion by 2050. This population growth has been accompanied by an increasing population density and infrastructure complexity in the major urban areas.

For at least 4000 years of human history, high-density cities were the historical exception and even as recently as 250 years ago, only 3% of the total human population lived in metropolitan areas. By the end of the 20th century this figure had risen to 47% with a good fraction of the world's population living in what are now called Megacities. These Megacities are defined as metropolitan areas with a total population in excess of 10-million people and a minimum population density of at least 2,000 persons per square kilometer.

To further complicate the situation, more than two-billion people now live around these megacities in ever-sprawling high-density "shanty towns" with unsanitary conditions, a lack of health care, insufficient housing, malnutrition, and minimal access to education and the regional economy. Such conditions are ideal for the spread of a contagious infectious disease. If these slum areas became infected with a future 1918-type of Influenza virus, the global death toll from this event could well be unimaginable.

Yet there is an even greater problem and it is one that remains largely hidden and only partially understood by the small number of mathematicians who study very complex systems.

Today in the United States, most large cities contain no more than a 72-hour supply of consumables for their population. The meat, fruit, milk, vegetables, bread, pasta, and rice do not just "magically" appear in the supermarkets and at the corner grocery stores. The availability of these items is dependent on a highly complex system of agricultural production, food manufacturing and processing, central wholesalers, regional distributors, and individual supermarkets. These in turn, are linked by a complicated system of timetables for cargo trains, ships, and trucks.

Consequently, the food delivery system of our cities depends on an even more complex fuel transportation network involving individual gasoline stations and truck stops. This in turn, is dependent upon fuel manufacturing by the refineries which are supplied with crude oil by another complex system involving some 187,000 miles of pipelines, ships at sea, and tanker trucks that themselves are dependent upon the fuel that is being refined.

All these systems are irrevocably interlinked and the "just in time" inventories of the necessary metropolitan commodities depend upon a reliable and functioning infrastructure and work force. What has emerged from the studies of complex systems is the premise that there is a critical point where a sudden percentage loss of a region's work force from either war or disease, could initiate a series of catastrophic infrastructure failures that would destroy a large metropolitan region's functionality. This would be followed by a sudden, rapid collapse to a lower degree of societal complexity.

Analogous events of this type were witnessed in 2005 during the tragedy of Hurricane Katrina and in 2017 after Hurricane Maria in Puerto Rico. While these involved only a localized infrastructure collapse that affected only a specific region, it helped to emphasize the dangers inherent with living inside a complex urban infrastructure. Most particularly, what could happen if such a collapse occurs over multiple large geographical areas as a result of a rapidly spreading lethal infectious disease. In this case, the surrounding states or regions may be unable to provide mutual assistance during and after such an event.

Primarily because their own infrastructures may have collapsed as well.

Aside from the dangers inherent in modern infrastructure complexity, there is another major difference between 1918 and today with respect to Influenza. In 1918, the Influenza pandemic spread by steam ship and by railroad. Consequently, it required a time span of some 11-months to completely encircle the globe. However, today a virus can be carried anywhere in the world within 24-hours. This is significant because the planning by the U.S. Government is under the assumption that there will be several-weeks warning that a global Influenza pandemic is underway. As a result, the WHO has established six Pandemic-Alert Levels (recently modified) to give national authorities time to prepare. The U.S. Government has developed an even more complicated color-coded pandemic warning chart. However, because of air travel, this type of a pandemic alert could be worthless if a highly pathogenic Influenza strain breaks out virtually everywhere at the same time.

Colorful Government charts, a stockpile of expired (but FDA extended drugs), and an abundance of overly optimistic paper plans, will not be able to provide the actual surge of medical resources that would enable a local community to manage a 1918-type event. As we will explain, under current doctrine, most cities and towns will be largely left to themselves to manage their outbreaks. Consequently, with no immediate vaccine or effective drug treatment, Americans will be forced to employ the same non-pharmaceutical public health countermeasures that were used during the 1918 Pandemic.

Finally, it is not only the Influenza virus that should provoke concern. The historic numeric expansion of our species has brought humans into an ever-increasing contact with previously unknown animal viruses. For centuries, these viruses were isolated deep inside vast forests and jungles, but they are now emerging into human populations at an alarming rate.

The current total world population is now estimated to be 7.5 billion people, and no other species of large mammal known to science, has ever achieved such an unnaturally high global population density. The net result is that everyone alive today, is participating in an on-going real-world biological experiment.

We cannot know for certain how this experiment will continue to play out, but with respect to an eventual severe pandemic of some type, it is reasonable to believe that it will not have a good outcome.

SECTION

I

AN INTRODUCTION TO VIRUSES AND EMERGING INFECTIOUS DISEASES

1

INFLUENZA AND OTHER RNA VIRUSES

TO BETTER UNDERSTAND THE PREVIOUS 1918 INFLUENZA PANDEMIC and its relevance for today, it is first necessary to understand a few things about viruses. More specifically, the viruses that fall under the Influenza Group A classification. This will help the reader to make their own judgement as to the seriousness of what is described in this book.

The first thing to understand about viruses is that although they are indeed a definite biological entity that can both replicate and change with time, a virus cannot be considered to be "alive." A virus of any type is simply a very small assembly of complicated molecules that include proteins, RNA molecules (or DNA molecules in some viruses), and sometimes fat and sugar molecules. Although these biological molecules are highly organized, a virus is incapable of any form of energy production or biochemical metabolism. A virus is simply an inert collection of chemicals until it penetrates and enters into a living cell of its host.

Once it is inside a suitable cell, viruses turn into the ultimate parasites of nature as they quickly subvert and force the infected cell to perform a series of virus-driven biochemical reactions which leads to the formation of hundreds of new viral particles. These new mature "daughter" viruses are released from the now damaged or dying cell, to infect even more cells within the host. As this process amplifies, these new daughter viruses are eventually shed out into the environment to find more individual hosts in which to replicate.

However, without the biochemical machinery already normally operating inside a living cell, viruses are nothing more than a precise collection of complex inanimate molecules. Indeed, viruses have been constructed in the laboratory by adding and incubating chemicals and specific proteins in the correct sequence. These "artificial" viruses are fully functional, and they replicate and even evolve when incubated together with suitable live cells in tissue culture.

VIRUSES ARE EXTREMELY SMALL

The viruses that use molecules of RNA as the material for their genetic "blueprints" are tiny in size, extremely tiny. They are 100 times smaller than bacteria and 1000 times smaller than a human cell. A human cell itself is 10 times smaller than the diameter of a single human hair.

As far back as 1892, scientists had realized that there were infectious disease-causing agents much smaller than bacteria that could not be seen with the microscopes of the time. This was discovered by passing the infectious fluid from the leaves of virus-infected and diseased tobacco plants through special porcelain filters that filtered out all bacteria. The scientists found that the strained and filtered fluid could still cause disease when it was applied to healthy tobacco plants. A century ago, what we now call "viruses" were known simply as "filterable agents."

By the early 1900's, scientists had discovered that the causative infectious agent of animal Foot-and-Mouth Disease was "filterable", as was the causative agent of Yellow Fever. In 1903, the causative agent of Rabies was determined to be "filterable", followed by the same discovery for Smallpox in 1906 and Polio in 1908. However, it took another 40-years for scientists to be able to actually see what these various viruses looked like. This was made possible by advances in physics, electronics, and manufacturing processes, together with a major 12-year effort by Dr. Ernst Ruska and his colleagues to create the first powerful electron microscopes. These experimental instruments could eventually resolve and photograph objects as small as 2 nanometers (or two billionths of a meter) in size.

The ability of scientists to finally grow viruses in cell culture and now to directly observe them, allowed a classification to be made based on their appearance. This quickly yielded numerous new and important discoveries, and from the 1970's onward, this knowledge exploded as the first tools of modern molecular biology were developed and expanded. Although there is still much to learn, scientists now understand a great deal about the structure of viruses and their epidemic potential. Particularly for the problems associated with the viruses that use ribonucleic acid (or RNA) as the chemical code for their genetic material. These RNA molecules contain the individual "blueprints" or "genes" that carry the instructions that allow viruses to replicate and complete their infectious life-cycle once they have infected a suitable cell.[1]

Viral Tropism

Different viruses can infect different life forms and specific viruses usually spread in specific ways. Some plant viruses are transmitted from plant to plant by insects that feed on infected plant sap. Some animal viruses are carried by different species of blood-sucking insects which transmit these viruses from animal to animal, from animal to man, and sometimes from human to human. Some human and animal viruses are transmitted by close contact, or they can enter the body through food or water. Some are transmitted by an exposure to infected blood or are sexually transmitted within a species. Some viruses are excreted out into the environment through an infected host's feces or urine. Some viruses like Influenza, are spread by infectious coughs and sneezes or through eye, or by hand contact with virus-contaminated surfaces. Some viruses like Smallpox and Ebola, may shed into the environment through the skin.

The ability of a virus to infect a certain type of animal or plant cell is known as *viral tropism,* and this is a critical factor in determining the outcome of any viral infection. Some viruses exhibit a broad tropism and they can infect many types of cells and tissues in several different species of animal. Other viruses may infect only a single type of tissue in a single species.[2] Most human viruses are not able to infect other animals, and most animal viruses cannot infect humans. This is termed the "*host range*" of a virus. A virus may have a narrow host range, meaning the virus is capable of infecting only one or a few species, or it may exhibit a broad host range and can infect many different types of animals. A few viruses are known that can even infect both plants and animals.[3]

Much of this tropism is caused by the fact that to enter a living cell and hijack its metabolism, a virus first must have a special "key" to pass through its host cell's outer protective cell membrane. This "key" is in the form of special proteins that protrude outward from the surface of the virus. Conversely, the receiving "lock" is made up of different molecules located on the outer surface of the host cell that is being attacked. If the protein "key" on the outside of the virus manages to fit into the surface molecule "lock" on the outside of a susceptible cell, the virus can attach itself and enter the cell to cause infection.

VIRUS REPLICATION INSIDE AN INFECTED CELL

The *RNA-dependent RNA polymerase* is a special viral protein enzyme that can read the RNA "blueprints" of a virus and create more copies of these "blueprints" using other normal molecules found inside the host's cells. From now on we will call this special molecule an "*RNA Replicase.*"[4] In the Influenza virus, this RNA Replicase is made up of three different, smaller, proteins called PB2, PB1, and PA. There is an RNA Replicase molecule attached to each one of the eight different RNA "blueprints" that the Influenza virus needs to make new copies of itself. This includes the actual instructions for making copies of the RNA Replicase itself once the virus is inside a suitable cell.

If the replication machinery is working optimally, new copies of the "blueprints" for the Influenza virus can be produced inside a host cell every 0.4 seconds. However, the RNA Replicase is not very accurate when it copies its RNA "blueprints" and it makes roughly one mistake in each copy it produces. In addition, unlike the very specialized Replicase proteins used by normal animal cells, the viral RNA Replicase lacks the ability to proofread the new blueprints it has created and check these against the original viral RNA instructions it has copied.

This means that every time any RNA virus makes a copy of itself, each of its daughter viruses may contain one random error (called a mutation), somewhere in every copy. This is called "Error-prone Replication" and it is important for understanding how Influenza, Ebola, and many other different RNA viruses, function in nature.[5]

Following their replication, the many copies of these viral "blueprints," are transported to sites in the cell where proteins are made. Here, the various component viral proteins are manufactured in quantity, and these self-assemble into new daughter viruses. The process is very quick, and the first new daughter viruses are released from the infected host cell within the first 6-hours after initial infection. In fact, a single infectious virus particle inside a cell may produce on average, some 100,000 daughter viruses within the first 10-hours. Within a few days, the number of viral particles in an infected animal or human, may be as high as 10.[12]

With respect to Influenza, these new viruses are first released from the damaged host cell, and then released outside the body into the environment by the coughing and sneezing droplets of virus-laden respiratory and nasal mucous. These escaped Influenza daughter viruses are now free to infect other healthy animals or humans.

ERROR-PRONE RNA VIRUS REPLICATION AND THE "QUASI-SPECIES" CONCEPT

Because of this error-prone viral replication, scientists now understand that a population of newly constructed RNA viruses are not made of daughter viruses with identical blueprints, but rather they contain large numbers of very slightly different viruses. These are called a "quasi-species".[6] The consequence of this is that viral infections are not initiated by a single virus, but by a swarm of daughter viruses each with slightly different properties because of the different mistakes in their "blueprints" that were made when they were first created. Thus, the new daughter viruses that are released from a host encompass a broad spectrum of mutants which may have very slightly different properties.[7]

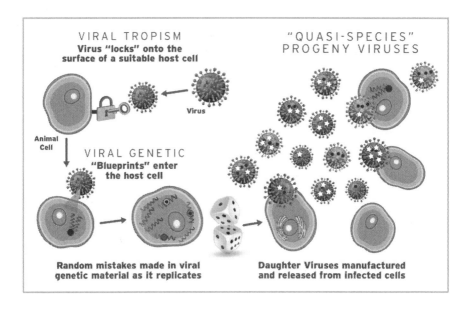

Figure 1. *Error-Prone RNA Virus Replication and Release from an Infected Cell.*

The ability of any RNA virus to produce a prodigious number of slightly different strains through mutation, provides a powerful advantage for survival. While some of the daughter viruses carry mutations that are not compatible with continued virus replication, other daughter viruses may have mutations that make them better selected to replicate in a new host.[8]

THE INFLUENZA VIRUS

The word *Influenza*, dates from the Middle Ages when the physicians of that time recognized that a mysterious fever and respiratory disease would appear every 20-30 years and spread across Europe. Physicians at the time thought that the heavens above them influenced these infectious disease outbreaks and the name Influenza means "Influence" in reference to the night-time stars overhead.

There are four Genera of Influenza virus termed A, B, C, and the newly discovered D group (which is an Influenza virus that only affects cattle). Of all these, the Influenza A group of viruses are the ones that worry scientists the most. Influenza A is a bird virus that over time, has repeatedly jumped into several different species of animal, including humans. Birds carry all but two of the known strains of the Influenza A, including several strains that have become well-adapted to man.

This process of a bird Influenza virus adapting to infect humans is not a straightforward proposition. A bird virus is designed to function at the higher body temperature commonly found in birds, not the cooler body temperature of humans. In addition, the host cell proteins that the Influenza virus uses to replicate inside birds are slightly different in humans, and the receptor molecules the virus uses to bind to the cells of a bird, may be different in human cells. All of this makes the transition of a normal bird influenza virus into a virus that can infect humans, difficult.

However, when this does happen, it may cause a highly lethal human infection. Fortunately, usually during this type of event, the virus has not fully adapted to man and it lacks the ability to be efficiently transmitted from human to human without further mutations. Consequently, while lethal, these types of "micro-outbreaks" usually die out fairly quickly.

In birds, most strains of the Influenza A virus do not make these animals ill. Rather than attack the upper respiratory tract, these avian Influenza strains infect the bird's intestines which then shed the virus into the environment through infected bird droppings. Waterfowl are notorious for transmitting the Influenza viruses this way, and when healthy birds ingest water or grass seeds contaminated with fresh bird droppings, they can become mildly infected. Sometimes the infected droppings can infect humans through a mechanism called "*viral spillover*." This will be discussed later.

To understand how a virus that infects the guts of birds can infect the cells lining the human airway, it is necessary to understand a little bit more about the Influenza A virus. For this we need to once again discuss the concept of *viral tropism*.

As previously mentioned, the ability of a mammalian virus is usually limited with respect to the types of cells and the species of animal that it can infect. In the Influenza virus, this tropism is caused by a sugar-containing protein called Hemagglutinin that is found on the outside structure of the virus (Figure 2). This Hemagglutinin protein acts as the special "key" that allows the virus to bind to and enter the live cells of a host animal.

The "lock" that the viral Hemagglutinin "key" recognizes on normal cells is called Sialic Acid. This is actually an entire family of nine-carbon acidic sugar molecules that are naturally present on the outside of some animal cells. These may be part of a larger outside sugar chain connected to the host cell's surface or attached to specific proteins on the cell surface. All Influenza A virus strains recognize a particular type of Sialic Acid as the specific "lock" for their viral Hemagglutinin "key."

Because there are different types of Sialic Acid, there are also numerous variants of the Influenza Hemagglutinin protein. This diversity is an important factor that determines which animal species a given strain of Influenza virus can successfully infect.

Until recently, scientists recognized only 16 different Hemagglutinin proteins named H1 through H16. Because Influenza is primarily a disease of birds, it is not surprising that different avian Influenza viruses use one of these H1 to H16 proteins.

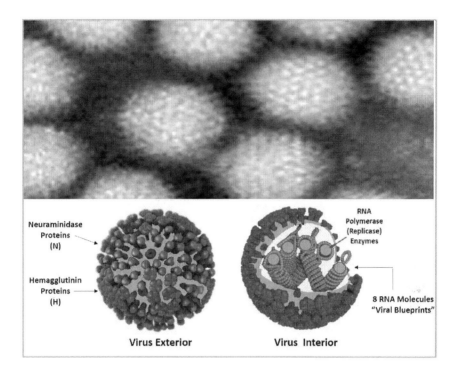

Figure 2. *Influenza electron microscope image and major virus components.*[9]

However, the H2 Hemagglutinin protein can also be found on Influenza strains that can infect both humans and birds, and the H3 Hemagglutinin protein is found in Influenza strains that can infect humans, pigs, horses, and birds. In this respect, the H1, H2, and H3 Influenza A viruses have all caused previous major human pandemics.

In 2012, an additional H17 Hemagglutinin protein was discovered in fruit bats. Then in 2013, a new H18 Hemagglutinin protein was discovered in a bat in Peru. Further studies have shown that bats have receptors in their respiratory and digestive tracts that can support the binding of both avian and human influenza viruses, and as in the case of ducks and pigs, it is thought that this may create conditions that enable the virus to share genetic information to create new strains that could infect humans.[10] This is a worry because the number of different bat species encompasses ¼ of all the known different species of mammal on the planet, and bats are already known to carry some of the most lethal viruses known to medical science.

There is a second major protein found on the surface of the Influenza A viruses that must be discussed, and this is called the Neuraminidase enzyme (NA or N), This helps the Influenza virus penetrate the protective mucous of the respiratory tract of its host animal during infection. Once the Influenza virus has entered a cell and it is replicating and self-assembling into new daughter viral "quasi-species", the Neuraminidase enzyme on the surface of the virus will also act to release the newly manufactured viruses from the host cell so they can spread to infect other cells.

There are 9 different types of numbered Neuraminidase proteins. As will be discussed later, these are the targets for the antiviral drugs Tamiflu and Relenza which bind to the Neuraminidase protein to inhibit the release of the new "quasi-species" of daughter virus.

Thus, the different strains of Influenza A can be classified by the type of Hemagglutinin and Neuraminidase proteins that are on the surface of the virus; such as H1N1, H1N2 or H2N1. Leaving out the Hemagglutinin proteins 17 and 18 which are found in Bats, the avian influenza viruses represent a diverse group that can be divided into 144 subtypes, based on different combinations of the 16 variants of the Hemagglutinin proteins and the 11 variants of the Neuraminidase proteins.

The Influenza A strain that caused the catastrophic 1918-pandemic carried the H1 Hemagglutinin protein. It can bind to the cells in the guts of birds and it can also bind to the type of Sialic Acid found on the cells of the human upper respiratory tract. It can also bind to human red blood cells and to the Sialic Acid molecules found in the upper respiratory tract of pigs. The 1918 virus also carried the N1 Neuraminidase protein on its outer surface. Therefore the 1918 virus has been classified as an H1N1 strain.

Following the severe 1918 H1N1 Pandemic, there was a much less severe 1957 pandemic caused by the H2N2 strain, a moderately severe 1968 pandemic involving an H3N2 strain originating out of Hong

Kong, and a 1977 Pandemic caused by a mild strain of the H1N1 virus. Most recently, a 2009 pandemic was caused by an H1N1 strain that appeared to have passed through pigs. This was incorrectly given the name "swine flu" by the national media. This 2009 pandemic was an important outbreak because initially there was a great worry that this particular H1N1 strain was a highly lethal virus. Although this did not prove to be the case, it dramatically showed that the United States was still unprepared for a 1918-type event. By the time a vaccine became available for this new H1N1 strain, the pandemic was essentially over.[11,12]

Why do we keep having influenza outbreaks, especially repeated seasonal outbreaks from strains such as H1N1? The major reason is because of the ability and propensity of the Influenza A viruses to modify (drift) or replace (shift) the structures of their H and N proteins. Because these two proteins are the main targets for the human immune system, any slight changes in the viral "blueprints" for these proteins can have an effect on how well an individual can fight off the virus after an exposure. In this respect, scientists have categorized the Influenza Group A viruses into both Seasonal and Pandemic types.

SEASONAL INFLUENZA

The annual seasonal strains of Influenza are created by the continuing small mutations that occur in the predominant Influenza viruses that are constantly circulating between humans and birds. This process is called *Antigenic Drift*. These mutations cause changes to the virus's genetic "blueprints" that result in small changes in the viral H or N proteins. Because of the virus's error prone Replicase enzyme, Antigenic Drift is a continuous ongoing process that results in the emergence of new strain variants. Eventually one of the new variant strains becomes dominant which usually lasts for a few years, until a new variant strain emerges and replaces it.

As mentioned, Antigenic Drift occurs in the Influenza viruses that are already in worldwide circulation. The new H and N protein mutations allow these viruses to re-infect humans that were previously immune to the virus the year before. These new viruses then circulate around the world as they are spread by migrating birds flying on their north-south flyways (or by the travel of infected humans). This creates the natural seasonal nature of these Influenza outbreaks. It is the reason that the Influenza virus strains in the annual vaccine must be updated each year.

A single IHD (Infectious Human Dose) of influenza virus might be between 100 and 1,000 viral particles and during Seasonal Influenza outbreaks, millions of virus particles are shed in the nasal secretions from a single infected human. A single 0.1 μl (microliter) mucous droplet can contain more than 100 Influenza virus particles. In addition, during the early course of influenza infection, the virus can be found also in the blood, feces, and other body fluids. This all serves to increase the chances for the spread of infection during a seasonal Influenza outbreak.

Technically, Seasonal Influenza is a pandemic because it spreads out from one country to affect others. However, because this involves Influenza virus strains that are already known and just recirculating in a minor altered new form, they are called "Seasonal Influenza." The term "Pandemic Influenza" is reserved to describe something that is much more serious.

PANDEMIC INFLUENZA

In contrast to *Antigenic Drift*, what are referred to as the Pandemic Influenza viruses normally arise through a process known as *Antigenic Shift*. In this case, the viral H and N proteins on the virus are not the result of simple mutations caused by the normal error-prone "blueprint" copying. Instead, an Antigenic Shift occurs when two much different Influenza A strains exchange their specific genetic "blueprints" like players in a card game. This can occur when certain animals like pigs become simultaneously co-infected with both a wild bird Influenza virus together with a different human-adapted Influenza virus. When the two different strains of virus replicate in the same animal, the different viral "blueprints" get mixed up, and they recombined to form a brand new "hybrid" Influenza virus. These hybrid viruses can be extremely lethal because humans may not have any pre-existing immunity to them.

In Asia, it is common to house domestic chickens and ducks above pig pens on the large agricultural farms. In addition, the farmers keep ducks around their large fishponds. This agricultural method is called "polyculture" and it is a highly efficient farming practice. However, it also makes a perfect environment for viral trafficking and viral hybridization (mixing of genetic material) when wild birds and especially wild waterfowl, come into contact with the domesticated farm animals.

Studies have shown that approximately one out of four wild birds are naturally infected with some strain of Influenza virus, and it is common to find two or more major strains of the Influenza virus in their gut at the same time. Inside the gut, these viruses trade their gene segments ("blueprints") back and forth and these segments may occasionally recombine to form a completely new hybrid Influenza virus.

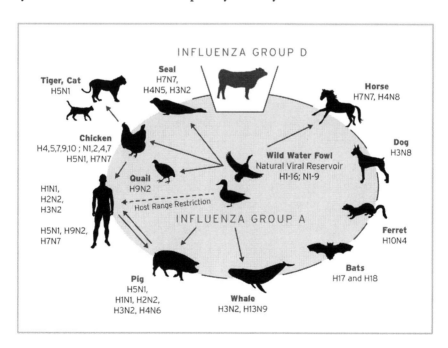

Figure 3. *Major Influenza Group A Subtypes. Species Jumps of Influenza A Virus Subtypes from Wild Waterfowl.*

Sometimes these new hybrid viruses may jump from wild waterfowl into domestic chickens with a lethal effect. These are called *Highly Pathogenic Avian Influenza* (HPAI) strains and they can occasionally be highly lethal to humans as well. Sometimes a new strain that is developed that can move from birds to pigs or horses and sometimes, a series of genetic recombination events can occur that create a multiple-hybrid Influenza virus containing a mixture of bird, human, and pig virus "blueprints." This can have particularly deadly consequences.

Again, the analogy is like a gambler who is rolling the dice. If the dice are thrown often enough, eventually a 7 or 11 will appear. If the gambler is throwing 10 dice at one, the chances of rolling a winning number are increased. The more Influenza virus strains there are circulating in nature and the more domestic chickens and pigs that there are being bred, the more chances there are for viral mixing, and the greater chance there is for a hybrid Influenza virus to be created with human pandemic potential.

This ability of the avian Influenza viruses to recombine to create new hybrid strains is a risk to man that might be being fueled by the current tremendous growth of the poultry industry.

Each year, some 51.4 billion chickens are artificially hatched, fattened up and slaughtered globally. In the United States alone, in less than 60 years, the number of broiler chickens raised yearly has skyrocketed from 580 million birds in the 1950s to nearly 9 billion today. Some farms contain as many as half a million birds living inside huge buildings or outdoors.[13,14,15] This transformation of the industry has been accompanied by a greater total load of Influenza A strains in the environment. With more of these RNA viruses circulating, there is an enormously greater chance for these viruses to recombine and adapt to man.[14]

As humans, it is important for us to realize that even though we are now heavily urbanized and greatly removed from natural wild areas, we still live in an ecological environment that we share with 62,305 other known species of vertebrate animals and possibly as many as 3,613,690 different types of viruses that can infect them. It is the nature of these viruses to constantly try to expand their host range and expand into different geographical areas. This is held in check by balanced animal populations and diverse ecological factors.

New strains of the Influenza A virus continue to emerge into man, and these are only one type of the many new viruses that have emerged into humans from the animal world in recent years. This will be discussed more in the next chapter.

Many different viruses other than Influenza are lurking in Nature with the potential to jump into humans. They are only waiting for the right conditions to make this leap.

NOTES FOR CHAPTER 1

[1] Crawford, Dorothy H. Viruses: Oxford University Press, USA; 2011. ISBN 0-19-957485-5.

[2] Raven, Peter H. (2008). "Biology 8th Edition". New York, McGraw-Hill.

[3] Hatfill, S.J., Von Wechmar, M.B., et.al. (1990) "Hybridization studies to localize a new insect picornavirus in aphid tissue sections". J. Inv. Path. 55;265-271.

[4] Vincent Racaniello, The error-prone ways of RNA synthesis, virology blog, http://www.virology.ws/2009/05/10/the-error-prone-ways-of-rna-synthesis/

[5] Domingo, E. (1978). Nucleotide sequence heterogeneity of an RNA phage population Cell, 13 (4), 735-744 DOI: 10.1016/0092-8674(78)90223-4

[6] Domingo E, Sobrino F., et.al. Quasispecies and molecular evolution of viruses. Rev Sci Tech. 2000 Apr; 19(1):55-63.

[7] Domingo, E. (1978). Nucleotide sequence heterogeneity of an RNA phage population Cell, 13 (4), 735-744 DOI: 10.1016/0092-8674(78)90223-4

[8] Nowak M., What is a quasispecies? Trends Ecol Evol. 1992 Apr; 7(4):118-21. doi: 10.1016/0169-5347(92)90145-2.

[9] https://www.cdc.gov/flu/professionals/laboratory/antigenic.htm

[10] Tong S., Donis, R. O., et.al. New World Bats Harbor Diverse Influenza A Viruses. PLOS: Pathogens. 9(10): e1003657

[11] 2009 GAO-10-73Monitoring and Assessing the Status of the National Pandemic Implementation Plan Needs Improvement.

[12] 2009 GAO-09-909T Gaps in Planning and Preparedness Need to be Addressed

[13] Big Chicken; Industrial Poultry Production in America http://www.pewtrusts.org/~/media/legacy/uploadedfiles/peg/publications/report/pegbigchickenjuly2011pdf.pdf

[14] "Free From Harm". https://freefromharm.org/animalagriculture/chicken-facts-industrydoesnt-want-know/

[15] Michael Greger. Bird Flu: A Virus of Our Own Hatching. 2006, Lantern Books ISBN 1590560981 (ISBN13: 9781590560983) http://birdflubook.com/

2

SOMETHING ALARMING
IS HAPPENING IN THE WORLD

FOLLOWING THE SECOND WORLD WAR, a series of rapid developments lulled medical science into an era of complacency for infectious disease research and public health. These developments included the discovery and use of antibiotics for bacterial infections, the polio vaccine, and the successful global program to eradicate smallpox.

For the next 40-years, medical science underwent a dramatic change as it now became focused on chronic conditions such as cancer, heart disease, and diabetes. The previous generations of infectious disease experts retired, infectious disease funding and research was reduced, and tropical medicine became a largely neglected curriculum in the medical schools. Then in the mid-70's, some unusual things began to happen.

In 1975, a cluster of cases thought to be Juvenile Rheumatoid Arthritis occurred in three towns in southeastern Connecticut. This included the towns of Lyme and Old Lyme. The condition turned out to be something much different and it took another 8-years to isolate the unusual bacteria that caused human "Lyme Disease" and discover that its transmission route was through ticks living on the blood of mice and deer. By 2017, Lyme Disease had spread out from its initial geographic area and it is now one of the most expanding infectious diseases in the United States.

One year after the first outbreak of Lyme Disease, a strange respiratory infection occurred in 221 people attending the US Bicentennial Convention held by the American Legion at the Bellevue Stratford Hotel in Philadelphia. A total of 33 people died and scientists at the Centers for Disease Control and Prevention (CDC) struggled for 6-months to isolate the unusual microorganism responsible for causing this "Legionnaires Disease". This was because the scientists involved in the search were mistakenly fixated on the idea that a virus was the cause of the disease. Eventually when chicken eggs were inoculated with preserved patient samples prepared without the normally added antibiotics, the bacteria that caused the disease were quickly isolated.

Then in 1976, the Ebola Virus was recognized after simultaneous outbreaks in Zaire (former Belgian Congo) and Sudan. The Ebola virus is highly lethal, and this first recognized outbreak was dramatic, and it received worldwide media attention. However, still unrecognized, another even-more lethal virus called HIV-1 was already silently spreading throughout the world. Unlike Ebola, the HIV-1 virus caused a slow progressive disease and it took years to kill its host. It would eventually be discovered that HIV-1 was the virus that caused AIDS.

By the mid-1990's, after decades of declining infectious disease mortality in the United States, increasing different types of bacteria began to develop a resistance to multiple antibiotics. Hospital-acquired infections become both more common and difficult to control, and the number of Americans dying from infectious diseases started to increase. On a global scale, the parasites that caused malaria were becoming increasingly drug-resistant, and the mosquitoes carrying this parasite became insecticide-resistant. The age-old scourge of Tuberculosis resurged in Russia accompanied by a resistance to most of the drugs able to treat this terrible malady. Even outbreaks of Whooping Cough (Pertussis) and Measles began to re-occur with an unusual frequency in the United States. Something serious seemed to be happening on a global scale. In response, a small number of scientists began to scramble to find the reasons for this apparent phenomenon.

The term EID or "Emerging Infectious Disease" refers to a previously unknown infectious microorganism that has suddenly appeared in a human population, or a known infectious disease that is rapidly increasing in its incidence or expanding its geographic range.[1] An EID usually has an identifiable source, which is most often a wild animal infected with a virus or bacterium that can infect humans, or in a worst case, one that has acquired the ability to efficiently transmit from person to person in a human population. An animal disease agent that can infect man is termed a *zoonosis,* and the RNA viruses represent the greatest risk for this type of event.

Of the 1,417 organisms (fungi, bacteria, parasites, protozoa, and viruses) that are known to infect humans, 58% of these are animal diseases that have jumped into man. Some 174 of these are considered newly emerging or reemerging infectious diseases. What is particularly worrying is that some 45 previously unknown new human infectious diseases have jumped from their normal animal hosts to man during the last 50-years. Recent historical reviews have confirmed this phenomenon and based on this data, some scientists estimate that 10–40 more new viruses may emerge into human populations over the next 20 years.[2,3] The pathogenic severity of these viruses and their epidemic potential are currently unknown.

Thus, the natural trafficking of infectious RNA viruses into man represents an ever-increasing strategic threat to the United States. It is one that could potentially cause massive civilian casualties, destroy national morale, initiate gross infrastructure disruption, and inhibit the nation's ability to produce the materials and services necessary for the proper functioning of its society.

The causes of this increase in EID are complex and they include an ever-expanding global human population, the fragmentation of natural animal habitats, intensive domestic animal breeding with an associated increase in the genetic mixing of wild viral strains, changes in insect vector numbers, and the migration of animal disease reservoirs. Modern air travel is another important factor and the global risk for an eventual serious global epidemic (pandemic) of some type is increasing.[1,4]

ANIMAL VIRUS SPILLOVERS AND SPECIES JUMPS

As previously explained, most animal viruses have a narrow, specific species host range. As a result, most animal viruses do not infect humans and most human viruses do not infect animals. However, as previously explained, the RNA viruses exist as "quasi-species" with slightly varying genetic makeups. If enough virus is present in the environment, the chances of it mutating to develop an enhanced transmission to another species is increased.[5]

It is thought animal viruses can jump into human populations by one of two methods. These are called *Spillover Events* and *Species Jumps*.[6] A Spillover Event occurs when an animal virus enters an environment that has susceptible humans who are rarely exposed to it. When this happens, it may cause a small devastating "Micro-Outbreak" but the virus is not well-adapted to man, and it spreads poorly from person-to-person. Therefore, a large epidemic fails to develop.

However, this is not the case in a *Species Jump*. Here, the original animal virus has previously cycled through a second different species of mammal. During this event, the virus acquires genetic changes which allow it to later be better transmitted to and between humans. As an analogy, the virus has "learned" how to efficiently use man as its new host. When this happens, the virus now has the potential to spread into an epidemic and under the right circumstances, to progress into a global pandemic. As the virus continues to cycle through humans, it may either increase or decrease its virulence to man. The reasons for this will be discussed later.

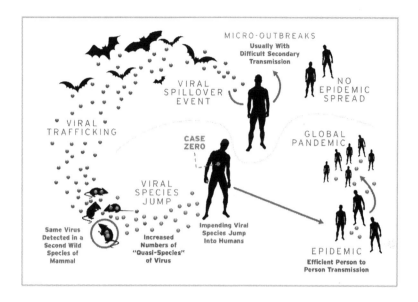

Figure 4. *Viral Spillover Events, Viral Trafficking, and Viral Species Jumps.*

Our current understanding of host–pathogen ecology and viral evolution is not yet sufficiently advanced to allow scientists to recognize all the processes and mechanisms that facilitate the jump of a virus into a new host species. However, there is enough information to indicate that it may be possible to predict if a virus has, or is acquiring, the ability to jump species into man. A recent multidisciplinary scientific workshop has affirmed that the detection of a wild-type virus in more than one species of mammal in the same environment, might be an indication of "viral trafficking" between species and an early warning for its possible jump into humans.[5,6] This will be discussed in detail in the last chapter.

H5N1 INFLUENZA STRAIN

In Mid-May of 1997, a critically ill little three-year old boy lay in the intensive care facility at the Queen Elizabeth Hospital in Hong Kong. What had started as an inflamed sore throat in the boy a few days earlier, had quickly degenerated into multiple organ failure. Unconscious in his hospital bed, a mechanical ventilator forced oxygen into the child's ravaged lungs as his kidneys and liver began to shut down. Finally, he began to bleed from his eyes and nose. Suspecting a case of viral hemorrhagic fever, virologists were called in, but the diagnosis remained a mystery. The boy died a few days later and autopsy samples were sent to the U.S. Centers for Disease Control in Atlanta and to the high-containment viral laboratories in Rotterdam, Holland and to Porton Down in the United Kingdom.

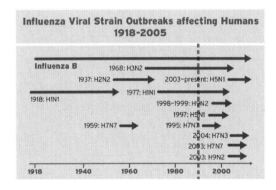

Figure 5. *New Influenza Strain Outbreaks.*[7] Modified by Authors

Within days, the boy's autopsy samples showed that a strain of Influenza virus of the H5N1 group A subtype could now cause human disease as well.[8] Scientists around the world were shocked because at the time only the H1, H2, and H3 strains of Influenza were known to infect humans. They were also alarmed because contrary to most bird Influenza viruses, this new strain was also killing domestic chickens. This highly pathogenic avian influenza A subtype H5N1 (HPAI H5N1) (now commonly known as "bird flu") was killing tens of millions of birds. This event spurred the intentional killing (culling) of hundreds of millions of Asian chickens in an attempt to try to halt its global spread.

Since that time, concerns over a severe avian influenza pandemic has only increased as small but fatal micro-outbreaks in humans continue to be caused by H5N1 spillover events from domestic chickens. These infections have caused a human case fatality rate estimated to be more than 50%.

With unprecedented numbers of chickens intensively bred and confined at record densities around the world, bird flu viruses are trying to adapt to humans in ways that have never been seen before. As seen in Figure 5, beginning in 1990, there has been a worrying, progressive increase in the number of "micro-outbreaks" of new Influenza A strains that have been attempting to emerge into humans. Some scientists have interpreted this recent proliferation as a sign that co-circulating Influenza viruses are increasingly exchanging their genetic material to form novel strains.

Beginning in December 2014 and continuing into mid-June 2015, the H5 bird flu virus was detected in 21 U.S. states, either in domestic poultry, captive birds, or in wild birds.[9,10] Although an H5N1 Influenza is severe, its person-to-person transmission rate has so far remained low and its adaptation to cause efficient human-to-human spread has not yet occurred. However, scientists remain worried as further research has shown that only small changes in this strain's H5 hemagglutinin protein can provide the virus with an ability to optimally bind to receptors in the human airway.

As already mentioned, in March of 2009, an outbreak of another Influenza strain occurred in Mexico. This involved a hybrid avian/pig/human H1N1 recombination virus. In response, the U.S. raced to develop and manufacture a vaccine for this new Human/Swine H1N1 strain. Despite its recognition and a WHO-directed global campaign, the virus quickly swept around the world infecting 10-20% of all humans living on the planet.[11]

The first doses of vaccine to this virus arrived very late because of a manufacturing delay, and this was compounded by the fact that the vaccine was only partially effective. During this pandemic, the Department of Health and Human Services allocated available vaccines to each state and territory by population size. It shipped vaccines directly to locations designated by each jurisdiction. Yet by October 14, only

5,885,900 doses had been shipped out from the 11,422,900 influenza vaccine doses allocated. California received 836,900 doses, the highest of any jurisdiction, while American Samoa and the Marshall Islands received no doses at all.

Compounding the problem is the fact that even if large amounts of vaccine can be manufactured for early distribution, each individual jurisdiction is responsible for deciding which of its residents will be vaccinated first. However, as witnessed in 2009, inadequate infrastructure, geographical or socioeconomic barriers and cultural differences, can all lead to inequitable access to vaccines. Even with the best intentions.

Although moderate in its overall lethality, the 2009 strain killed an estimated 250,000 people worldwide and the 2009 Mexico outbreak was yet another warning that the United States remained ill-prepared for another 1918-type event.[10,11] It is important to understand that Mother Nature will give us only so many warnings.

When scientists analyzed the new H1N1 virus, they found that it was a recombination of five different known flu viruses and that the new hybrid had probably been circulating for some time in pigs. Sometime in the 2008-2009 timeframe, a final recombination event took place involving a different Euro-Asia Influenza virus and this new hybrid jumped into humans in Mexico.[12]

H7N9 INFLUENZA IN HORSES AND BIRDS

In March of 2013, an H7N9 avian virus was first reported to have infected humans in China as the result of another spillover event. The ability of any new Influenza strain to cause major lung pathology in humans is always a major concern, and human H7N9 infections show a distinct pathological, immunological, and tissue tropism different from the other Influenza A strains.[13] The H7N9 bird flu virus has continued to sicken and kill several hundred people in China over the last few years with the occasional sporadic bursts of cases that have overtaken those caused by the H5N1 strain that has been causing sporadic human infections a decade longer.

Influenza experts find these changes unsettling. In addition, there has been reports that some of the "quasi-species" of the H7N9 virus have already developed a resistance to the antiviral drug Tamiflu. In addition, infection with the H7N9 strain is accompanied by a high death rate. During China's previous four annual epidemics, about 40 percent of people confirmed with H7N9 virus infection have died. Other changes in the virus are also worrying, and the Asian lineage H7N9 virus is rated by many scientists as having the greatest potential to cause a future pandemic.

At present, the potentially most dangerous of these new Influenza strains have shown only poor human to human transmission, but as Figure Five shows, it is an ominous sign that something is seriously wrong with the ecology of our planet. It is also an indirect indication that in addition to Influenza, other types of animal RNA viruses will continue to emerge into human populations.

Notes for Chapter 2

[1] Morse, S.S. Factors in the emergence of infectious disease. Emerg Infect Dis. 1995; 1:7-15.

[2] Jones KE, Patel NG, Levy MA, Storeygard A, Balk D, Gittleman JL, Daszak P. Global trends in emerging infectious diseases. Nature. 2008; 451:990–993. [PubMed]

[3] Smith, KF, Goldberg, M. et.al., Global Rise in Infectious Disease Outbreaks. 2014; J.R. Soc. Interface 11: 21140950. http://dx.doi.org/10.1098/rsif.2014.0950.

[4] Taylor LH, Latham SM, Woolhouse ME. Risk factors for human disease emergence. Philos Trans R Soc Lond B Biol Sci. 2001; 356: 983–989. [PMC free article] [PubMed]

[5] Parrish, C.R., Edward C. Holmes, et.al. Cross-Species Virus Transmission and the Emergence of New Epidemic Diseases, Micro and Mol Bio. Rev.2008.

[6] Morse, S., Mazet, J.A.K., Daszak, P. et.al., Prediction and prevention of the next pandemic zoonosis, Lancet. 2012 Dec 1; 380(9857): 1956–1965.

[7] WHO 2005; Avian Influenza, Assessing the Pandemic Threat.

[8] Subbarao K, Klimov A, et al. Characterization of an avian Influenza A (H5N1) virus isolated from a child with a fatal respiratory illness. Science. 1998; 279:393–6.

[9] Claas EC, Osterhaus AD, et al. Human influenza A H5N1 virus related to a highly pathogenic avian influenza virus. Lancet. 1998; 351:472–7.

[10] Check, Hayden Erica (5 May 2009). "The turbulent history of the A(H1N1) virus". Nature. 459 (7243): 14–5. ISSN 1744-7933. PMID 19424121. Doi:10.1038/459014a.

[11] 2009 GAO-09-909TGaps in Planning and Preparedness Need to be Addressed. 11. 2011 GAO-11-632 Lessons from the H1N1 Pandemic Should Be Incorporated into Planning.

[12] Vijaykrishna, D., Guan Y et.al., Reassortment of pandemic H1N1/2009 influenza A virus in swine". (18 June 2010). Science. 328 (5985): 1529. PMID 20558710. doi:10.1126/science.1189132.

[13] Peiris, M., Yuen KY, et al. Human infection with influenza H7N9. Lancet. 1999; 354:916–7.

SECTION

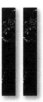

THE HISTORICAL THREAT
OF PANDEMIC INFLUENZA

3

HUMAN SOCIOLOGY
AND EPIDEMIC VIRAL DISEASE

AS PREVIOUSLY MENTIONED, the major factors for the increase in new human viral diseases are complex and interlinked.[1,2,3,4,5] It is also recognized that changing human social structures and collective behavior can also have a major effect in determining if an infectious new virus produces only a localized "micro-outbreak" of cases, or if it progresses into a major global pandemic affecting millions of people in multiple regions and nations (pandemic).

A poignant example of this is the HIV-1 virus, the causative agent of human AIDS. Molecular studies indicate that HIV-1 was first transmitted from chimpanzees to humans near the Sangha River in the southeastern African rain forests of Cameroon. This may have occurred as early as 1915 during the time when Africa was undergoing its major colonization by multiple European nations.[6,7]

Before 1910, no town in Central Africa had more than 10,000 people. As large local labor forces were raised to build towns, roads, rail infrastructures, and operate mines and plantations, the rural Africans moved into these ever-expanding urban areas. This large-scale recruitment of indigenous labor acted to separate families, disrupt traditional tribal values, and it precipitated an unprecedented increase in the movement of people across portions of the continent. This culminated in the establishment of the major African cities and the epidemic emergence of HIV-1 farther south in the city of Léopoldville (now Kinshasa) in the Belgian Congo.

A combination of additional social factors then came into play. Starting in 1956, these included the rapid large-scale European decolonization of Africa with the loss of existing European-style public health systems. This combined with an unsustainable indigenous population growth rate of almost 3 per cent per annum throughout much of the continent.

Additional human factors driving the expanding epidemic included the Uganda–Tanzania war of 1978–1979 which helped drive AIDS into Southern Africa along the major north/south trucking routes, and the indigenous practice of multiple simultaneous long-term heterosexual relationships extending across large areas.[8] These factors combined with the fact that HIV-1 positive individuals remain infectious during the prolonged time that it takes them to develop noticeable signs and symptoms.

Consequently, the HIV-1/AIDS pandemic had been underway for decades before it was first recognized in a small cluster of cases in San Francisco in 1981. The HIV-1 virus was eventually isolated in 1984 and since its discovery it has caused an additional 36 million deaths globally with an additional 35.3 million people thought to be currently infected.

In 1918, as the HIV-1 virus was transforming itself into an eventual major human infectious disease, some 7000 miles away, another type of animal virus was undergoing a change in a sparsely populated corner of the U.S. Midwest.

The placid rural geographical area of Haskell County in Kansas represented an unlikely spot for the outbreak of a major global pandemic.

Founded in 1887, the almost exclusively agricultural county was flat, treeless, and scattered with individual landholdings, crop fields, and livestock in the form of hogs, cattle, and poultry. Sometime late in January 1918, a new strain of a bird Influenza virus arrived in the county where it infected some of the area farmers. These cases presented with a general malaise and muscle aches followed by a high fever, the onset of a severe dry cough, and the development of an unusually severe headache.

A local physician in the County began to see multiple cases of Influenza, but one with an unusual virulence that was accompanied by a secondary bacterial pneumonia and death. It was also peculiar in the fact that in contrast to the usual seasonal outbreaks of Influenza that affected the very old and the very young, the most severe cases were occurring in the young healthy adults in the area.[9]

In addition to making house calls with his horse and buggy, the local area physician was also the Health Officer for the 24 by 24-square mile Haskell County region. Greatly alarmed, he reported this unusual outbreak to the U.S. Public Health Service.[10] Subsequently, his notification was published in the Government's weekly Public Health Reports. There is no mention of any other Influenza outbreak in the United States at that time.

Then, almost as quick as it had appeared, the number of new cases started to drop and by March the unusual event seemed to be over. The low total area population and its relative isolation from a major metropolitan area seemed to have caused the event to be contained. However, the effects of collective human behavior still had their role to play. This was in the form of the sudden rushed entry of the United States into World War One. This action would soon precipitate one of the three greatest biological catastrophes in recorded human history. During the next 12 months, between 3 to 5% of all the people on the planet would die from this new Influenza strain. As a comparison and without any adjustment for population growth, the 1918 Influenza pandemic would kill more people in a year than HIV-1/AIDS has killed during the last 24 years.

Scientists have now determined that the deadly 1918 virus did not originate through a recombination event involving a bird and a human Influenza virus. All eight of the "blueprints" of the H1N1 virus that caused this lethal pandemic are most closely related to avian Influenza viruses than to Influenza from any other species, including man. This indicates that an avian virus may have directly infected humans and then adapted without a major genetic recombination event.[10]

This is a very worrying prospect for the future.

THE SEED AND THE SOIL

Just as a seed requires the proper soil conditions to germinate and grow, so does the outbreak of an infectious disease. With respect to the 1918 influenza event, the Haskell County outbreak would provide the seed in the form of a mutated strain of the Influenza virus. The date of 28 July in 1914, would provide the soil in the form of the beginning of the First World War.

During the following months, the United States stood on the sidelines as this conflict in Europe erupted and amplified. It continued to watch as the absolute carnage on the battlefields settled into a stalemate in the form of protracted trench warfare. While the U.S. assisted the British by selling and shipping them armaments, America refused to participate in any form of actual ground combat.

However, Germany's resumption of unrestricted submarine warfare and the sinking of seven U.S. merchant ships, together with the interception of the famous Zimmermann telegram that outlined a plan for Germany and Mexico to seize territory on America's southern border, was a defining point. President Woodrow Wilson asked Congress for a Declaration of War against Germany on 6 April 1917. This was granted and overnight the U.S. entered World War One as an associated Allied power.

In 1917, the U.S. had only a small professional army of 100,000 men supported by an additional 112,000 members of the National Guard. Five-weeks later, Congress passed the Selective Service Act. This authorized the Federal government to quickly raise a large standing national army by compulsory civilian enlistment into the Armed Forces. Under the new law, all males aged 21 to 30 were required to register for military service and a draft of some 2.8 million men for training and overseas service began. Many additional volunteers would also enlist. Consequently, thousands upon thousands of fit young men began to pour into the large military training camps that were quickly set up throughout the United States.

Two hundred and sixty miles northeast of the rural area of Haskell County in Kansas, lay the Army installation of Fort Riley. Urgently expanded by America's sudden entry into the war, in 1917 a large training cantonment named Camp Funston had been constructed five miles east of the main Fort. Made up of some 1,400 buildings on 2,000 acres, the camp was named after the Medal of Honor holder U.S. Army Major General Frederick Funston, who was best known for his roles in the previous Spanish American War and the Philippine–American War.[11]

Camp Funston was the largest of sixteen Divisional Training Camps erected across the United States. Originally designed to accommodate roughly 40,000 men, it was soon overcrowded with more than 56,000 soldiers in training. These men would be part of the initial Divisions sent to France the following spring.[2]

The winter of 1917-1918, was typified by extreme cold weather in Kansas and the coal-heated tents and formal barracks at the Camp Funston cantonment were not only overcrowded but also poorly ventilated. In addition to the low humidity created by the cold weather, this created the perfect environmental conditions for the spread of any airborne respiratory virus.

A small number of men undergoing the training at the Camp had been inducted from Haskell County, and a few of them had returned home on leave. They returned to camp during the time of the unusual Influenza outbreak in that county. Influenza came with them and it subsequently broke out at Camp Funston in early March of 1918.

Recently returned from Haskell County, was a young butcher. Just before breakfast on the morning of March 11, he presented to the hospital at Fort Riley complaining of a sore throat. Within hours more than 100 other soldiers presented with this and other symptoms of Influenza. Over the next 3-weeks more than 1100 cases were admitted to the Camp's overcrowded hospital. This outbreak was highly infectious and hundreds more soldiers now presented to the various infirmaries scattered around the base. This local epidemic was unusual in that it was associated with a secondary pneumonia in roughly 20% of cases.

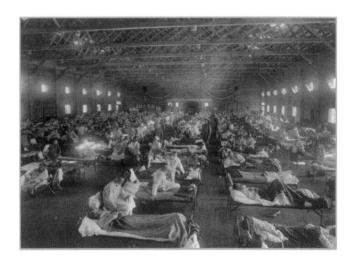

Figure 6. *Emergency Care Facility at Camp Funston, 1918.* Source: Otis Historical Archives, National Museum of Health and Medicine, Silver Spring, MD, USA (photographer unknown).

In a modern retrospective note, the disease appeared to be milder than what had struck Haskell County a few weeks before and only 46 soldiers died during this outbreak.[12]

All during this epidemic, freshly trained soldiers were constantly being transferred in and out of Camp Funston and Fort Riley, with destinations to other large Army bases in the United States. The results were entirely predictable.

Within two-weeks of the outbreak at Camp Funston, the Influenza virus had spread to two separate military camps in Georgia where it infected some 10% of the personnel stationed there. By the end of March, some 24 of the 36 largest military training camps in the United States were experiencing Influenza outbreaks. In addition, some 30 cities near these Army camps, were also suffering from outbreaks of Influenza. Yet the disease continued to maintain a relatively moderate virulence. In spite of the cases of secondary bacterial pneumonia, the overall death rates remained relatively low.[12]

Predictably, Influenza also broke out across the Atlantic at the site of the American troop disembarkation point. This was at the major receiving port in Brest, France. By early April, the infection was spreading through the French Naval Command at the port. The epidemic was now technically considered to be a pandemic because it was affecting more than one country. By mid-April, outbreaks were occurring in both the French and British Army and by the end of that month, Influenza outbreaks were occurring in the suburbs of Paris.[11]

Then the pandemic exploded. In May, the British First Army suffered 36,000 hospital admissions from Influenza with thousands more less-serious cases. This was followed by large outbreaks in the British Second and Third Armies. Although highly infectious, the disease appeared to remain moderate and most soldiers made a full recovery.[11]

By June, troops returning from Europe carried the Influenza virus to England. Somehow the disease also found its way to Germany and neutral Spain. It reached Denmark and Norway in July, and it arrived in India by ship where it spread along the rail lines to Calcutta and Rangoon. It would soon arrive in Shanghai and rapidly sweep through the population of China.

From the first of June to the end of July, roughly 200,800 soldiers out of the 2-million men fighting in France had contracted had suffered an attack of Influenza.[11]Yet despite its continuing spread, the causative Influenza virus seemed to show an apparent progressive decrease in its virulence. Among 40,000 French Army hospital admissions, there were less than 100 deaths.

One outbreak in the British Navy infected over 10,000 sailors, yet it was accompanied by only 4 deaths. By August, the disease had become limited to an infection of the lining of the upper airways with a classical 3 to 4-day duration of symptoms. Some military physicians began to wonder if the disease was still Influenza.[11]

While outbreaks were still occurring among the new recruits in the military cantonments on the US mainland and in some surrounding urban areas, the disease failed to sweep across North America as it had in Europe and Asia. Consequently, most military doctors were convinced that the Influenza pandemic was generally over.[9,11]

The process of RNA virus infection of a human or animal host is complicated, and it involves multiples factors operating in both the host and the virus. These include the type and number of specific cells in the host that are susceptible to infection by the virus (skin, eyes, upper airway, lower airway, etc.) as well as how well the virus can use the existing proteins of its host's cells to help it replicate. Additional factors involve whether the viral replication kills the host's cells and the various properties of the differing "quasi-species" of daughter viruses that are generated. In addition, the host itself is fighting back and the blood stream of infected individuals are quickly flooded with various antiviral and inflammatory chemicals generated by their own activated immune systems.

All these factors interact to exert a selection process that determines which viral mutants in the "quasi-species" swarms will be able to survive and go on to infect and replicate inside more of the host's cells and then spill outside the body to infect other individual humans or animals.

To better understand what can happen during an RNA viral epidemic, scientists in the 1950's developed a laboratory technique called *Serial Passage*. This involved inoculating a particular virus into an animal which may or not, be naturally susceptible to the infection. The pathogen is allowed time to replicate in the animal before a blood sample is removed and injected into another fresh animal, or a nasal swab taken and used for the transfer. This process is repeated for multiple animals; hence the name *Serial Passage*.[12]

During these studies, scientists soon found something very strange. It appeared that the serial passage of an RNA virus could have several different possible outcomes. Often the virus being passaged could be observed to show an increase in its virulence. For example, when the polio virus was serially passed through mice, it progressively adapted to be able to produce an ever-increasing amount of virus in the mice with an earlier onset of muscle paralysis.[13]

Scientists also observed that during a serial passage, a virus could evolve to become adapted to a completely different host than that the one in which it is was naturally found. In more recent times this has been observed when laboratory Guinea Pigs were inoculated with infectious material from human Ebola virus cases. Normally these animals develop only a mild, non-lethal, illness. However, if the virus is sequentially passed from animal to animal, the virus undergoes a progressive increase in its virulence and the Ebola virus develops into a strain that can cause a 100% lethality in Guinea Pigs.[14,15] The same was found when Ebola was serially passaged in mice and many other examples exist of different RNA viruses increasing their virulence in a new species during a serial transfer.[16]

However, to further complicate matters, other experiments showed that the virulence of an RNA virus could sometimes decrease during serial animal passage. One experiment with a highly virulent pig-adapted Foot-and-Mouth Disease virus showed a drastic reduction of virulence after only 14 serial passages in pigs. Upon further passage, the virulence of the passaged virus decreased to point where it was only able to cause an asymptomatic infection in the animals. Although the virus could be isolated from tonsil and nasal swabs, it had transformed itself into a natural carrier state. The virus was still in the pigs, it just did not cause overt disease while it reproduced. It had become perfectly adapted to the animals.[17]

The same thing can be observed with the Influenza A virus.

Occasionally new Highly Pathogenic Avian Influenza (HPAI) strains emerge to cause lethal epidemics in wild birds and domestic chickens (*in 2014-2015 some 48 million domestic chickens and turkeys had to be culled in the United States due to a HPAI strain outbreak*). However, for the most part, the Influenza Group A viruses cause no overt disease in waterfowl although live virus can be recovered in their droppings.

Some type of a similar virulence reduction now appeared to be happening with the 1918 Influenza virus in man. Reports from the U.S. camps overseas indicated that the severity of the Influenza and the number of cases with a severe associated pneumonia were diminishing. Yet, medical communications in 1918 were not the same as today, and it was difficult to determine exactly what was happening in Europe. Some military doctors knew of reports of recent Influenza cases that had suffered a more severe disease and death. One isolated report described an outbreak in a remote French Army Camp with a 5% mortality rate. Other scattered reports described recent cases of Influenza with fulminating pneumonias and extensive hemorrhagic lung damage.[9,11] A few unofficial reports from doctors in France were also reporting that some Influenza cases were being first misdiagnosed as meningitis (a serious inflammation of the membranes that surround the brain).[11] All of this should have served as an ominous warning, but it did not.

By the mid-summer of 1918, the United States was transporting some 10,000 newly trained soldiers to France each day from its crowded military staging areas. At the same time, the Influenza virus was experimenting......trying to find the right set of mutations that would let it adapt further and replicate at higher numbers with more chances for spread. The many soldiers and sailors in the abnormal high-density living conditions of the First World War, served as numerous and readily available test subjects for this purpose.

QUASI-SPECIES, BOTTLENECKS AND MULLER'S RATCHET

As discussed before, the replication of an Influenza virus creates "showers" of slightly different "quasi-species" of daughter Influenza viruses, each one with a random mutation. This helps the virus meet the challenges of replicating in different environments such as a new host species, or to survive an attack by the host's immune response.

It is not always the most virulent or rapidly reproducing strains in the "quasi-species" that are selected by this process. If the host's selection pressures on a virus are severe, then only a few of the "quasi-species" that enter the host can survive and replicate. If this selection pressure is maintained during virus transmission from human to human, the further mutations generated by the error-prone RNA Replicase enzyme continue to be selected against. This is known as a *genetic bottleneck*. This is even more pronounced during aerosol droplet infection because the number of different quasi-species that are transferred to a new host through the air may be reduced by the additional requirement of having to survive for a period outside the body.

In addition, these propagating viral strains will begin to accumulate "genetic garbage" in the form of mutations that neither hurt nor help the virus survive in its host. Consequently, the "quasi-species" that are being generated are now slowly accumulating random mutations and losing their general fitness. This process is called *Muller's Ratchet*, and it can account for a change in disease severity during RNA virus outbreaks.[18,19]

There are two ways for a virus to escape such a genetic bottleneck. The first method is simple. Because the RNA Replicase enzyme of the Influenza virus is constantly making random mutations as the virus replicates, a genetic bottleneck it is just as likely to generate mutations that cause it to revert back to some form of a pre-bottleneck strain.[20,21]

The other method is more complicated, and it involves the process of genetic recombination when a host becomes simultaneously co-infected with "quasi-species" from different outside Influenza strains and this genetic material recombines to form novel hybrid Influenza viruses.

Scientists currently do not have any virus samples from the first pandemic wave that broke out in Camp Funston to compare these with the more lethal secondary wave of Influenza that was soon to come. However, irrespective of the mechanisms in play; by June 1918 the Influenza virus found itself constrained and bottlenecked by the normal defenses of the human body. Desperate to find new combinations of mutations that would allow it to continue to spread and with the high-density of humans everywhere around it, it did not matter if the virus killed its host quickly or not. There were no constraints against the virus developing a new lethality.

Some scientists now believe that the virus started to accumulate mutations in the "blueprints" of its most treasured and conserved protein, one that could tolerate only few mutations and still remain functional. This was in the RNA Replicase enzyme itself.[22,23]

If the handle of a gambling slot machine is pulled down enough times, it may take millions of pulls, but eventually its spinning wheels will stop in the configuration of a jackpot. For the Influenza virus, its spinning wheels stopped sometime between the end of June and the first week of July in 1918.

Notes for Chapter 3

1 Jones KE, Patel NG, Daszak P., et.al. Global trends in emerging infectious diseases. Nature. 2008; 451:990–993. [PubMed].

2 Smith, KF, Goldberg, M. et.al. Global Rise in Infectious Disease Outbreaks. 2014; J.R.Soc. Interface 11: 21140950. http://dx.doi.org/10.1098/rsif.2014.0950.

3 Morse, S.S. Factors in the emergence of infectious disease. Emerg Infect Dis. 1995; 1:715. [PMC free article] [PubMed]

4 Taubenberger, Jeffery K., et.al. (2006). "1918 Influenza: the mother of all pandemics". Emerging Infectious Diseases. 12 (1): 15–22. doi:10.3201/eid1201.050979. PMC 3291398. PMID 16494711.

5 Taylor LH, Latham SM, et.al. Risk factors for human disease emergence. Philos Trans R Soc Lond B Biol Sci. 2001; 356: 983–989. 2005; 11:1822–1827. [PMC free article] [PubMed]

6 Sharp, P., Bailes, E., et. al. "The Origins of Acquired Immune Deficiency Syndrome Viruses: Where and When?" The Royal Society (2001): 867-76. Print.

7 Keele BF, Bailes E, et.al."Chimpanzee Reservoirs of Pandemic and Nonpandemic HIV-1" Science. 313 (5786): 523–6.Bibcode:2006 Sci.313.523K. PMC 2442710 . PMID 16728595. doi:10.1126/science.1126531.

8 http://discovermagazine.com/2004/feb/why-aids-worse-in-africa

9 The Great Influenza: The Story of the Deadliest Pandemic in History, John M. Barry Paperback, Revised Edition, 560 pages Published October 4th, 2005. by Penguin Books (first published 2004) ISBN 0143036491 (ISBN13: 9780143036494).

10 Robert B. Belshe. The Origins of Pandemic Influenza — Lessons from the 1918 Virus. N Engl J Med 2005; 353:2209-2211 DOI: 10.1056/NEJMp058281

11 America's Forgotten Pandemic: The Influenza of 1918, Alfred W. Crosby Paperback. Second Edition, 2003 by Cambridge University Press. (ISBN0-521-54175-1).

12 Woo, H. J., & Reifman, J. (2014). Quantitative Modeling of Virus Evolutionary Dynamics and Adaptation in Serial Passages Using Empirically Inferred Fitness Landscapes. Journal of Virology, 88 (2), 1039-1050.

13 John D. Ainslie Increase in Virulence of the Lansing Strain of Poliomyelitis Virus with Passage in Mice J Immunol October 1, 1951, 67 (4) 331-337.

14 Bowen E, Platt G, et.al. A comparative study of strains of Ebola virus isolated from southern Sudan and northern Zaire, J Med Virol. 1980, vol. 6 (pg. 129-38)

15 Connolly BM, Steele KE, et al. Pathogenesis of experimental Ebola virus infection in guinea pigs, J Infect Dis. 1999, vol. 179 suppl. 1 (pg. S203-17).

[16] Mike Bray, John Huggins, et.al. A Mouse Model for Evaluation of Prophylaxis and Therapy of Ebola Hemorrhagic Fever J Infect Dis (1999) 179 (Supplement 1): S248-S258. DOI https://doi.org/10.1086/514292

[17] C. Carrillo, Z. Lu, M. V. Borca, et.al., Genetic and phenotypic variation of foot-and-mouthdisease virus during serial passages in a natural host Journal of Virology, 81:20 2007,11341-11351http://dx.doi.org/10.1128/JVI.00930-07

[18] Duarte E, Clarke D, et.al. Rapid fitness losses in mammalian RNA virus clones due to Muller's ratchet. Proc Natl Acad Sci U S A. 1992 Jul 1;89(13):6015-9. PMID: 1321432 PMCID: PMC402129

[19] Serafín Gutiérrez. Yannis Michalakis, et.al. Virus population bottlenecks during within-host progression and host-to-host transmission, Current Opinion in Virology, Issue 5, October 2012, Pages 546-555.https://doi.org/10.1016/j.coviro.2012.08.001

[20] Novella IS, Elena SF, et.al. Size of genetic bottlenecks leading to virus fitness loss isdetermined by mean initial population fitness. J Virol. 1995 May;69(5):2869-72. PMID:7707510PMCID: PMC188983

[21] Clarke DK, Duarte EA, et.al. Genetic bottlenecks and population passages cause profound fitness differences in RNA viruses. J Virol. 1993 Jan; 67(1):222-8. PMID: 8380072 PMCID:

[22] Jeffery K. Taubenberger, et.al. Characterization of the 1918 influenza virus polymerase genes Nature 437, 889-893 (6 October 2005) | doi:10.1038/nature04230.

[23] Special Report; The 1918 flu virus is resurrected, Nature 437, 794-795 (6 October 2005) doi: 10.1038/437794a. 33

4

WILDFIRE

I N 1918, THERE WAS LITTLE SCIENTIFIC UNDERSTANDING of viruses, no vaccine for the prevention of Influenza infection and no antiviral drug treatment. Scientists did know however, that Influenza was contagious and that limiting social contact could reduce the chances of infection. Today these measures are called Non-Pharmaceutical Interventions or NPI. As we shall outline in this book, during a similar 1918-type Influenza pandemic today, roughly 1/3 of the American population will not have access to effective antiviral drug therapy or a vaccine until the pandemic is near or past its peak. This faction of the population will be relegated to almost the same NPI as was used a century ago.

In the next few chapters we will examine how severe such a scenario might be. In this respect, we found that trying to reconstruct what the 1918 pandemic was like, was difficult and we were aided greatly in our understanding by two outstanding authors and their painstakingly researched books. These books are *The Great Influenza: The Story of the Deadliest Pandemic in History*, by John M. Barry published in 2004, and *America's Forgotten Pandemic: The Influenza of 1918*, by Alfred W. Crosby, Second Edition, published in 2003. These writings greatly helped us to understand the severity of the events a century ago and we have heavily referenced these works in the next few chapters to help the reader understand how important it is for the United States to have an effective pandemic influenza plan.

Every major human crisis has some type of a preliminary starting point and the one involving America's disaster with Influenza began on June 30, 1918 when a British cargo ship named the "City of Exeter" docked in Philadelphia.

Upon retrospective examination, although the first wave of the 1918 pandemic seemed to have ended several weeks earlier, an unusual outbreak of Influenza had broken out among this ship's crew during their transatlantic voyage from England. This outbreak was marked both by the severity of its onset and the catastrophic pneumonia that it caused. There were other strange signs and symptoms in the infected crew members as well. This included epistaxis (bleeding from the nose). While nosebleeds are a rather common occurrence, when they are severe and when they occur in patients suffering from an infectious disease, it can be a very serious sign. There were also some central nervous system signs. Again, very worrying because of the possibility of meningitis. This is a very serious, potentially lethal infection of the membranes around the brain.

While in transit, the City of Exeter had radioed its developing medical problem back to England and when the ship docked in Philadelphia, the British Consulate had arranged for a special U.S. quarantine team to meet it. The dock had been cleared and the entire crew were taken off and placed in a special isolation ward in a hospital. There, more crewmembers died.[1,2]

This should have prompted the U.S. health authorities to rapidly spin up into overdrive to initiate strict quarantine inspections as well as other arrangements for future incidents of this type. In addition, the conditions at the ship's point of departure should have been immediately investigated with possibly blocking future departures from this British port. None of this was apparently done.

In 1918, Dr. Rupert Blue was the 4th Surgeon General and as such, he was the head of the U.S. Public Health Service. He had extensive experience in epidemic control and had been involved in containing an outbreak of Bubonic Plague in San Francisco during 1900-1904. He was also a skilled diplomat and that may have been the problem.[1,2] Most likely pressured by President Wilson, he issued no instructions with respect to ordering ships with suspected Influenza cases to be quarantined. The Surgeon General would continue to demonstrate an almost complete lack of leadership throughout the events that would soon transpire. He would step down from his post in 1920.

The doctors at the quarantine hospital attending the ill sailors suspected that something unusual was occurring and their suspicions would soon prove to be correct. Through trial and error, the Influenza virus had finally found its way out of the confining genetic bottleneck that developed after its first lethal outbreak months earlier in Haskell County, Kansas. The predominant quasi-species of the virus that was now circulating had become fully human-adapted. Precisely how this process occurred and whether it was due to mutations in the viral RNA Replicase enzyme or to a new plasticity in the Influenza hemagglutinin protein, would be a question that scientists would still be trying to answer a 100-years later.[3]

Across the Atlantic, fatal cases of Influenza were now appearing in London. Many of these cases were typified by the victims dying from an unusually rapid disease course that ended in massive respiratory failure.[2] Over the next few days, an additional 120 victims died in the important English industrial center of Birmingham.[1,2] The autopsies performed on these cases revealed a severe type of lung damage never before seen with Influenza. Clinical records showed that before dying, the patients had turned blue from a buildup of carbon dioxide in their blood. This condition is called cyanosis and it was caused by the victim's lungs losing their ability to perform a normal gas exchange with the air.[1,2]

On July 8, England reported the severe nature of the Birmingham outbreak to the U.S. Public Health Service. In response, the U.S. Surgeon General issued an urgent national warning to all State Public Health departments. However, he did little else and his alert would have no impact on the biological carnage that was soon to come.[1]

Already a focal point for the previous milder Influenza outbreak during the first part of April, by late July the French seaport of Brest was infected with this new modified strain of the Influenza virus. By mid-August, its large port naval hospital was overwhelmed with cases. Incredibly, there were few measures put in place for infection control and the disease quickly spread to the entire civilian region around the port. At the same time, thousands of American soldiers continued to flow into Brest before being quickly shipped off to the front lines, predictably transporting this new lethal Influenza strain with them.[4]

During the end of August, an ever-increasing number of troop transport and cargo ships suffered lethal Influenza outbreaks during their Atlantic transit. The virus spread through the British Commonwealth to countries as far away as South Africa and New Zealand. In late August, an infected troop transport docked for coal at Freetown in Sierra Leone. A few weeks later some 3-6% of the African population in the area were dead from Influenza.[5]

With America's direct involvement in the fighting of the First World War, a single mindedness had taken over President Woodrow Wilson. Following his own divine inspiration, he determined that the fighting in Europe would take place over everything else. He ignored the American Bill of Rights, ruthlessly controlled the press, and he directed an extensive national propaganda campaign. An ineffective

Congress let this happen. Wilson's Justice Department established the Enemy Alien Bureau, which was authorized to arrest and jail allegedly disloyal foreigners without trial. The first job of the controversial J. Edgar Hoover after his completion of law school was to head this effort.[2,6] Hoover would later to go on to be the first and only life-time Director of the new Federal Bureau of Investigation (FBI). Based on his abuses of power, FBI directors are now limited to one 10–year term, subject to extension by the United States Senate. Even this has been shown to be problematic in recent times.

Throughout 1918, thousands of American soldiers continued to cross the Atlantic and disembark into the middle of this new lethal Influenza outbreak in Europe. The new seed had now found its ideal soil. With the high density of humans around it, the new Influenza strain was free to reproduce as fast as possible without any worry over killing its host before it could spread further. Wilson's fixation would result in more deaths of American soldiers due to Influenza than would be killed by enemy weapons.

Long-distance passenger air travel across the United States or to Europe was unknown in 1918 (Charles Lindbergh would not make his historic solo flight across the Atlantic until 9-years later). Therefore, long-distance continental travel was mainly by lengthy railroad journeys. This factor had helped to minimize the earlier spread of the more moderate Influenza pandemic that had swept the world earlier in April through July. Outside of the Influenza cases in the military cantonment camps and their surrounding urban areas, the civilian population of the United States had been largely spared. However, at the end of August, America's luck finally ran out.

As discussed previously, on Tuesday, August 27, 1918, a transport ship ferrying U.S. soldiers back from Europe docked in Boston Harbor. There the soldiers were transferred over to the Receiving Ship at the Commonwealth Pier building. The Receiving Ship was in fact, the dockside barracks that served as a central point for both freight and passenger traffic, with nearby transportation by rail, truck, and bus. Here, these soldiers were given temporary overcrowded accommodations while they awaited their transfer to other destinations all over the United States.

Over the next two days, 58 cases of the new Influenza developed among the arriving soldiers and they were transferred to the nearby Chelsea Naval Hospital.[7] Within 48-hours, the three medical officers who had seen these patients also fell ill. Influenza had arrived back in the United States in a new, mutated, and much more deadly form.

Although the infected men were immediately isolated at the Naval Hospital, it was already too late. On the 3rd of September, a civilian was admitted to the Boston City Hospital suffering from severe Influenza. The next day, military students attending a specialized Naval Radio School also began falling ill.[8] This was the start of a severe Influenza epidemic in Boston that would expand for another six-weeks, generating a horrific final death toll in the city. Schools and draft boards were closed, and stores reduced their business hours. The congested subways and above-ground rail transportation system helped spread the airborne Influenza virus among Boston's civilian population.

On September 7, as the Boston epidemic continued to increase, some 300 sailors at the Commonwealth Pier were transported from Boston to the Philadelphia Navy Yard. The new Influenza strain would accompany them on this journey. Unlike its narrow escape at the end of June, the City of Philadelphia would soon feel the full wrath of this new Influenza, more so than any other major metropolitan area in the United States.

As the epidemic began to rage in Boston and transfer to Philadelphia, a large 5,000-acre military cantonment area lay just thirty-five miles north of the city. Formally named Camp Devens, it was named after the Civil War General Charles Devens. Initially constructed to hold 36,000 soldiers, the Camp was severely overcrowded with over 45,000 men.[9]

On September 8, the new Influenza struck with a vengeance. Over the next 10-days it infected almost 20% of the soldiers in the Camp. Some 75% of these cases were serious enough to be hospitalized. This was clearly not a normal Influenza outbreak. In one single day, some 1500 soldiers were admitted to the Camp's large and efficient hospital.[10]

Several hundred Army doctors, nurses and support staff were quickly brought in by train to assist with the developing crisis, and they worked until they themselves became ill with some dying from Influenza. Overwhelmed by the developing civilian outbreak in Boston, the Red Cross could only send 12 nurses to Camp Devens to assist. Within a few days, eight of these nurses were severely ill with Influenza, and two quickly died.[1]

A few days later, a small but expert Army medical/scientific team was sent to Camp Devens to investigate the situation. Leading this team was Dr. William Welch, one of the most distinguished pathologists of the early 20th century. Welsh had been on the Board of the pioneering Rockefeller Institute. Highly patriotic, he had left this position to join the staff of the Army Surgeon General where he had been given the rank of Colonel.[1]

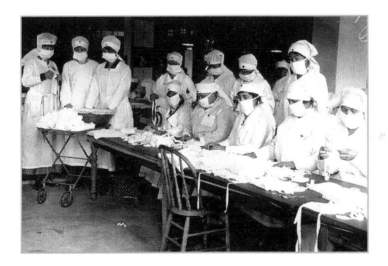

Figure 7. *Boston Red Cross volunteers assemble gauze influenza masks for use at Camp Devens. Eight of these Nurses would soon become infected and two would die from Influenza.* 1918 Historical Image Gallery | Pandemic Influenza (Flu) | CDC.

Sixty-three soldiers died the day Colonel Welsh and his team arrived at Camp Devens and what they found was horrendous.

The camp was falling apart, and the large military hospital designed to hold 1200 patients was overflowing with over 6000 cases of Influenza.[1,2] All hospital beds were filled. Hundreds of sick and dying soldiers were lying on cots in the hospital's hallways and porches. Out of the 200 nurses in the Camp, 70 of them were severely ill and medical care for any of the patients was almost nonexistent.[1] The grounds of Camp Devens had become a biological battlefield with an enemy that was invisible to the microscopes of the time.

Inside the hospital, the scene was reminiscent of the "Vestibule of Hell" in Dante's Inferno. Lying in dirty bedding and bloodied clothing, many of the patients were crying out in delirium. Previously fit, active, healthy young men just a few days before were now bleeding from their noses, coughing blood, and turning blue from cyanosis. Corpses could be found in every hallway and dead bodies were stacked on top of each other outside of the overflowing hospital morgue.

Amid the increasing chaos around them, the investigative team poured over the records of the first victims, made when record keeping was still possible. They visited the hospital laboratory and ignoring the danger, they went to the wards to interview and examine patients.[2]

Desperate to understand what was happening, Colonel Welsh and his team began to conduct autopsies in their frantic search for clues. As highly trained doctors and scientists, what they found inside the dead far surpassed the horrors they had witnessed on the wards. Blood-tinged fluid poured from the body openings of the cadavers and upon cutting open the chest cavity, it was the shocking appearance of the lungs that attracted the team's first attention.

Normal lung tissue is light in weight, spongy, and a relaxing pale pink in color. In the patients that had died quickly from the disease, the scientists found evidence of rampant tissue destruction. The normal pink color of the lungs was replaced by multiple large, angry, dark red and purple hemorrhagic areas of destroyed tissue. A foamy tan-colored froth exuded from the lung tissue when it was cut open with a knife. Inside, the air passages had been stripped of their normal lining of epithelial cells.

The entire pulmonary system appeared to have been damaged by an acute inflammatory process generated by the body's own defenses. The lungs were heavy and filled with fluid, blood, and damaged tissue debris that blocked the normal exchange of oxygen with carbon dioxide. To-day, this condition would be called ARDS, or the Acute/ Adult Respiratory Distress Syndrome. Even with modern intensive care, ARDS can lead to death in 40-60% of cases.

There were other unusual signs as well in the victims. The heart muscle in some of the cases appeared to have been severely damaged and the tough pale-grey membranous sack that enclosed the heart (called the pericardium), was red and inflamed. In every case, there was damage to the kidneys. Highly unusual for a respiratory disease. The small adrenal glands located above each kidney also showed areas of destruction with tiny hemorrhages. The liver in some patients was damaged and, in some cases, the brain as well. Whatever was causing this disease was affecting the major organs throughout the body.[11]

Shaking their heads in wonder, the team struggled to put together what is now called a *Case Definition*. This included the symptoms and timelines of the disease combined with what they had learned from the autopsies. They found that the victims of the new disease had a variety of different symptoms. Some developed excruciating pain in their joints along with fever, chills, and intense headaches. Some 41% of cases had a severe infection of the middle ear, and 5-15% of cases developed severe nosebleeds while the victims were still alive. Some patients had signs of brain damage with paralyzed eye movements or partial body paralysis in the final stages of their disease. Bleeding from the mucous membranes was common and intestinal bleeding with bloody diarrhea could also be a part of the death process.

One shocking thing was soon apparent......the disease appeared to affect the younger adults the worse. Men in their late teens and early 20's were the cases struck the most violently by the infection. These were the ones that died within 48-hours of their first cough.[12]

What the team was seeing was a complete reversal of everything that was known about Influenza at that time. Even today, Influenza normally causes only a mild to moderate illness in adults in the 19 to 35-year old age group. Somehow the biological agent causing the 1918 outbreak had become adapted to the specific age group of the population that was facilitating its spread. The investigative team were in total agreement on one thing. If this was Influenza, it was a type that had never been seen before.

That evening, the team consolidated their findings and Colonel Welsh contacted the Office of the Army Surgeon General to outline their data. He recommended that Camp Devens be quarantined and he gave his team's recommendations for other immediate actions that needed to be taken. In response, Welsh learned that it was already too late. Similar large Influenza outbreaks in other military cantonment camps had already begun. The spillover of infection into the major metropolitan areas of the United States was now inevitable.

Promoted by war and facilitated by the global movement of humans in the form of transcontinental trains and international ocean transport, this new lethal Influenza strain would now sweep around the world in a matter of weeks. Without a vaccine or treatment, the death toll would be unremitting. In South Africa, some 4% of the city of Cape Town's population were dead within 30-days. Entire villages were annihilated in West Africa with the bodies left unburied. In Germany, Influenza would demonstrate a shocking fatality rate of 27% in some cities. In Paris, 10% of all who contracted the infection died. Areas of Mexico would lose 10% of their total population within days. In South America, 50% the population in the capital of Argentina contracted the new disease.[1]

The new Influenza also struck China and while there are no precise known statistics, it is estimated that half the population in the city of Chungking contracted the infection. However, the infection seemed to have had a much lower mortality in China. One explanation is that Influenza had struck the nation hard during the first milder pandemic wave that occurred weeks before and this had provided the population some degree of immunity. This makes sense, especially because scientists now know that China is a site of constant new Influenza virus generation because of its agricultural practices. Therefore, the population of China may have had some cross-immunity to the new, lethal, 1918 Influenza strain.[13]

Elsewhere, even the isolated Pacific islands were not safe. In Fiji, 14% of the population died within 14-days and it became impossible to bury the dead. In contrast, the American Territory of Eastern Samoa initiated immediate total quarantine measures and suffered no cases for weeks. At the same time, Western Samoa lost 22% of its total population.[1,2]

Although Influenza reached most American communities by late September of 1918, the disease did not hit Alaska until late in the fall. This was due to the foresight of the territorial governor, Thomas Riggs Jr., who imposed a strict maritime quarantine. He stationed US Marshals at all ports to ensure the disease did not reach the territory's widely dispersed towns and settlements. However, it would only take one mistake to cause a catastrophe. That mistake occurred on October 20, when a small ship arrived in Nome. The doctor on duty placed the passengers and its crew under a quarantine in the local hospital as per the new regulation. However, after five days, only one person had fallen ill. After an examination, the doctor dismissed this case as nothing more than a case of tonsillitis and he lifted the quarantine. Four days later, one of the hospital workers came down with a lethal case of the new Influenza. The virus was now loose in Nome.[14]

At the same time, a ship named the *SS Victoria* arrived and docked at the port so that its crew could unload bundles of mail. Although the bundles had been fumigated, some of the crew may have come into direct contact with the local mail carriers as they packed their dogsleds. These mail carriers may have picked up the viral infection at that time. Alternatively, the method used to decontaminate the mail before it was unloaded has been lost to time and it is possible that live virus still contaminated the letters in the bundles. Most viruses exhibit a prolonged survival time outside the body if very cold, dehumidified air is present. Whatever the exact mechanism, as these carriers rode out of Nome on their dog sleds that day, they unwittingly delivered both the mail and the new deadly new strain of Influenza to the villages across western Alaska.[14]

Two-days later, the city of Nome was under quarantine and its inhabitants were ordered not to leave the city limits. It made no difference. A major Influenza outbreak was already well underway in the nearby Eskimo village. Over the next few weeks, half of Nome's white population fell ill. The nearby Eskimos suffered tremendously with ten to twenty of their number dying each day until more than half the population of the village expired.[14]

In a desperate response to the pandemic, local leaders and doctors across Alaska now ordered the closure of churches, schools, and theatres. Traveling was prohibited between villages. Traditional Native assemblies were banned. Armed guards took up positions outside some communities to establish a reverse quarantine. It made no difference. Within days, all contact with the villages across the Seward Peninsula was lost. Back in Nome, the local government now asked miners to take their dog sleds out to inspect the backcountry. As these teams traveled up the coast, they found that the Influenza epidemic had struck the villages at roughly the same time as it broke out in Nome.[14]

In the little settlement of Brevig Mission, the virus had struck quickly and brutally, killing 90 percent of the town's population in five days, leaving scores of corpses frozen and unburied. These dead bodies would provide important clues to scientists 80-years later. The situation was even worse in a tiny town called Wales.[2] Rescuers from Nome reached this settlement three weeks after the flu had struck the village. They found orphaned babies trying to suckle their dead mothers and a shivering girl keeping tins of milk warm against her body to feed her siblings. The rest of the survivors were sheltering in the local schoolhouse, living on reindeer broth.[14] In some cases, upon entering a Native igloo, children were found huddling together for warmth and living between their dead parents.

Because subsistence living was common throughout the area, influenza killed the native Alaskans both directly and indirectly. When a family became ill with the virus, no one was left to tend the fires and many simply froze to death in their homes or found themselves unable to hunt large game or set and harvest their traps. They died of exposure from the lack of calories.[14] Yet none of this compared to the truly apocalyptic effect that the new Influenza virus created on the other side of the world.

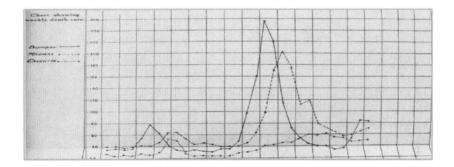

Figure 8. *Chart showing the Weekly Death Rate in Bombay, Madras, and Calcutta, 1918.*[15]

On the Indian subcontinent the mortality of the 1918 influenza epidemic was higher than anywhere else on the planet and the descriptions that survive of this event are almost inconceivable today. Following the rail lines, the new Influenza virus swept across India in roughly three months. In the poor, high-density, low resource communities in Bombay, the Central Provinces and Berar, its impact was horrendous. There, the death demographics was the same as in Europe with the 20 to 29-year old age group affected the worst. The total number of fatalities in the Central and Berar regions reached 17.9% of the population within days. One estimate has suggested that India suffered some 18.5 to 22.5 million deaths.[16,17] Other estimates have placed the total death rate at a lower 17.4 to 18.5 million, but even this number dead in a single country, is overwhelming.[18]

Whatever the precise figure, death was everywhere in India. Trains would arrive at their destination with passengers having died on board during their trip.[1,2] In the Punjab, the hospitals were so overwhelmed that the dead could not be removed quick enough and both the streets and alleys became littered with corpses. Bodies were simply collected and placed into pits for large-scale cremation and the ashes put into the river. When the firewood ran out, the bodies themselves were dumped into the river.[2]

———

By 1918, medical science had recognized that Influenza was a specific infectious disease, but most scientists were of the conviction that it was caused by a still unknown type of bacteria. Yet scientists could not consistently isolate bacteria from the lungs in many of the cases. As the 1918 pandemic began its exponential rise to its full lethality, the Medical Research Council (MRC) in England felt that some attention should be turned to the possible role of a 'filterable agent' causing the disease.

At the time, small teams of physicians and pathologists did most of the wartime medical research in England. Consequently, in November of 1918, two teams of MRC scientists were sent to France. Both teams discovered that a 'filterable agent' did indeed seem to be present in soldiers suffering from the classical signs and symptoms of Influenza.[19] Using filters to remove the bacteria from the bronchial secretions of an influenza patient, they injected this cleared filtrate into the eyes and noses of experimental animals that in turn, developed a fever. This same filtrate was later administered to a brave volunteer by subcutaneous injection who went on to developed some of the signs of Influenza.[20]

However, the team's findings remained controversial. The so-called 'filterable agent' could not be seen with the microscopes of the time, and it could not be cultured, so its presence was inferred. In addition, with the First World War still raging, medical science was already overstressed by the treatment challenges posed by thousands of poison gas injuries, traumatic brain injuries ("shell shock"), trench foot, facial reconstruction surgery, epidemic typhus in the trenches, and overwhelmingly staggering numbers of infected wounds and gangrene. The 1918 Influenza outbreak simply joined the long list of the suffering and horrors inherent in the First World War.

Perhaps a more important factor was that scientists had already become fixated on the false clues that were attributing bacteria to be the cause of Influenza. The scientists involved had failed to keep an open inquiring mind. Work towards developing a specific vaccine as had been done previously for other 'filterable agents' never occurred. Indeed, it took until 1933 for scientists to conclusively prove the existence of the human Influenza virus by using ferrets as an animal model of the disease. The actual direct visual observation of the Influenza virus did not occur until years later, and this had to wait until several diverse technologies had matured and combined.

The first breakthrough in visualizing the virus came in 1931, when scientists managed to grow influenza and several other viruses inside fertilized chickens' eggs. This allowed the first pure cultures of the filterable "Influenza agent" to be made. By 1939, these pure cultures could be analyzed by ultracentrifugation using special centrifuges with high-speed steel rotors capable of concentrating the virus by spinning at 65,000 rpm. This made it possible to study the invisible "filterable agent" in solution and it gave scientists a rough estimate for the general size of a virus.

All during this time, the electron microscope was being developed into a practical instrument for research. Invented in 1931, this type of microscope used a beam of accelerated electrons for illumination instead of visible light.

In 1937, the physicist Ernst Ruska built one that exceeded the resolution of the normal optical (light) microscope and in 1939, a 'filterable agent' called the Tobacco Mosaic Virus was first imaged. By 1943, these three technologies came together, allowing scientists for the first time to make a visual observation of the Influenza virus.[21]

More recently, the actual genetic blueprints for the deadly 1918 strain of Influenza have been recovered from preserved tissue sections archived from soldiers that had died from Influenza during World War I. In conjunction with other frozen tissue samples taken from Eskimo bodies buried in the Arctic permafrost at the time, the complete instructions for making the 1918 pandemic virus was determined (Figure 9).

Consequently in 2005, an influenza virus bearing all 8 gene segments of the pandemic virus was artificially constructed in the laboratory using reverse genetics. The first studies on this recreated 1918 Influenza virus showed that it was an H1N1 strain and that it retained the "blueprints" of Influenza viruses that are primarily found in birds.

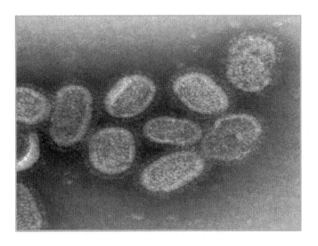

Figure 9. *This negative-stained transmission electron micrograph shows the recreated 1918 Influenza virus replicating in infected Madin-Darby Canine Kidney (MDCK) cells cultured for 18-hours after infection.*

In contrast to the human influenza H1N1 viruses found today, the 1918 strain has the ability to cause death in mice and it shows an extremely high replication rate when cultured in the type of cells that line the human airways.

Alarmingly, further research suggests that it may take fewer genetic adaptations than it was once thought for a bird Influenza virus to jump into man and efficiently spread from person to person.

This has serious and ominous implications for the future.

Notes for Chapter 4

[1] The Great Influenza: The Story of the Deadliest Pandemic in History, John M. Barry Paperback, Revised Edition, 560 pages. Published October 4th, 2005 by Penguin Books (first published 2004) ISBN 0143036491 (ISBN13: 9780143036494).

[2] America's Forgotten Pandemic: The Influenza of 1918, Alfred W. Crosby Paperback, Second Edition, 2003 by Cambridge University Press. (ISBN0-521-54175-1).

[3] Gerard Kian-Meng Goh, Vladimir N. Uversky et.al. Protein intrinsic disorder and influenza virulence: the 1918 H1N1 and H5N1 viruses. Virology Journal 2009 6:69 DOI: 10.1186/1743-422X-6-69.

[4] Vaughan, Victor C., Influenza and pneumonia in Brest, France. Journal of Laboratory and Clinical Medicine, vol. 4, (Jan 1919, p223).

[5] Dudley, Sheldon F., The biology of epidemic Influenza, illustrated by Naval experience, Proc. Royal Soc of Medicine, vol14, War Section (9 May1921) pp.44-45

[6] Weiner, Tim (2012). "Anarchy". Enemies a history of the FBI (1 ed.). New York: Random House. ISBN 978-0-679-64389-0

[7] Department of the Navy (US) Annual Report, 1919. Washington: U.S. Government Printing Office; 1920 (p. 2473–4)

[8] Monthly Bulletin of the Health Department of the City of Boston, Vol. 7 (September 1918) 42

[9] The epidemic of Influenza at Camp Devens, Massachusetts, Journal of Laboratory and Clinical Medicine vol.4 March 1919; Wooley PC. Box 84, Entry 31, RG 112. College Park, MD: National Archives and Records Administration; 1918. Sep 16, to Surgeon General.

[10] War Department (US) Office of the Surgeon General, Medical Department of the United States Army in the World War, vol. 4, activities concerning mobilization camps and ports of embarkation. Washington: U.S. Government Printing Office; 1926. pp. 49–50.

[11] Wolbach, S., Comments on the Pathology and Bacteriology of Fatal Influenza Cases, as observed at Comp Devens Massachusetts Johns Hopkins Bulletin, vol. 30 (April 1919)

[12] Symmers, Douglas, Pathological Similarities Between Pneumonia of Bubonic Plague and of Pandemic Influenza, Journal of the American Medical Association, Vol. 71 (2 November 1918

[13] K.F. Cheng, P.C. Leung, What Happened to China During the 1918 Pandemic? International Journal of Infectious Diseases (2007) 11, 360-364. doi: 10.1016/j.ijid.2006.07.009

[14] Alaska and the 1918 "Spanish Flu", Colleen Pustola, http://alaskaweb.org (with permission).

[15] Siddharth Chandra and Eva Kassens-Noor; The evolution of pandemic influenza: evidence from India, 1918–19 BMC Infectious Diseases: 510, 19 September 2014. https://bmcinfectdis.biomedcentral.com/articles/10.1186/1471-2334-14-510

[16] Phipson, E. S., The Pandemic of Influenza in India in the Year 1918 (With Special Reference to the City of Bombay). Indian Medical Gazette 1923 Vol.58 No.11 pp.509-524 ref.13

[17] Davis K., The Population of India and Pakistan. 1951, Princeton: Princeton University Press.

[18] Mills, I. D., Influenza in India during 1918-19. Chapter 8 in T. Dyson (ed.) India's Historical Demography: Studies in Famine, Disease and Society. 1989, London: Curzon Press.

[19] Nicolle and Le Bailly, BMJ, 11/2/1918.

[20] JAMA. 1918; 71(26):2154-2155. doi:10.1001/jama.1918.02600520040012

[21] A. R. Taylor, D. G. Sharp, Dorothy Beard, J. W. Beard, John H. Dingle and A. E. Feller Isolation and Characterization of Influenza A Virus (PR8 Strain) J. Immunol. September 1, 1943, 47 (3) 261-282.

5

THE CITY OF PHILADELPHIA

ALL COMMUNITIES WILL EXPERIENCE a global Influenza pandemic as their own individual local epidemic. If they can successfully manage the medical effects of the outbreak in their area, then the community is free to work on the other problems that may be associated with the event. These could involve the loss of family incomes, a reduced food supply to the locality, the loss of mass transit services, maintaining the community's electricity and water supply, its garbage collection services, and helping families already dealing with non-epidemic related medical issues. An important factor that must always be considered, is the dignified disposal of the dead.

This requires knowledgeable and intelligent community leaders along with some degree of pre-planning and preparation. Such planning does not require a great expense, but it does require time and careful thought. It also requires an application of the science of Public Health.

Public Health refers to the practice of medicine on an entire population rather on just individuals. It is one of the major factors that allow millions of people to continue to safely live and work under our modern unnaturally high population densities.

When examining the possible effects that a 1918-type event might exert today in the United States, it is useful to examine what a worst-case scenario looked like in the past. In this respect it is recognized that in 1918, the city of Philadelphia, Pennsylvania, was the most seriously affected major urban center in the United States. It is therefore reasonable to examine if there were any factors that made this city different from the other U.S. cities affected by Influenza at the time, and to look at how Philadelphia managed its event. There are important lessons to be learned for today.

One factor that immediately stands out was Philadelphia's rapid and uncontrolled increase in its population. Federal estimates in 1918 give the official civilian population of Philadelphia as 1,700,000. However, as the U.S. prepared for the First World War, the city experienced an unprecedented surge in population as new transient workers (many poor immigrants) flocked to the rapidly expanding war-time industries of steel production, shipbuilding, and munitions manufacturing). In 1918, the Philadelphia Department of Public Health and Charities had estimated that these transient workers and their families added an additional 300,000 people to the official city population.[1,2]

Consequently, most homes in the non-affluent areas had lodgers and the rapid influx of workers and families created its own public health crisis. This was in the form of inadequate, unsanitary, and overcrowded urban housing areas. Multiple large high-density immigrant slums and tenement districts quickly developed. Many had public outhouses that served dozens of families and multiple families crowded into small two-room or three-room apartments. "Rooming Houses" often shared beds among different single men sleeping in shifts.[1,2]

The most difficult conditions were found in South Philadelphia in the southern part of the Seventh Ward running along Lombard and South

Streets, together with the whole Thirtieth Ward. This was Philadelphia's first slum and it was one of the largest in the northern U.S.[3] These slum and tenement areas provided an ideal setting for the spread of any infectious disease and it would be these communities that would soon suffer the worst.[4] We will discuss this Public Health aspect further on in this book when we look at the problem of the high-density economically-disadvantaged urban areas of the 120 largest cities in the United States.

Compounding the problems created by these 1918 high-density population areas, was a chronic shortage of health care workers. During the previous 12-months, over 26% of Philadelphia's doctors and even more nurses, had left to become part of the war effort. The Pennsylvania General Hospital in Philadelphia itself had three-quarters of its staff called overseas to France.[2,5]

While these are all major factors, the biggest reason for the soon-to-occur catastrophe lay in the utter lack of leadership provided by a corrupt Philadelphia city government and its combination with an incompetent City Public Health Department. As we have noted previously, human behavior plays a major role in every epidemic and in the case of Philadelphia this was in the form of the original Sins of "Greed and Power."

In 1918, the City government was run by the dominating and corrupt Senator Edwin Vare who had amassed a huge wealth, apparently generated by contractor kickbacks. The Mayor of Philadelphia acted as Vare's deputy and the Mayor himself would be eventually indicted for conspiracy to murder but was never charged.[1,2]

The Director of Public Health and Charities at the time was a physician and while basically a good man, he had little understanding of Public Health and he was serving under the Mayor's discretion. This, plus the rest of the list of hack political appointees to the city government, assured that Philadelphia would be incapable of responding to any serious large public health emergency.

The city had dodged its first bullet back on June 30, 1918, when the Influenza riddled British cargo ship the "City of Exeter" had arrived at the Philadelphia docks with its dying sailors onboard. However,

Philadelphia's luck only lasted for another month. As previously described, in August 27, 1918, a new lethal mutated Influenza virus arrived in the United States when a group of American soldiers returned to Boston Harbor. In mid-September with the Boston epidemic already underway, some 300 Navy personnel were transported out of the city and shipped by train to the Navy Yard in Philadelphia.[1,2] This quickly led to an outbreak of the new Influenza strain in the Philadelphia Navy Yard, and within a few days, the first civilian infections in Philadelphia itself were underway.

The public health authorities had missed their chance and they compounded this by issuing only a pathetically weak public warning and health campaign that advised against coughing, spitting, and sneezing in public. It made no serious public health preparations and it was only at the end of September when Philadelphia decided to make Influenza a notifiable disease in the city.[6] The Director of Public Health stated there was little chance of the Influenza outbreak spreading.[1] Just as today, the National Press demonstrated their usual ignorance of medical matters. Philadelphia's major newspapers falsely reported that the cause of Influenza was a recently discovered bacterium (*Hemophilus influenzae*) and that doctors now had a causative organism on which to base their campaign against the disease.[2]

Incredibly, on September 28th, the Philadelphia city government allowed a massive Liberty Loan Drive to take place in the downtown area. Some 200,000 residents crowded the city streets to watch the marchers and listen to the bands on parade (Figure 10).[1,2] At the same time, primitive military biplanes flew overhead. When the parade halted, people would gather close together to hear patriotic speeches. In another part of town, a large audience packed into the Willow Grove Park to hear the martial music performed by John Philip Sousa and his Naval Reserve Band. Within three-days of this event, the appearance of 635 new civilian cases of serious Influenza signaled the beginning of a catastrophic explosion of the Influenza epidemic in the city.

It first became noticeable in the Hog Island Shipyard in Philadelphia. This was the largest shipyard in the world with some 35,000 workers. Three days after the Liberty Drive, some 2800 workers at the Yard came down with Influenza.[2] By October 3, the outbreak was out of control. Doctors in the city became so overworked with patients that the mandatory case reporting was not done. At the same time, Influenza was spreading through the other cities of the state.

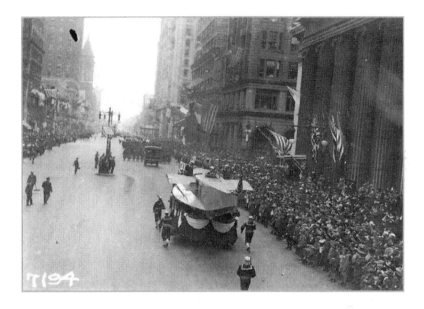

Figure 10. *Rally down Broad Street on Sept. 28, 1918 helped spread Influenza among the general population of Philadelphia.*

On October 3, the Acting State Commissioner of Health issued an emergency order for all bars and places of 'public amusement' throughout the state be closed.[1,2,7] The next day, Philadelphia closed all bars, schools, theaters, churches, and other public mixing places. At the same time the ineffective Surgeon General of the United States, sent out telegrams to all the states recommending the same actions.

However, the narrow window had already closed for any mandated social distancing measures to have any effect in Philadelphia. This window for *Non-Pharmaceutical Interventions* to be effective was missed in other large U.S. cities as well.

INFRASTRUCTURE DISRUPTION IN THE CITY

By the end of the first week of October, the Philadelphia General Hospital was at its full capacity of 2,000 patients and it struggled to find room for 1,400 more seriously ill cases. By the end of the following week, 52 of the hospital's nurses had contracted Influenza and an additional 2,600 deaths had been registered in the city. At the same time, doctors were falling ill and some were dying. Over the following week, an additional 4,500 people deaths from Influenza were recorded. The epidemic by now become a plague and it was impossible to manage this number of dead. At the same time, the number of people with incapacitating Influenza infections began to rise into the hundreds of thousands. These cases continued to overflow the area hospitals filling the empty beds left by the dead. At the small Lebanon Hospital, there would soon be only 3 nurses to care for 125 seriously ill patients.[8]

At the same time, doctors were falling ill and some were dying. Over the following week, an additional 4,500 people deaths from Influenza were recorded. The epidemic by now become a true plague and it was impossible to manage this number of dead. At the same time, the number of people with incapacitating Influenza infections began to rise into the hundreds of thousands. These cases continued to flood the area hospitals filling the empty beds left by the dead.

The infrastructure of the city began to falter when some 850 employees of the city telephone company failed to report for work and the telephones had to be restricted to essential calls only.[9] Over the next two weeks, thousands more city workers fell ill, with some dying. Records show that 487 police officers became too ill to work. Although not clearly documented in the records of the time, the absentee rate for other essential city personnel such as firefighters, clerks, transport drivers, bank staff, grocery store workers, and garbage collectors, must have been equally as high.[2]

The organization that today would be known as Child Services, quickly became overloaded with hundreds of children whose parents were either too ill to care for them or had tragically died. This is a factor that must be remembered when creating future local authority and state pandemic plans. Yet, there is another even more critical factor that must be pre-planned for when considering a future 1918-type pandemic.

Before the Philadelphia outbreak, only a handful of doctors, nurses, and social workers had a responsibility to work in the slum areas of the city. It would be there, like in all the other cities of the world, that the highest infection and death rates from Influenza would occur. For Philadelphia, the statistics would show that its poor communities suffered some 1,500 more total deaths than any other area of the city. Nurses entering the slum areas witnessed almost the same scenes as described 500-years earlier during the outbreak of the "Black Death" in the Europe.[1,2] Throughout the slums and tenements, dead bodies began to putrefy in the streets or in the cramped housing areas still occupied by living family members too ill and weak to do anything about the situation.[1,2] Un-embalmed bodies piled up outside Philadelphia's only morgue at Thirteenth and Wood Streets.[2,10]

With the hospitals inundated, the corrupt city government turned to the local Public Health Boards to set up soup kitchens and turn churches, schools, and armories into makeshift emergency care facilities. However, most of these Health Boards were understaffed with poor leadership and little coordination. In addition, there was still a severe shortage of health care workers.

The lack of effective city leadership was evident as the bodies continued to pile up and more essential services began to break down. While some extremely courageous volunteers could still be found in the religious and civic associations, most of the public were afraid of contracting the disease and bringing it home to their families. The population became demoralized and afraid. Neighbors refused to help or even talk to each other for fear of infection.

As witnessed during the previous historical times of plague, the native-born residents of the city quickly turned their blame towards the immigrant sector of the population. Looking for a scapegoat, Public Health officials blamed the hygiene habits of the immigrants as the cause of the outbreak.

During the European Bubonic Plague pandemic some 500-years earlier, the immigrant population of Paris had been accused of poisoning the city and they were dragged into the streets and burnt alive. In 1918, the overall social behavior was milder and in Philadelphia, the authorities only issued city fines for spitting on the sidewalks which added to the corrupt city coffers.[2] The city government did little else to provide effective leadership against the expanding epidemic.

Never at any time did any branch of the Federal government, make an attempt to help Philadelphia. The one exception was when the U.S. military sent 10 Army morticians to the city to assist with the dead.[2]

The death toll from Influenza now continued to mount as Philadelphia moved closer to a complete infrastructure collapse. Only one thing saved the city, and this was the result of an unintended consequence of the war. This needs to be described because there are lessons to be learned here that are applicable for metropolitan pandemic management today.

In 1916, anticipating the eventual involvement of the United States in World War One, President Wilson's representatives met with the most prominent leaders in labor and industry throughout the United States. The purpose was to form a *Council for National Defense* to prepare the U.S. economy for war should it be necessary.

At the time, the US Government could not simply print more money when it needed it, so the money for any war had to be raised from its citizens. As part of this national plan, smaller versions of the *Council* were set up as committees in America's largest cities. These daughter organizations were composed of the most prominent, educated, leading citizens of each city and their job was to politicize the population and lead Liberty Loan Drives to raise money for the war effort. These Liberty Loan Drives not only raised money, but they helped to create a feeling of national unity among the donors who felt that they were now part of the war effort as well.

Fortunately, the local chapter in Philadelphia was composed of some very strong personalities, some of them women which was highly unusual for the time. Dissatisfied with the pandemic response by

Philadelphia's City government, some of these leading figures resigned from their positions in the Philadelphia Council of National Defense and they banded together to supply the leadership and organizational ability needed to save the city.[2] These individuals were not useless politicians, nor were they in the medical profession. Instead, they were experienced business leaders with private money and influence on other organizations with resources and money. They combined all these under an umbrella *Emergency Aid Committee* and quickly started to coordinate and add to the existing pandemic efforts underway.

HOW THE CITY WAS SAVED

On October 10 as its first task, the new Emergency Aid Committee established a Bureau of Information with twenty telephones available to receive calls 24-hours a day. This "Help-Line" was widely advertised on posters, local radio broadcasts and in newspapers. It was a focal point and the single number to call for Influenza information and assistance. The number was "Filbert 100" and it served as what today would be called an Emergency Medical 911 number or a *Nurse Triage Line* which will be discussed later.[2,9]

The women on the Emergency Aid Committee were previously involved in the Women's Division of the Council of National Defense, and they were just as formidable as their husbands at organizing. Using the structures already established for raising War Bonds they already had their local residential leaders, and this included leaders inside the slum areas. These individuals were recruited for local community efforts.[2,9]

From the local Philadelphia Chapter of the Red Cross, volunteers were recruited by the female leaders of the Emergency Aid Committee who quickly motivated them for assignments. They used the list prepared from their time with the Council, to contact and recruit all the retired doctors and nurses in the city that were willing and still healthy enough to serve. This was truly heroic individual behavior as these medical volunteers now prepared to fight a highly contagious disease with no treatment or vaccine.[10,11] The Deans of the city's five medical schools at the time, were contacted and brave senior students and interns were sent out of the classrooms and into the hospitals.[2,12] The same was done with the nursing students.

To help direct needed resources, the Emergency Aid Committee divided Philadelphia into seven districts. Whenever a citizen called in to the Help Line, one of their volunteers would be dispatched to the caller's residence for a preliminary assessment of the situation.[2]

Surprisingly, the Director of the Philadelphia Department of Health now rose to the occasion and he began to show true leadership. He relinquished control of the nurses who worked for the city and appropriated unauthorized city funds to set up multiple emergency Alternate Care Sites in the closed schools and churches. The active and retired physicians that had been mobilized, were sent to every police station in the disadvantaged south part of the city. These police stations would serve as Forward Operating Bases for the community visitation teams. Street cleaners were tasked to clean the garbage out of the slum areas and accessory morgues were created in buildings of opportunity. One of these was in a requisitioned cold storage plant. (Today, there are plans to use freezer trucks for this purpose, providing that fuel still remains available in the high-density metropolitan areas).

The Director also ordered the city police to work with the Bureau of Information and the Help Lines along with priests sent out by the Catholic Church. Their job was to collect the dead bodies in the streets. Local furniture stores involved in making cabinetry and furniture were contracted to build cheap wooden coffins. City municipal workers were sent into the cemeteries to dig mass graves. At Holy Cross Cemetery alone, the local seminarians became grave diggers as they buried an average of 200 bodies a day (Figure 11).[2,13]

The Bureau of Highways eventually supplied a steam shovel to the city to dig large trenches, and hundreds of coffins were put into large common graves. The firm leadership and rapid actions taken by the Emergency Aid Committee provided a focal point for additional volunteers and resources to be efficiently directed. Consequently,

Philadelphia's population started to rally. Schoolteachers (inactive because of the school closures), volunteered to answer telephones, work in the hospital laundries and some bravely acted as nursing assistant on the wards.[1,2]

The Emergency Aid Committee opened and provisioned the kitchens of the closed public schools. These quickly began preparing tens of thousands of calorie and vitamin-concentrated stews, for the families in the slums that had no adults healthy enough to cook food or their breadwinner had tragically died. Volunteers brought the food to the incapacitated residents in the slums and tenements.

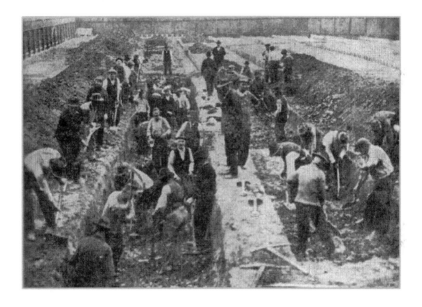

Figure 11. *Mass grave being prepared for victims of the 1918 Flu Epidemic taken by a student at St. Charles Borromeo Seminary.* 1918 Historical Image Gallery | Pandemic Influenza (Flu) | CDC www.cdc.gov

Modern pandemic planning today seems to ignore the faith-based organizations but in 1918, they played a major role in the pandemic response. The Catholic Archbishop assigned 200 nuns to the emergency Alternate Care Sites to assist the few nurses that were available. Priests worked with squads of off-duty policemen who were mobilized as stretcher bearers to help transport the critically ill from homes to these Alternate Care Sites.[14,15] Although they wore surgical masks, 33 of these police officers died from the Influenza they contracted by going into homes to remove the ill and the dead.[2] More would follow.

Little was understood at the time about how Influenza was transmitted, and it was only after the pandemic that it was realized that the wearing of surgical face masks did not provide complete protection from contracting the disease. If worn by infected patients, surgical masks could indeed have some effect on Influenza transmission by reducing the amount of aerosol droplets generated by a patient's sneezing and coughing. However, when worn by healthy individuals to prevent infection, surgical face masks showed a mixed protective ability.[16] The reasons for this will be discussed later.

Transportation was vital for all these community efforts and hundreds of vehicles were donated by auto dealers. These were used to transport doctors and nurses on their "Filbert 100" calls, to take volunteers on their food delivery runs, to make supply runs for the Alternate Treatment Centers, and they were even used as ambulances to collect the ill and take them to the treatment centers and hospitals (Figure 12).

Gradually, Philadelphia began to gain control of its epidemic and the city morgue was eventually emptied of bodies. By the end of October, the epidemic was burning itself out and the "Filbert 100" hotline was closed.

On the 11th day of the 11th Month at the 11th hour, the First World War officially ended and by the start of December, the weekly deaths caused by influenza and pneumonia in Philadelphia had dipped to under 100 for the first time in three-months. Fear among the population may have caused individuals to limit their contact with others and this new selection pressure was affecting the proliferating strain of the H1N1 Influenza virus. This may have led to some reduction in its virulence. As previously discussed, this can occur with RNA viruses undergoing serial passage. In fact, some of the seasonal strains of H1N1 Influenza that occur today are actually mutated viral remnants of the original 1918 lethal strain.

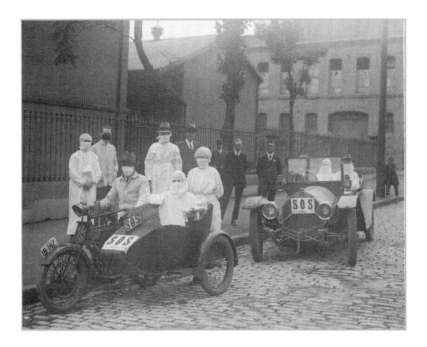

Figure 12. *Dispatched Community Outreach Health Teams.*

The final death toll in Philadelphia from the three waves of pandemic Influenza was estimated to have been 16,000 deaths with 12,191 deaths in the second wave alone. This was out of a population of 1.7 million, with unknown thousands of people in the city severely ill.[17,18] The age distribution of these deaths resembled that of the soldiers in Europe with a preponderance of fatalities in the 25-34 age group and a relatively low number of deaths in people over 65-years of age.[2]

It was also clear that while the disease had struck everywhere, the slums of Philadelphia had been affected the most. This was evident in the other large cities of the United States as well, and it will also be a feature of the next severe Influenza pandemic that will eventually occur.

These statistics do not begin to describe the staggering loss of life and the grief that overwhelmed the population of Philadelphia during such a short period. This poses the question of what effect such an outbreak would generate today in the urbanized interconnected high-density populations of the United States. A variety of computer models have been developed in an attempt to answer this question, but the answers have been variable.

Despite the horrors described in this chapter, it must be emphasized that in 1918, over 80% of influenza infections in the industrialized nations were moderate. Although secondary pneumonias complicated roughly 20% of these cases, the majority were similar to some of the annual seasonal influenza outbreaks seen today.[19]

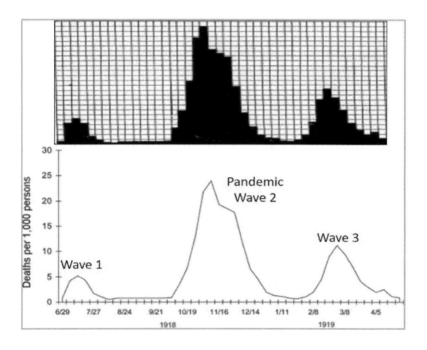

Figure 13. *Pandemic Graph of England and Wales. Jordan, Oakes.* Epidemic Influenza: A survey. Chicago American Medical Association, 1927

However, what distinguished the 1918 outbreak was the actual second pandemic wave of infection that came back from Europe to Boston and Philadelphia and quickly spread throughout the United States and the rest of the world (Figure 13). This second wave was lethal, and it killed young adults quickly. Case fatality rates rose above 2.5%, compared to the less than 0.1% seen in other influenza pandemics.[20,21] This new mutated strain was a product of the intense overcrowding of the soldiers during the First World War. Natural selection became reversed and it did not matter how fast the virus killed, as there were plentiful new victims wherever these deadlier mutated "quasi-species" went.

This second wave of infection caused a global death toll initially estimated at around 50 million. A recent study has suggested that the total death toll may have been as high as *100 million.*[22]

Most of those who recovered from the first-wave infections earlier in the year appeared to have some degree of immunity to the new mutated strain present in the second wave. This was illustrated in Copenhagen, which escaped with a combined mortality rate of just 0.29% (0.02% in the first wave and 0.27% in the second wave) because of exposure to the less-lethal first wave.[23]

As mentioned, there has recently been great progress in characterizing the 1918 influenza virus and its mechanism for causing severe disease. The complete blueprints of the 1918 virus have been recovered and the virus present in the second lethal pandemic wave has been recreated in the laboratory. Recent findings on this 1918 strain of Influenza A, have identified a small number of mutations in the highly conserved "blueprints" for the 1918 viral "Replicase" RNA polymerase genes in addition to changes in the viral nucleoprotein. These may have enabled the 1918-strain to better adapt to man.[24] However, the history of the 1918 pandemic leaves some unresolved paradoxes, particularly with respect to its infectiousness.

When studying epidemics, scientists use the concept of a basic reproduction number to compare how infectious one disease is with respect to other infectious disease. For convenience, the basic reproduction number is written as Ro. The Ro number is the average number of people that each infected person would infect over the course of their illness in a susceptible population. This comparison is useful because it helps determine how well an infectious disease can spread through a population. If the Ro number is less than 1, the infection will die out in the long run. If the Ro is greater than one, the outbreak has the potential to spread as an epidemic and eventually as a pandemic. In this respect, Measles is currently the most highly contagious viral disease known to science and it has a Ro number of 12-18. Smallpox has a Ro of 6-7, Mumps 4-7 and during its 2014 outbreak, the Ebola virus showed a Ro of 1.5-2.5. For the 1918 Influenza strain, it's estimated that the Ro number was 2 to 3.23.[25]

One paradox is that despite the social measures introduced in 1918 to disrupt the spread of the virus, these failed to reduce its transmission by the 60% needed to gain control of the local epidemic. This is important because most of the social interventions tried in 1918, are nearly identical to the measures that would be implemented today.

In the next few chapters, we will examine some additional factors of modern civilization that make it difficult to accurately predict the effects of a future 1918-type pandemic event.

NOTES FOR CHAPTER 5

[1] Crosby, Alfred W. America's Forgotten Pandemic: The Influenza of 1918. New York: Cambridge University Press, 1989.

[2] Barry, John M. The Great Influenza: The Epic Story of the Deadliest Plague in History. New York: Viking, 2004.

[3] The Philadelphia Negro, A Social Study by W.E.B. Dubois, 1899 Schocken Books

[4] Monthly Bulletin of the Department of Public Health and Charities of the City of Philadelphia, Vol 3 (December 1918).

[5] Philadelphia Inquirer, 6 September 1918.

[6] Philadelphia Inquirer, 19 and 20 September 1918.

[7] New York Times, 4 October 1918.

[8] Philadelphia Inquirer, 8 and 13 October 1918.

[9] Philadelphia Inquirer 7,8,10, October 1918.

[10] Southeastern Pennsylvania Chapter of the ARC. Report, September–October 1918. NARACP, Epidemic, Flu, 803.11; Emergency Service of the Pennsylvania Council of National Defense in the Influenza Crisis.

[11] Arlene W. Keeling, Alert to the Necessities of the Emergency: U.S. Nursing During the 1918 Influenza Pandemic, Public Health Rep. 2010; 125(Suppl 3): 105–112. doi: 10.1177/00333549101250S313PMCID: PMC2862339

[12] Journal of the American Medical Association, Vol 71, (9 November), 1918 pp. 1592. https://babel.hathitrust.org/cgi/pt?id=mdp.39015082605638;view=1up;seq=

[13] Brennan, Thomas C. "The Story of the Seminarians and their Relief Work during the Influenza Epidemic." Records of the American Catholic Historical Society of Philadelphia 30 (2) (June 1919): 115-177.

[14] Journal of the American Medical Association, Vol 71, (26 October), 1918https://babel.hathitrust.org/cgi/pt?id=mdp.39015082605638;view=1up;seq=7

[15] Starr, Isaac. "Influenza in 1918: Recollections of the Epidemic in Philadelphia." Annals of Internal Medicine 85 (4) (October 1, 1976): 516-518.

[16] Benjamin J. Cowling, Editorial Commentary: Airborne Transmission of Influenza: Implications for Control in Healthcare and Community Settings., Clin Infect Dis. 2012 Jun 1; 54(11): 1578–1580.

[17] Marks G, Beatty WK. Epidemics. New York: Scribners, 1976.

[18] Ministry of Health. "Report on the Pandemic of Influenza, 1918-19" in Reports on Public Health and Medical Subjects (No. 4). London: His Majesty's Stationery Office, 1920.

[19] Taubenberger JK, Morens DM. 1918 Influenza: the mother of all pandemics. Emerg Infect Dis2006;12:20. http://wwwnc.cdc.gov/eid/article/12/1/pdfs/05-0979.pdf

[20] Rosenau MJ, Last JM. Preventative medicine and public health. New York: Appleton Century-Crofts; 1980.

[21] Patterson KD, Pyle GF. The geography and mortality of the 1918 influenza pandemic. Bull Hist Med. 1991; 65:4–21.

[22] Johnson N, Mueller J. Updating the accounts: global mortality of the 1918–1920 "Spanish" influenza pandemic. Bull Hist Med 2002; 76: 105–15

[23] Viggo Andreasen, Cécile Viboud, and Lone Simonsen, Epidemiologic Characterization of the 1918 Influenza Pandemic Summer Wave in Copenhagen: Implications for Pandemic Control Strategies, J Infect Dis. 2008 January 15; 197(2): 270–278.

[24] Tokiko Watanabea, Shinji Watanabea, Kyoko Shinyab, et.al., Viral RNA polymerase complex promotes optimal growth of 1918 virus in the lower respiratory tract of ferrets PNAS. January 13, 2009 vol. 106 no. 2, 588–592. doi10.1073, pnas.0806959106

[25] Mills CE; Robins JM; Lipsitch M (2004). "Transmissibility of 1918 pandemic influenza" (PDF). Nature. 432 (7019): 904–6. PMID 15602562. doi:10.1038/nature03063.

SECTION

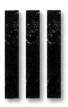

PANDEMICS AND THE PROBLEM OF MODERN INFRASTRUCTURE COMPLEXITY

6

THE COMPLEXITY OF MODERN URBAN INFRASTRUCTURES

THE TERM "INFRASTRUCTURE" REFERS TO THE ROADS, schools, power plants, highways, streets, roads, railways, bridges, telecommunications, mass transit services, airports and airways, along with the water supply, dams, levees, electric power generation and transmission, food and fuel distribution, finances, law enforcement, health care, emergency services, and regional government, together with the operating procedures that allow humans to live under extreme high-density conditions.

Infrastructure also entails the management practices and policies that interact together with societal needs, and the physical transport of people and goods, water, waste disposal, energy, and information transmission within and between communities.[1]

Consequently, a modern urban infrastructure is more complex than any system that has ever been fully analyzed and there are no widely accepted mathematical models for infrastructure interdependency. This is important because a disruption in one infrastructure area has the potential to cause a cascading degrading effect on multiple other infrastructure areas.

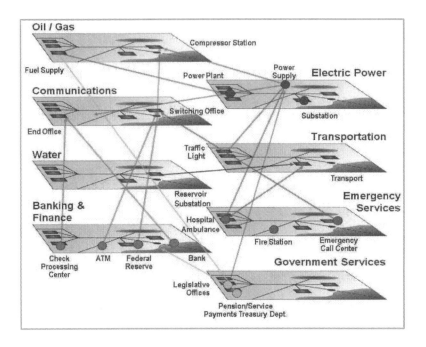

Figure 14. Modified from Infrastructure Interconnections and Complexity. Department of Homeland Security, National Infrastructure Protection Plan.[2]

As Figure 14 depicts, a metropolitan infrastructure is a highly complex and interdependent system and the lack of accurate computer models make it a challenge to make realistic estimates on what could happen with a sudden loss of workers due to illness or death. It is much more complicated now than back in 1918. What is understood however, is that complexity can only grow to a certain threshold limit without failures constantly occurring. The limit to this growth is called the *"critical complexity point."* Once any system approaches critical complexity, it becomes fragile with a tendency to deliver unexpected behavior.

Because the individual infrastructure areas are dependent on other infrastructure areas working properly, once a level of critical complexity is reached, cascading failures are highly probable.

There are multiple examples of real-world cascading system failures and the most common is the electric system blackout.[3] In August of 2003, a squirrel chewed through a wire to cause a cascading series of failures on the US and Canadian Northeastern Power grid. Some 55 million people were suddenly without electricity. Sewage systems quickly began to overflow, rail service disintegrated, gas stations shut down, communications systems began to fail, the loss of home refrigeration caused food to spoil, and the food processing and distribution systems to the supermarkets ceased operation.[4] This example illustrates the reliance of the food sector on electrical power and other interdependent infrastructure systems.

EPIDEMIC-INDUCED INFRASTRUCTURE COLLAPSE

During a pandemic, the impact to critical infrastructures arises not from the disease itself but from its effects on the workforce that is needed to maintain and operate the different critical components and supply chains (including medical supplies and food). However, not all infectious viral disease pandemics are the same.

A pandemic's effect on an urban infrastructure will vary depending on the transmissibility of the virus involved as well as its infectiousness (R_0 Number). Also important is the viruses' incubation period, its replication rate inside human cells, the severity of the disease it produces, the need for prolonged hospitalization or intensive care, as well as the demographics of the workforce, their behavior during a pandemic, and the ability of the healthcare and public health system to take rapid appropriate consequence management measures.

Based on the 1918-event, a serious influenza pandemic is likely to occur as several waves, each lasting several months, with outbreaks occurring simultaneously across the United States. As the U.S. population density continues to grow and the movement of people increases, the probability of a national pandemic in some form increases.

Furthermore, in the high-density populated urban areas, the growing population of the poor are collecting in larger numbers creating an ideal breeding ground for any highly infectious viral disease.

As mentioned, most cities contain no more than 72 hours-worth of food and fuel for their inhabitants and millions of urban humans are totally dependent upon the complex systems of agricultural production, food manufacturing, and supermarket delivery. The delivery trucks themselves are dependent on an even more complex system of fuel transport to individual gasoline stations and truck stops that in turn are dependent upon manufactured fuel from the refineries. All these systems are irrevocably interlinked.

Thus, the normal function of modern urbanized society is dependent upon a reliable constant infrastructure and work force numbers. In a pandemic, the seriously sick do not go to work. Nor do individuals fleeing infection, or those remaining in their houses to avoid contact by adhering to "social distancing" proclamations by federal health agencies. Fear of infection, illness, or caretaker demands for ill family members, could cause an estimated workforce absenteeism as high as an estimated 40% during the peak weeks of a national pandemic.

Another problem are the Suburbs where many people live a considerable distance away from their place of work. Recent U.S. Census Bureau data indicates that the average U.S. commute time is approximately 25-minutes each way. A pandemic-induced lack of fuel or a reduction in the mass transit capability of an urban area, could prevent individuals from getting to their jobs.

There are also some indications that a severe influenza pandemic could conceivably lead to a prolonged partial failure of the US electrical power grid. Most power production in the US is coal fired, and these power plants depend upon regular delivery of coal by rail. Industry guidelines call for generating plants to keep a 25-day coal stockpile onsite to ensure uninterrupted power production in the event of a supply disruption.[3] However, these coal stockpile guidelines are voluntary and are not well adhered to.

The delivery of coal by rail may well be of the weakest links in the resilience of the U.S. electric power grid. The dependence of bulk power systems on the Big 7 Class I Railroad corporations is a significant factor for the continuity of electricity generation. The illness or absence of 30% of key workers at any point from the coal mines to the power plants could dramatically affect coal deliveries. These workers are highly trained, some require licensure to perform their duties, and none are easily replaced. With little reserve coal in stockpiles, this could cause the shutdown of the affected plants. If enough of these shut down, it would affect the national power grid with brownouts and blackouts in large regions of the US.

Nuclear, solar, geothermal, and hydroelectric power generating facilities are not dependent on frequent supplies of fuel. Hence, these power providers might remain online if there were sufficient workers to operate these plants safely. However, even combined, these will not be able to supply sufficient power to the United States avoid large-scale infrastructure disruptions.

THE PROBLEM OF THE MEGAREGIONS

A megaregion is a large network of metropolitan regions that share some of the following: environmental systems and topography, infrastructure systems, economic linkages, settlement and land use patterns, culture, and history.

More than 70 percent of the population and jobs within the United States are located within the 11 megaregions identified by the Regional Plan Association (RPA) America 2050.[5] Because megaregions are defined by connections such as interlocking economies, transportation links, shared topography, or a common culture, it is difficult to define precise boundaries for these areas (Figure 15).

The commonality of high-density human communities sharing common lifelines presents a major pandemic risk. What the implications will be if the major critical infrastructure components of these regions break down due to workforce illness or supply disruptions caused by a highly contagious disease outbreak, should be a subject of great concern.

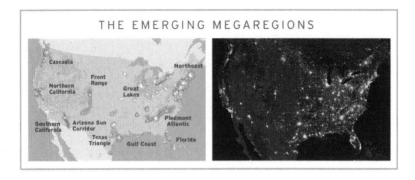

Figure 15. *The Emerging Megaregions in the United States are at a Particular Risk for Pandemic Infrastructure Collapse.* Source: Night Photo NASA.gov.[6]

THE GLOBAL PROBLEM OF THE MEGACITIES

As mentioned, in 1800, only 3% of the world's population lived in cities. This figure rose to 47% by the end of the twentieth century. A recent United Nations forecast predicts the planet's urban population of 3.2 billion will rise to nearly 5 billion by 2030 with most of the growth in the developing world. By 2030, cities will account for 60% of the world's population and 70% of the worlds GDP. [7] Many people will live in what are termed "Megacities". A Megacity is defined by the United Nations as a city with a 10-million or more population, or an average population density of 2000 persons per square kilometer.

Due to their high concentration of people, the Megacities represent a significant global risk area for communicable infectious disease. They are also prone to infrastructure disruption by just-in-time supply crises, social disorganization, and natural disasters. Like the federal government, many Megacities have a multitude of administrative bodies with overlapping and poorly defined responsibilities, making a rapid and decisive disaster response difficult.

As of 2015, there were 37 confirmed megacities in existence with Tokyo and Shanghai the largest.[8] Each with a population of over 30-million inhabitants. The United States has two Megacities; New York with a population of 22 million including parts of northern New Jersey, and Los Angeles with a population of 18 million including the contiguous parts of Riverside and Orange Counties. The unprecedented size of these Megacities serves to magnify the risks associated with the lesser cities. These include, pollution, poverty, food shortages, limited access to water or fuel, escalating crime, and ongoing social tensions, in addition to potential small and large infrastructure failures.

Looking internationally, the Megacities are growing and becoming more interconnected. The ability of governments to effectively deal with their explosive growth and maintain law and order, is in many cases, diminishing. Of significant note is the fact that some two-billion disadvantaged people now live in overcrowded, unsanitary, "shanty towns" created around these foreign Megacities, with limited access to health care. These conditions facilitate the amplification of a communicable disease placing the actual Megacity residents themselves at risk. Not only are more people directly at risk but should a large disaster befall a Megacity, the repercussions of the event will be felt by many individuals well outside the area due to the interconnectedness between the infrastructure networks.[9]

Healthy skilled people are essential to effectively operate and maintain many infrastructures that without constant maintenance will fall into disrepair, some quite quickly. Because the Megacity is a relatively recent phenomenon, it is not easy to assess the risks and develop emergency plans.

In this respect, a contemporary study by the U.S. Army Strategic Studies Group noted that every city has a unique way of organizing, equipping, and connecting with the resources required to maintain its infrastructure. This study also noted that cities differ widely on their ability to adapt to volatility and stress. Some cities respond poorly, making bad situations worse. Others quickly return to a normal state, expending the necessary resources to minimizing the impact of the problem or disaster. A comparison of Texas with Puerto Rico during the 2017 Hurricane season is illustrative of this.

What is good for the Goose—is not always good for the Gander, and understanding the individual surge capacity of any city (emergency planning and response, material resources and reserve, and mobilization capability) is essential to forecasting a Megaregion or Megacity's ability to return to a normal state after a large-scale disaster and how much external assistance (including military support to civil authorities), may be necessary to help it do so.[10]

THE GLOBAL PROBLEM OF FERAL CITIES

In 2004, the national security experts Peter Liotta and James Miskel outlined that the concept of the "failed state," is now being supplemented by the emergence of "failed cities", where normal civil order and interlinked infrastructures disappear and are succeeded by large criminal or terrorist groups.

In this respect, the term "*Feral Cities*" refer to major urban sprawls that lack adequate governance. This has been seen in recent times in the Mideast and Africa when warlords, gangs or terrorist groups occupy a major metropolitan area. This area soon begins to operate at a lower complexity filled with sewage and trash, with packs of wild dogs and a failed or failing normal infrastructure.[11]

Mogadishu is a prime example of a fully feral city as was Falluja and Najaf in Iraq before their reoccupation. Cities with the potential to become feral include Johannesburg, South Africa. At present, much of downtown and the Hillbrow area, including the original stock exchange, has been abandoned to squatters and drug gangs. In another example, crime is out of control in Mexico City and the region is surrounded by high-density shanty towns. Although it is premature to predict that either of these urban centers will inevitably become feral, under certain circumstances this is a possibility. Another example is Karachi, Pakistan, where 40% of the population live in slums with gangland violence and operative Al Qaeda cells.

These Feral cities present not only a problem for US military forces who may have to fight in these environments, but they are also a huge problem for global public health. A new pathogen or a strain of an existing disease could easily breed or mutate in these areas without detection before it escapes to the outside world with little warning.

City-derived pandemics are not a new phenomenon. The SARS outbreak in 2003 is an example of a city (Guangdong, China) serving as an origin and pathogen incubator for a later intercontinental pandemic. In the case of SARS, Guangdong is a modern city with a functional infrastructure. Fortunately, the existence of the new SARS virus was identified, its outbreak origin was traced, and a medical offensive was mounted in time to bring the pandemic to a halt.[12] Had this new infectious disease originated in a feral city with minimal or no medical facilities and an absence of Public Health infrastructure, it is likely that this process would have been more complicated and lengthier with a wider international dispersion of the virus.

Cities have descended into savagery in the past, usually as a result of war or civil conflict, and armed groups have been associated with metropolitan areas before. But feral cities are a new phenomenon and they may pose security and health threats on a scale never encountered before.

It is questionable whether the necessary tools,
resources and strategies required to deal with this threat exist at
this present time.[13]

NOTES FOR CHAPTER 6

[1] Infrastructure for the 21st Century, Washington, D.C.: National Academy Press, 1987.

[2] http://www.dhs.gov/xprevprot/programs/editorial_0827.shtm

[3] Dobson, I., B.A. Carreras, V.E. Lynch, D.E. Newman DE, Complex systems analysis of series of blackouts: cascading failure, critical points, and self-organization. 2007; Chaos 17:1–13.

[4] Fisher, Travis, "Assessing Emerging Policy Threats to the U.S. Power Grid", Institute for Energy Research, Washington, D.C., February 2015, Accessed on 30 July 2017 at http://instituteforenergyresearch.org/wp-content/uploads/2015/02/Threats-to-U.S.Power Grid.compressed.pdf

[5] "About Us - America 2050". America2050. USA: Regional Plan Association. Accessed on 29 June 2017.

[6] https://commons.wikimedia.org/w/index.php?curid=7761887)

[7] United Nations. 2011. World Urbanization Prospects, 2011. Department of Economic and Social Affairs. New York. http://esa.un.org/unup/pdf/WUP2011_Highlights.pdf

[8] Accessed on 30 July 2017 at http://www.newgeography.com/content/005593-thelargest-cities-demographia-world-urban-areas-2017

[9] Economic Intelligence Unit, Globe-Scan and MRC McLean Hazel, Megacity Challenges: A Stakeholder Perspective, 2006.

[10] Megacities and the US Army, preparing for a complex and uncertain future, June 2014. Chief of Staff of the Army, Strategic Studies Group. https://www.army.mil/e2/c/downloads/351235.pdf

[11] James F.Miskeland, Richard J. Norton, "Spotting Trouble: Identifying Faltering and Failing States," Naval War College Review 50, no.2 (Spring1997), pp.79–91.

[12] China Criticized for Dragging Feet on Outbreak," News in Science, 7 April 2003, p. 1

[13] Stanley D. Brunn, Jack F. Williams, and Donald J. Zeigler, Cities of the World: World Regional Urban Development (Lanham, Md.: Rowman & Littlefield, 2003), pp. 5–14.

7

THE PANDEMIC RISK
TO MEGAREGION FOOD SUPPLIES

I**T IS ACKNOWLEDGED** that worker absenteeism can place significant stress on critical manufacturing, energy production, and transportation systems.[1,2,3] However, there is a distinct lack of research focused on the possible higher-order effects of a severe pandemic such as food availability.

A recent landmark study used a system dynamics model to demonstrate the possible effects of a pandemic on the U.S. food system. This model indicated that a severe pandemic with greater than a 25% reduction in the workforce could create a significant, widespread food shortage in the United States. This reduction in the amount of available food would obviously have severe consequences on American society.[1]

Globally, the situation could be even worse. The United Nations Food and Agriculture Organization reports that 925-million humans are already significantly malnourished. This compounds the problem because poor nutrition can be a major risk factor for infectious disease outbreaks because of reduced resistance to bacterial and viral infections.[4]

The global food system is yet another example of the dependency on multiple other critical infrastructures and without a healthy workforce, supply chains operate below optimal capacity or shut down altogether. Sick employees, changes in product demand because of population illness, or inventory shortages, can affect multiple different supply chains, not only those for food but for the medical supplies needed to combat a pandemic as well.[5,6]

Typical food supply chains are large, vertically integrated, and owned by multinational public and private corporations, and they feature an enormous product diversity.[7] If this is in doubt, simply look at the number of different breakfast cereals offered on the supermarket shelves. Over 80% of this food is delivered through the global supply chains with a major focus on low-cost and high efficiency. Driven by the small profit margins within the industry, the pressures to reduce cost has led to a progressive merger and consolidation of the national and international food companies. Incredibly, only a few entities now control most of the volume of food that is constantly flowing through the global food system (e.g., Archer Daniels Midland, Cargill, Kraft, Nestle, PepsiCo, Unilever, and Walmart).[8] The economies of scale created by these companies have blocked the market entry for new smaller competitors.[9] In addition, the food system is totally dependent on a normal transportation infrastructure to deliver its products over long distances via intercity trucking and by rail. On average, the food sold in the United States travels 1,300 miles from farm to fork.[10]

Studies have shown that a shut-down of the food delivery system during a pandemic is an actual possibility in some scenarios.[11] The effects of such a shut-down would be made worse by the just-in-time supermarket inventories. These inventories are kept at low levels intentionally and are completely dependent on a resupply by daily or twice-daily delivery trucks. This provides increased efficiency but results in low supermarket inventories with a vulnerability to unanticipated demand. Food stocks cost money and may be taxed, and businesses are reluctant to build any type of resilience by significant stockpiling. To appreciate the fragility of transportation services to food security, consider two real-world cases that demonstrated the impact of an interruption in transportation on food supply.[12]

In 2000, truck owners and operators in the United Kingdom blocked major roads and fuel distribution depots for 3-days. If the blockade had lasted one day more, food retailers in the UK would have run out of food. The volume of retail traffic dropped to 10–12% below average and the national industrial output decreased by 10%. This experience demonstrated that even relatively minor disruptions in transportation can cause large problems if they persist.[13] In simulations of the effect due to a total loss of trucking, it is likely that all bread would be gone within 2-days from supermarkets.[13]

A second study conducted by the United Nations Food and Agricultural Organization, indicated that the worker absenteeism caused by the large 2014 African Ebola virus outbreak shut down food production and food supply chains in Western Africa. In November 2014, the World Food Program estimated that 460,000 additional individuals became "food insecure" in Liberia, Sierra Leone, and Guinea, because of lost production and trade reductions.[14]

These real-world events in addition to computer simulations, highlight the fragile nature of the global food system and the interconnectedness of food supply and transportation. These dense, complex supply chains are highly vulnerable to disruptions and the continuing trend for the consolidation of retail distribution could increase the consequences of any severe pandemic.

In the USA, our food system's critical points are in the processing plants, packaging plants, and in the large distribution centers within the supply chain.[15] These "choke" points create a vulnerability to the point that a disruption of the food system's workforce could conceivably adversely impact the entire food supply chain.

Another potential problem is the fact that of all the total food consumed in the USA, anywhere from 10–15% is imported.[16] In this instance, localized epidemics or a global pandemic could slow or stop deliveries to the continental U.S. and American companies are completely un-prepared for the possibility that some U.S. borders may be closed during a pandemic.[12]

Consumers also do not typically store large amounts of food at home. With the projections of increasing global urbanization, this will likely exacerbate the problem of any event that disrupts the food supply chain.[17] During the 2002–2004 SARS outbreak in Asia, most people had very little food stored at home. The combination of a disruption of the food supply chain due to the SARS outbreak combined with minimal individual stores of food, did in fact create a situation where many people had difficulty. It is of note that the SARS situation was only considered to be a small pandemic. A severe pandemic will most certainly alter consumer behavior by creating uncertainty, last minute panic buying, and volatility in consumer demand. All of which make it difficult to maintain normally predictable food inventories.[18]

To help clarify the situation, the *National Infrastructure Simulation and Analysis Center* created a model to evaluate the potential impacts of a pandemic on numerous sectors of the US economy. Although there would be select food shortages with a workforce loss of 10%, the food supply system would remain operational. However, a 25% reduction in the workforce would cause a 49% reduction in food production.[19] It is of note that absenteeism in a severe pandemic has been estimated to be as high as 20–40 percent of the workforce in some economic sectors.[20]

Worker absenteeism can also have *indirect* effects on food systems. An example is when a pandemic-induced workforce reduction causes the interruption of waste removal. In a survey, one retail distributor stated: "food production operations would cease within 36-hours if (production) waste could not be disposed of."

The previously mentioned system dynamics model of the U.S. food system in a severe pandemic revealed that a 25% reduction in labor availability can create very significant and widespread food shortages.[1] The 2,000 simulations conducted in this study, indicate that even with augmented food storage at farms, there would likely be substantial disruptions to the food system due to pandemic labor shortages. This study also indicated that even if the transportation infrastructure could maintain its functionality, there might still not be enough food available in the system to prevent people from going hungry due to limited production.

The time of year when a pandemic occurs will have a drastically different effect on the food system and the number of resulting hunger-days, because of the inherent seasonality of food production. Increasing the food stored at farms to 200–500 days did not significantly reduce hunger-days (i.e., food deficits) in simulations. The hunger-day statistics in the study assumed that that the burden of hunger was the same across the US population. However, in reality, when food becomes scarce, it is likely that the lower social economic portion of the US population will suffer more hunger-days than the population with a higher social economic status.

One area of uncertainty in the study was the epidemiologic characteristics of a future pandemic. Infectious diseases that rapidly burn through the US population in less than 30-days will likely not have a great impact on supply chains. In contrast, diseases that moderately sustain themselves in the population over longer periods are likely to have greater consequences in terms of worker absenteeism. Pandemic Influenza is an example of this last category.

In 1918, America as a nation was much more self-sufficient. Today, with the corporate triumph of free trade and the concept of just-in-time inventory management, the problems accompanying a 1918-type pandemic event are likely to be far worse. When considering the Megacities and Megaregions, the possibility of widespread infrastructure disruption, the sprawling urban shanty towns or ghettos in some areas, and modern air travel; a lethal Influenza pandemic could today be many times worse globally than the pandemic of 1918. Especially with respect to food availability.

Today, the total world grain reserves stand at roughly 800-million tons. While this is considerable, the countries of the Middle East and North Africa have doubled their human populations over the last 27-years. Consequently, these nations import anywhere from 66 % to 90% of their grain requirements. Based on a stocks-to-use ratio, if a disruption of global crop distribution occurs as the result of a pandemic-induced workforce loss, the world grain reserves would only feed these regions for 97-days before the onset of mass starvation.

This implies an increased risk for global social disruption

Notes for Chapter 7

[1] Huff, Andrew G., Walter E. Beyeler, Nicholas S. Kelley, and Joseph A. McNitt, Published online: 6 June 2015 # AESS 2015, 338. J Environ Stud Sci (2015) 5:337–347.

[2] Kumar S, Chandra C (2010) Supply chain disruption by avian flu pandemic for U.S. companies: a case study. Transp J 49:61–73.

[3] Osterholm M.T., N.S. Kelley, Energy and the public's health making the connection, 2009, Public Health Rep 124:20.

[4] Food and Agriculture Organization of the United Nations, Global hunger declining, but still unacceptably high. Economic and Social Development Department, Policy Brief, September2010; Accessed 28 July 2017. http://www.fao.org/docrep/012/al390e/al390e00.pdf.

[5] Hessell, Pandemic influenza vaccines: meeting the supply, distribution and deployment challenges, 2009, Influenza 3:165–170.

[6] Osterholm M.T., Preparing for the next pandemic; 2005; N Engl J Med 352:1839–1842

[7] Roth A.V., A.A. Tsay, M.E. Pullman, and J.V. Gray, Unraveling the food supply chain: strategic insights from China and the 2007 recalls; 2008; J Supply Chain Manag 44:22–39.

[8] Beck, M., A. Bruins, t. Fox, F. Gayl, D. Giordano, D. Holmes, D.A. Morgan, Agribusiness industry, 2006; Industrial College of the Armed Forces Washington, D.C

[9] Nikou S.H., H. Selamat H (2013) Risk management capability within Malaysian food supply chains, 2013; Int J of Agr and Econ Dev; Accessed 27 July 2017 at http://www.gsmiijgb.com/Documents/IJAED%20V1%20N1%20P02%20Seyed%20hossein%20Nikou%20Food%20supply.pdf

[10] Zsidisin GA, Ritchie B (2009) Supply chain risk management—developments, issues and challenges; 2009; Supply chain risk, Springer, U.S.

[11] Luke T.C., and J.P. Rodrigue, Protecting public health and global freight transportation systems during an influenza pandemic, 2008, Am J Disaster 3:99–107.

[12] Meuwissen, M., K. Burger, A.O. Lansink, Resilience of food companies to calamities—perceptions in the Netherlands; 2010; Accessed 29 July 2017 at http://commodityplatform.org/wp/wp-content/uploads/2011/05/resilience-web.pdf.

[13] McKinnon, A., Life without trucks: the impact of a temporary disruption of road freight transport on a national economy, 2006, J, Bus.Logist. 27:227–250. 14. United Nations Food and Agricultural Organization, 2014

[14] Burger K., J. Warner, and E. Derix, Governance of the world food system and crisis prevention. http://www.stuurgroepta.nl/rapporten/;2010;Foodshock-web.pdf. Accessed 29 July 2017.

[15] McDonald B., Growing a global food system: agriculture, environment and power in America, 1945–1995; 2013; Accessed 29 July 2017 at http://www.ecotippingpoints.org/resources/presentation-foodresilience/presentations-foodresilience.pdf.

[16] Lederman R, Kurnia S, Lederman J (2009) Designing supply chain systems to cope with catastrophes. PACIS 2009 Proceedings 1–12.

[17] Vo, T.L.H. and D. Thiel D., A system dynamics model of the chicken meat supply chain faced with bird flu; 2006; University of Nantes and ENITIAA Nantes, LEM-LARGECIA, Accessed 27 July 2017 http://www.systemdynamics.org/conferences/2008/proceed/papers/VO153.pdf.

[18] Vo, T.L.H. and D. Thiel D., A system dynamics model of the chicken meat supply chain faced with bird flu; 2006; University of Nantes and ENITIAA Nantes, LEM-LARGECIA, Accessed 27 July 2017 http://www.systemdynamics.org/conferences/2008/proceed/papers/VO153.pdf.

[19] Federal Financial Institutions Examination Council, Interagency statement on pandemic planning, 2007, Washington, D.C., Accessed 21 July 2017 at http://www.fdic.gov/news/news/financial/2008/fil08006a.pdf.

[20] Peck, H., Resilience in the food chain: a study of business continuity management in the food and drink industry. Final Report to the Dep. for Environment, Food and Rural Affairs, Dep. of Defense Management & Security Analysis, Cranfield University, Shrivenham; 2006; Accessed 29 July 2017 at; http://randd.defra.gov.uk/Document.aspx?Document=FT0352_4705_FRP.doc.

8

PANDEMIC-INDUCED DISRUPTION OF THE HEALTH CARE INFRASTRUCTURE

WE HAVE DISCUSSED HOW A SEVERE pandemic could adversely impact some high-density urban infrastructures such as those involving power generation and food supply. While there are still some uncertainties as to the level these infrastructures will be degraded, there is little doubt that a severe global pandemic will severely affect the medical infrastructure of the major metropolitan areas. This will be due to a combination of reduced personnel numbers, lack of medical supplies, and lowered standards of care.

Today, the combined U.S. Healthcare and Public Health sectors employ more than 14-million workers. This represents more than 10 percent of the total American workforce and it includes the doctors, nurses, technicians, and orderlies who provide services directly to patients. In addition, it includes the personnel in supporting roles such as administrators and their staff, local and state health departments, and state emergency health organizations. In addition, there are the private health insurance companies as well as the national programs for Medicare, Medicaid, and the Children's Health Insurance programs which cover more than 100-million, or roughly one-third, of the American population. Also included is the pharmaceutical and vaccine manufacturers.[1]

With respect to direct patient care, the American Hospital Association reports that nationwide there are a total of 897,961 staffed beds in 5,686 U.S. registered hospitals. Over 35.4 million citizens are admitted to these facilities annually.[2] Most of these U.S. hospitals, (78 percent), are privately owned and 22 percent are owned by the Federal, State, or local governments. Collectively in 2013, these hospitals alone employed about 4.83 million people.[3]

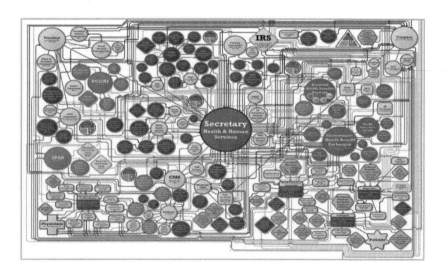

Figure 16. *Bureaucratic Complexity of the U.S. Health Care System.* Source: Congressional Chart Used for Health Care Hearing.[4]

All of these hospitals are supported by the medical equipment and supply manufacturers and distributors who employ approximately

600,000 people in the United States. Supporting this direct patient care is an extensive system of medical laboratories, drug store chains, pharmacists' associations, laboratory associations, and blood banks. In addition, the healthcare system is becoming ever more dependent on information technology to make them more efficient. This includes the electronic health records system vendors. In 2014, approximately 70% of physicians were e-prescribing using electronic health records and 75.5 percent of hospitals adopted at least a basic electronic health records system. This represents a 66.1 percent increase in health information technology within a 6-year span.

Hospitals also rely on radio, telephone, and data communications for a wide variety of operations (i.e., emergency operations, interoperable communications with emergency services organizations, and business operations). In fact, the current U.S. Healthcare system is undergirded by a vast interconnected labyrinth of information technology, data centers and communications networks with no real defining "central node" or command and control hub. For healthcare alone in the United States, there are more than 150 bureaucracies, agencies, boards, commissions, and programs just to control this one aspect of society (Figure 16).

The Death Management Services include the cemeteries and crematorium facilities and the mortuary and funeral home services. These employ approximately 133,000 Americans, mostly in small businesses. Approximately 86% of funeral homes are owned by families, individuals, or closely held companies, with an average of three to five full-time employees.[5]

Finally, the Emergency Services Sector is also an integral part of the overall healthcare infrastructure. This includes more than 2.5 million personnel organized into 5 distinct disciplines which include Law Enforcement, Fire and Rescue Services, Emergency Medical Services, Emergency Management, and Public Works.[6] This sector provides specialized services such as 9-1-1 call centers, poison control centers and Hazardous Material Teams. In addition, specialized Aviation Units (i.e., police and medevac helicopters) are highly dependent on communications, information technology and transportation systems.

In a 1918-type event involving an Influenza A virus with the same transmissibility and lethality, the disease attack rate could range anywhere between 20% to 40% within the overall population of the United States. While not all communities will experience clusters of Influenza simultaneously, near-simultaneous clusters will likely occur in many communities across the United States, This will be more likely in large urban centers or megaregions with dense populations and it may limit the ability of any one jurisdiction to support and assist other jurisdictions. Morbidity and mortality may also vary between age groups.[7]

	Severe (1918-like)	Total U.S. Hospital Capacity	Percentage of Available Capacity
Illness	90 million		
Outpatient	45 million		
Hospitalization	9, 900,000	946,997 beds	191% of non-ICU beds
ICU care	1,485,000	87,400 ICU beds	461% of ICU beds
Mechanical ventilation	745,500	53,000- 105,000 ventilators (5000→7500 in SNS)	198% of ventilators
Deaths	1,903,000		

Figure 17. *Projection of Average Impact on Hospitals; Estimated Illness, Types of Medical Care, & Deaths from a Very Severe Flu Pandemic at Peak (week 5 of 8) with 25% Attack Rate.* (CDC Flu-Surge model)

With respect to projections, Figure 17 provides estimates of illness, outpatient medical care, hospitalizations, intensive care unit requirements, and deaths for a severe 1918-type Influenza pandemic. These estimates are based on DHHS scenarios that are unmitigated (no effective drug therapy or vaccine) and with the cities using the same non-pharmaceutical public health measures that were used in 1918.[8] Of those who become ill with influenza, up to 50% will seek care and it has been estimated that most of these cases can be managed by outpatient/home medical care. The number of hospitalizations and deaths will depend on both the severity of the disease, and the success of steps designed to mitigate its transmission. Nonetheless, these estimates could differ by as much as a factor of 10 between the severe and less severe scenarios.

Even a brief examination of the numbers of projected hospitalizations and ICU patients is daunting, but if the percentages of the infected population reach 30% or higher, absenteeism in the general workforce could greatly increase the risk for cascading infrastructure failures in the high-density urban megaregions of the United States.

One example can be seen in the medical infrastructure of the New York / New Jersey Megaregion. This area serves over 10 million people. The American Hospital Directory (AHD) reports that all of New York State has a total of 56,972 staffed beds across an aggregate of 196 hospitals statewide. New Jersey can provide another 20,553 staffed beds from 74 hospitals statewide.[9]

Considering a 1918-type Influenza pandemic with a 25% infection rate, this would produce 2,500,000 sick Americans in the New York/New Jersey Megaregion. Many of these individuals would be unable to function in their places of employment or serve as emergency responders. Of these, some 275,000 would require hospitalization and over 5,000 patients would require specialized Intensive Care Unit treatment. That itself would require over 2000 ventilators and unprecedented supplies of specialized induction drugs and sedatives.

With respect to mortuary services, in Philadelphia during the 1918 pandemic, this city suffered 12,191 deaths in the second wave of infection, out of a population of 1.7 million.[10] With respect to the same 1918-type event occurring in the New York Megaregion today, this would equate to 17,928 deaths within a matter of weeks. Without pre-planning this will overwhelm the existing morgues and mortuary facilities in the area.

In a partial planning response, the U.S. Department of Health and Human Services (DHHS), has promoted and facilitated the development of Health Care Coalitions. These Coalitions have been defined as a regional system of emergency preparedness involving a minimum of four contiguous state counties with cooperative agreements between at least two Hospitals and EMS Agencies in the region, together with their Emergency Management Organizations and Local Public Health Agencies. The purpose of these coalitions is primarily as planning organizations, with a main responsibility to develop regional emergency plans and proposed budgets and developing regional training. This has connected more than 28,000 health care personnel to help coordinate regional medical responses and to serve as a hub for common communication and coordination of a public health efforts.[6]

At present, it is uncertain what role this will have in a severe pandemic, and what tangible product this might eventually produce. The problem with this is that in a modern 1918-type pandemic, a near-simultaneous regional Influenza outbreak throughout the United States may limit the ability of any one municipal jurisdiction to support and assist other jurisdictions.

As mentioned, during a pandemic, infection in a regional area is expected to last between three to six weeks and most scientists believe that at least two pandemic disease waves will occur, possibly three. Irrespective of the details, an emerging 1918-type pandemic Influenza virus will place profound and prolonged demands on public health, the health care system, and on the providers of essential community services across the United States.

Medical Supply Chain Problems

The image of empty shelves and debris strewn along grocery store aisles is often telecast by the media as a prelude to the arrival of a hurricane along the U.S. coast. It is a stark reminder of the fragile just-in-time supply chain that characterizes most U.S. retail and manufacturing operations. The unsettling truth is that the U.S. healthcare system operates in much the same manner, with limited medical stockpiles and an enormous dependency on remote resource, just-in-time manufacturing, and complex logistical systems to assure that there is item delivery on demand. This just-in-time manufacturing requires a close coordination between suppliers and transportation resources so that parts arrive at the factory just before they are needed. While this increases efficiency, it also increases the vulnerability and a risk for disruption of the manufacturing supply, transportation, and the communications necessary for coordination. While not maintaining a large inventory reduces costs, the drawback is that a single component not arriving on time can bring a modern medical item production line to a grinding halt.

Another vulnerability is cutting down the number of suppliers to reduce the administrative costs of managing multiple contracts and vendor agreements. This tends to drive smaller suppliers out of business, and an industry with fewer suppliers also means fewer alternatives if things go wrong.

As hospitals and other healthcare facilities face tighter profit margins tied to patient care costs and cuts in reimbursement rates, more organizations are turning to a just-in-time inventory management system to keep supplies at a minimum and costs low.[11] However, this approach comes with risks. While just-in-time purchasing certainly benefits the Healthcare industry by lowering the carrying cost of inventory, there is an inadequate amount of medical supplies that are vital to pandemic preparedness and response.[12]

During a severe global Influenza pandemic, can our hospitals, clinics, pharmacies, and medical retail outlets meet the enormous spike in demand for anti-viral drugs, antibiotics for secondary pneumonias, personal protective equipment, and supplies? This seems unlikely given the fact that our supply chains are simply not robust enough to warehouse adequately for catastrophic events. An example was the lack of availability of the protective suits needed for the 2014 Ebola virus pandemic and the lack of simple IV fluids in some parts of the U.S. during the 2018 Influenza season. This was a direct result of the hurricane Irma that struck the IV manufacturing plants in Puerto Rico months before.

Market-driven forces and competitive survival simply do not afford the pharmaceutical companies the luxury of storing vast quantities of low-probability of use products. It is not rational to believe that those states that maintain their own stockpiles will share with adjacent states when an outbreak occurs, even in the spirit of the *Emergency Management Assistance Compact* which encourages interstate support to emergency response by formal agreement among all 50 states. If key supplies are unable to reach the private sector healthcare providers and the hospitals, or if reach-back (backup, surge capacity) support is eliminated, patients will be directly impacted by supply disruptions and delays in care.

The Healthcare sector cannot continue to operate for long without the networks of interconnected infrastructures dependent upon the effective performance of millions of our fellow citizens. As an example, the *Joint Commission on Accreditation of Healthcare Organizations* (JCAHO) accredits and certifies more than 20,500 health care organizations and programs in the United States.[13] For a hospital to remain open, it must be able to prove to JCAHO that it has sufficient capabilities to sustain itself (independently through backups or by the local community) for 96-hours (including fuel capacity, water for drinking and patient care and water for process equipment and sanitation). For example, if water and wastewater operations are significantly degraded for more than 48-hours, hospital standards may require the hospital to shut down and evacuate. Also, the loss of water in support of the building's fire suppression systems may necessitate a complete shutdown much sooner.[14]

The 2009 H1N1 pandemic served to highlight the importance of the medical supply chain in providing the drugs, vaccines, medical devices, and personal protective equipment needed for workforce protection.[15]

Notes for Chapter 8

[1] Department of Homeland Security and Health and Human Services. (2016). "Healthcare and Public Health Sector-Specific Plan. https://www.dhs.gov/sites/default/files/publications/nipp-ssp-healthcare-public-health2015-508.pdf. p. 5. Accessed June 26, 2017.

[2] American Hospital Association (AHA), "Fast Facts on U.S. Hospitals, 2014, www.aha.org/research/rc/stat-studies/fast-facts.shtml/, accessed June 10, 2014.

[3] IBISWorld, "Industry Report 62211: Hospitals in the U.S.," 2014, www.ibisworld.com/industry/default.aspx?indid=1587, accessed July 1, 2017.

[4] http://www.economplex.org/complexity-science/complex-vs-complicated/

[5] Department of Homeland Security and Health and Human Services. (2016). "Healthcare and Public Health Sector-Specific Plan." https://www.dhs.gov/sites/default/files/publications/nipp-ssp-healthcare-public-health2015-508.pdf. p. 5. Accessed June 26, 2017.

[6] Emergency Service Sector totals are approximations from a combination of U.S. Department of Labor, Bureau of Labor and Statistics data and discipline association Websites.

[7] U.S. Department of Health & Human Services, Pandemic Influenza Plan – 2017 Update, June 2017 DRAFT, Washington, D.C.

[8] Eric Toner and Richard Waldhor. Perspective; What Hospitals Should Do to Prepare for an Influenza Pandemic Biosecurity and Bioterrorism: Biodefense Strategy, Practice, and Science Volume 4, Number 4, 2006.

[9] American Hospital Directory, accessed on July 1, 2017 at https://www.ahd.com/state_statistics.html

[10] Pennsylvania Historical and Museum Commission. 1918 Influenza Epidemic Records http://www.phmc.pa.gov/Archives/Research-Online/Pages/1918-InfluenzaEpidemic.aspx

[11] Green, Chuck, "Hospitals turn to just-in-time buying to control supply chain costs", Healthcare Finance, May 06, 2015, http://www.healthcarefinancenews.com/news/hospitals-turn-just-time-buying-controlsupply-chain-costs

[12] Adalja A.A., T.V. Inglesby, et.al. The globalization of US medical countermeasure production and its implications for national security; 2012; Biosecur Bioterror 10:255– 257.

[13] The Joint Commission, "National Patient Safety Goals," January 1, 2014, www.jointcommission.org/assets/1/6/HAP_NPSG_Chapter_2014.pdf, accessed July 1, 2017.

[14] HHS, Hospital Evacuation Decision Guide, May 2010.
http://archive.ahrq.gov/prep/hospevacguide/hospevac.pdf, accessed July 2, 2017.

[15] Bush, Haydn (2011). Reliance on Overseas Manufacturers Worries Supply Chain
Experts. Hospital and Health Networks Journal.

SECTION

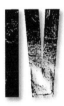

CURRENT UNITED STATES PANDEMIC
INFLUENZA PLANNING

9

THE NATIONAL PANDEMIC INFLUENZA
RESPONSE PLAN

IN 1976, A MICRO-OUTBREAK OF "SWINE FLU" occurred among the soldiers at Fort Dix located near Trenton, New Jersey. The outbreak was caused by a strain of the H1N1 Influenza virus and it killed one soldier and hospitalized 13 others. The outbreak lasted only from January 19 to February 9, and never spread outside of Fort Dix.[1]

The National Press served to quickly inflame public concern and based on the limited understanding of the Influenza A viruses at the time, the CDC recommended that every person in the U.S. be vaccinated against this viral strain. From the onset, the mass vaccination program was plagued by delays and it was eventually halted after it became associated with the occasional side-effect of a paralyzing medical condition called the Guillain–Barré Syndrome.

This fiasco prompted the U.S. government to begin creating a National Pandemic Influenza Response Plan. Various revised drafts of this plan were made in 1978 and 1983, but these were never finalized or subjected to widespread review and simulation exercises. Another attempt was made in 1993 but there was difficulty in outlining the responsibilities and coordinating the actions of the vast Federal bureaucracy.

Essentially, the approach taken for a National Pandemic Response was from the "top-down" rather than trying to formulate an action plan from the level of the local communities upwards to the individual counties and states, and then up to the level of the Federal government. For years, scientists have waited patiently for a detailed, rational, operational blueprint for a neighborhood by neighborhood and county by county plan for a pandemic Influenza response. They are still waiting. The *Government Accountability Office* (GAO), acts as the watchdog arm of Congress. Year after year it has continued to repeatedly criticize the Department of Health and Human Services for failing to develop a credible national Influenza response plan, despite many years of effort.

Following the September 11 World Trade Center terror attack and the widely publicized concerns over the overseas outbreaks of the lethal H5N1 strain of the Influenza A virus, the Bush Administration rushed to formulate a new pandemic plan. In November of 2005, amid much fanfare, President G.W. Bush spoke at the National Institutes of Health to announce a national strategy for Pandemic Influenza Preparedness and Response. However, by itself, the document that was released was almost worthless.[2]

A little later, the Department of Health and Human Services (DHHS) released their own Pandemic Influenza Plan. This identified the key roles of DHHS and its agencies in responding to a pandemic. It was based on rapidly detecting an outbreak, the stockpiling of antiviral drugs, creating new methods to rapidly produce effective vaccines, and ensuring a ready pandemic response at all federal, state and local levels.[3] The second section of the DHHS document was devoted to providing general guidance to state and local public health departments for what it considered to be 11 critical areas. The actual Operational Plans for this are still undergoing review and revision over a decade later.

The document also outlined a very basic 1918-type Influenza scenario to be used for planning by federal, state, local governments, and public health authorities. The criteria used was a pandemic with an infection rate of 30% of the US population resulting in 1.9 million deaths. However, this was only a guess and it was modelled on the H1N1 Influenza A strain. If a human-to-human transmissible H5N1 or H7N9 Avian strain becomes involved in a future Influenza pandemic, some scientists believe that the mortality could possibly be as high as 50% of all infections if an effective drug treatment or vaccine is lacking. This would quickly collapse the entire plan.

Basically, both the White House and the DHHS documents are simply federal recommendations to the state and local authorities. *Written into the fine print is the fact that the local authorities themselves are responsible for dealing with the mass hospitalizations and fatalities of a pandemic.* In addition, the local governments are also responsible for minimizing any infrastructure disruptions due to worker absenteeism. This would be expected to last for about 2-weeks at the height of the pandemic, with a lower workforce loss for a few weeks on either side of the peak.

Almost immediately, many experts began to describe the 2005 plan as "disturbingly incomplete," because it passed the most critical problems of a pandemic response directly on to the state and local authorities; none of which will have adequate resources for such a response. A distinguished Professor of Health Policy at Columbia University called the plan "The mother of all unfunded mandates."

Six-months later, a follow-on National Strategy for Pandemic Influenza Implementation Plan was unveiled based on three pillars of Preparedness and Communication; Surveillance and Detection; and Response / Containment.[4] This document clearly states that the Federal Government will only bear primary responsibility for certain critical functions, including:

- Support overseas containment efforts to delay the arrival of a pandemic to the US.
- Provide guidance to US state/local authorities related to protective measures to be taken.
- Review laws and regulations to facilitate a national pandemic response.
- Modify monetary policy to mitigate the economic impact of a pandemic.
- Procurement and distribution of vaccine and antiviral medications.
- Accelerate research and the development of vaccines and therapies for Influenza.

Following the release of the National Pandemic Plan, there was a flurry of general guidelines published by numerous Federal agencies. However, the actual usefulness of some of these documents is open to debate. For example, the Emergency Medical Services (EMS) Pandemic Guidelines for Statewide Adoption was written by the Department of Transportation, an agency with little or no experience in EMS.[5]

The problem is that 85% of the critical infrastructure resources of the United States reside in the private sector which in general, lacks individual and system-wide business continuity plans for workforce-loss due to a severe pandemic. Recognizing this threat to city infrastructures, the U.S. Department of Homeland Security prepared a document titled *"Pandemic Influenza Preparedness, Response, and Recovery Guide for Critical Infrastructure and Key Resources."*[6] Released in September 2006, the document was designed to fulfill the DHS responsibility to inform America's businesses and 17 critical infrastructure sectors, with the actions needed to prepare and recover from a severe pandemic. This document was followed by Interim Updates released in June 2006, November 2006, and January 2009.

Pursuant to the National Pandemic Response Plans, the Homeland

Security Presidential Directive-5 (HSPD-5), made the Department of Homeland Security (DHS) responsible for the coordination of Federal pandemic operations, resources, and communications with Federal, state, local, and tribal governments, the private sector, and Non-Government Organizations such as the Red Cross. This made both the DHS and DHHS responsible for pandemic preparedness and it required these two large Federal bureaucracies to closely work together.

Yet, incredibly, the DHS wasted no time in formulating its own differing response plan. For example, in an actual pandemic, the original DHS pandemic strategy called for using antiviral drugs only for treatment. In contrast, the DHHS pandemic plan called for the use of antivirals for both treatment and prophylaxis. This is important, because if antiviral drugs are going to be used for both prophylaxis and treatment, more than twice the existing stockpile of 81-million drug doses will be needed.

It is these types of inconsistencies that cast doubt on the ability of the Federal leadership to function in the swift and coordinated matter that would be necessary to impact a 1918-type pandemic event. Even the New York Times managed to get something right when it editorialized that the Plan "looks like a prescription for failure" and it continued to comment on how poorly prepared the U.S. is for a pandemic. In addition, for over a decade, a series of GAO Reports has remained constantly critical of the level of U.S. pandemic preparedness.[7,8,9,10,11]

The major involvement of the Department of Homeland Security in the National Pandemic Plan was particularly troubling. Especially because of this Department's wide-ranging mandate to stockpile drugs and medical equipment, formulate a distribution plan for this, communicate with the WHO and other international organizations, protect commerce and infrastructure, and assure governmental and economic continuity.

In 2006, Congress appropriated $47 million in supplemental funding for DHS to acquire the necessary medical items and protective equipment to safeguard its own employees during a major pandemic event. In August 2014, an independent DHS Office of Inspector

General (OIG) reviewed the ability of DHS to perform its essential pandemic functions and its report was scathing:[11]

- DHS failed to determine what it needed before purchasing pandemic supplies.
- DHS purchased 350,000 protective suits without justification.
- DHS purchased 16-million surgical masks without demonstrating a need.
- A stockpile of 200,000 respirators were past their 5-year shelf-life. This stock will be maintained for "employee comfort."
- Thousands of bottles of hand sanitizer expired in 2010.
- DHS failed to properly manage its stockpile of antiviral drugs for DHS use (81% expired).
- Drugs were missing from the stockpile along with many of other items.
- No contractor performance oversight mechanism was in place.
- Improper storage resulted in $5-million dollars of antibiotics with now questionable effectiveness.

Managing stockpiles and inventory is a basic procedure for even a small business, notwithstanding that the DHS stockpile is critical for the life and safety of its employees during a pandemic. DHS did not develop and implement stockpile replenishment plans, conduct proper inventory controls to monitor stockpiles, or provide adequate oversight for outside contracts. As a result, DHS has no assurance that it has sufficient personal protective equipment and antiviral medical countermeasures for its own personnel during a pandemic response.

A few months later, this incompetence reached a National level during the 2014 Ebola virus outbreak when the DHS proved that it could not implement even a simple syndromic surveillance system at 5 International U.S. airports. It failed to implement any coordination between DHHS and the CDC while spending $4-million dollars for outside contractors to take the temperature of select arriving passengers. In addition, not all the screeners wore the required Personal Protective Equipment. To top it off, roughly 12% of Ebola-infected individuals never even run a temperature (Chapter 20).

In January 2016, the DHS Office of the Inspector General released an audit report regarding the department's response to Ebola. Rather than being in control of a potentially major pandemic incident, the DHS was a major impediment and distraction for any type of successful, organized, U.S. Ebola Response. According to the Office of the Inspector General, the DHS Office of Health Affairs then impeded the OIG investigation.[12] In October 2016, DHS OIG released a report, entitled "*DHS Pandemic Planning Needs Better Oversight, Training, and Execution,*" (OIG-17-02). The report identified some progress made from its audit 2-years previously but stated that DHS cannot be assured that its preparedness plans can be executed effectively during a pandemic event. The 2016 DHS OIG report identified seven recommendations to improve oversight, readiness, timeframes, training, and exercises. The full implementation of these recommendations by DHS has not yet been reported. Apparently major changes are taking place. Hopefully, these include bringing DHHS and the CDC to be in primary control of a national pandemic response.

It must be remembered that the more complicated a plan is, the less likely it is to work properly when needed. It is our understanding that the roles of the Department of Homeland Security in a severe pandemic is now being reassessed and modified.

Notes for Chapter 9

[1] Gaydos JC, Top FH, Hodder RA, Russell PK (January 2006). "Swine influenza an outbreak, Fort Dix, New Jersey, 1976". Emerging Infectious Diseases. 12 (1): 23–28. PMID 16494712. doi:10.3201/eid1201.050965.

[2] National Strategy for Pandemic Influenza https://www.cdc.gov/flu/pandemicresources/pdf/pandemic-influenza-strategy-2005.pd

[3] HHS Pandemic Influenza Plan https://www.cdc.gov/flu/pandemic resources/pdf/hhspandemicinfluenzaplan.pdf

[4] https://www.cdc.gov/flu/pandemic-resources/pdf/pandemic-influenzaimplementation.pdf

[5] https://icsw.nhtsa.gov/people/injury/ems/PandemicInfluenzaGuidelines/

[6] https://www.dhs.gov/sites/default/files/publications/cikrpandemicinfluenzaguide.pdf

[7] 2009 GAO-10-73Monitoring and Assessing the Status of the National Pandemic Implementation Plan Needs Improvement.

[8] 2009 GAO-09-909T Gaps in Planning / Preparedness Need to be Addressed.

[9] 2011 GAO-11-632 Lessons from the H1N1 Pandemic Should Be Incorporated into Future Planning.

[10] 2013 GAO-13-278 National Preparedness: Improvements Needed for Awardee Performance in Meeting Preparedness Goals.

[11] 2014 DHS OIG 14-129 DHS has not managed PPE or antivirals.

[12] 2016 DHS OIG 16-18 Ebola Response Needs Better Coordination, Training, Execution.

10

THE STRATEGIC NATIONAL STOCKPILE

I N 1999, AN EXPENSIVE NATIONAL PHARMACEUTICAL STOCKPILE PROGRAM was created to ensure the nation's readiness against biological warfare agents such as botulinum toxin, anthrax, smallpox, bubonic plague, and tularemia. The mission was to assemble large quantities of essential medical supplies that could be delivered to states and communities during a biological weapon or chemical warfare emergency within 12-hours of a Federal decision to use the stockpile.

The Homeland Security Act of 2002 tasked the Department of Homeland Security (DHS) with defining goals for this stockpile, as well as distributing its assets. In 2003, the National Pharmaceutical Stockpile was renamed the Strategic National Stockpile (SNS) and in 2004, it was placed under the Department of Health & Human Services for general oversight. Under a funding arrangement, the SNS is stockpiled by the DHS, but managed by the DHHS (Department of Health and Human Services) and the CDC, with support from other agencies in the U.S. Government.[1] There is a disconnect here.

A complex bureaucracy is involved in deciding what goes into the stockpile warehouses. The location of these storage warehouses is secret as supposedly is their number (which has been inadvertently released), and they contain a total inventory valued at over $7 billion. However, there are a variety of other associated hidden costs. These include a now mandatory annual inventory that examines manufacturer lot numbers and drug expiration dates and then removing the constantly expiring drugs and having them certified for life-extension by the Food and Drug Administration.

This testing typically adds 12-months of extended shelf life and the costs for drug stockpile maintenance is more than half a billion dollars a year.[2] In addition, most states have their own stockpiles of medicines and supplies that were purchased either with partial federal funding or with state funds. State-maintained stockpiles are not currently eligible for participation in the Stockpile Life Extension Program.

The federal SNS stockpile inventory includes millions of doses of vaccines against various disease-causing agents like smallpox, an ever-expanding stockpile of antiviral drugs, medications for radiation sickness and burns, wound care supplies, IV fluids, hand sanitizer, chemical agent antidotes, mechanical ventilators that undergo yearly outside maintenance, and a range of antibiotics, HEPA surgical masks and narcotic pain medications. Inside the warehouses, giant freezers store highly perishable items.[3]

To facilitate getting components of the stockpile to where they are needed in an emergency, some of the items are stored in compact shipping containers collectively called a 12-hour Push Package, designed to arrive in any U.S. city within hours. These Push Packages are strategically located around the United States (6% of the Stockpile assets assets). Each contains various prepackaged, individual 10-day regiments for over 300,000 people, bulk drug stores, intravenous drugs and supplies for their administration, chemical antidotes and related supplies, airway management and other medical/surgical supplies. These can be delivered anywhere in the U.S. within 12-hours of a federal order to deploy. Each package weighs over 50 tons and it will arrive on nine semi-tractor trailers or one wide-body jet. Each Push Package requires some 12,000 square feet of on-site floor space for proper receiving, staging, and storing.

In addition to these rapid Push-Packs, if an event requires specific or additional medicines and supplies, a deployment from managed inventory (MI) supplies is delivered within 24-36 hours.[3] Medicines and supplies in an MI-deployed stockpile can be modified depending on the nature of the emergency and the suspected or confirmed biological agent involved.

However, the SNS is not a first response tool, but rather a support resource to enhance the response efforts of the local authorities. Federal personnel will work in conjunction with state and local officials to determine if and what components of the SNS are needed. Ultimately, however, the federal government is responsible for making the decision to deploy the SNS.[4] Upon approval, the items are shipped by ground or air and the SNS pandemic supplies are delivered to one pre-designated location in each state. Managed Inventory items will arrive by semi-trailer truck using commercial shipping agencies. Security for the materiel is provided by the U.S. Marshals Service and a small federal assistance team of 7 individuals (Technical Advisory Response Unit) is deployed with all SNS packages.

Each state or U.S. territory is then responsible for the command and control of its own pandemic response. Once authorized state personnel sign for receipt of the SNS assets, the materiel becomes the responsibility of that state.[4] The state is then responsible for the security of the SNS assets and their storage, as well as unpacking the shipment, re-packaging, staging, inventory control, and distributing the supplies to the local authorities in the cities and towns according state and local plans. It is this last item, the Local Authorities, that is the most critical aspect of the pandemic plan. At present, it is also the most problematic.

THE PROBLEM OF LOCAL AUTHORITY PANDEMIC PREPAREDNESS

Central to effective pandemic preparedness is getting the National

Stockpile medical products quickly to the people who need them most during a severe Influenza outbreak. This requires advanced planning at the local levels not only county by county, but even neighborhood by neighborhood. Local health departments are responsible for understanding the SNS system and assets. They are responsible for monitoring the population of their community during a disease outbreak, assessing resources, making predictions of what supplies and extra materials are needed, and informing the state of their SNS requirements as a biological event unfolds. When the drugs, supplies, and vaccines arrive, the local authorities are then responsible for establishing local warehousing and the security of the delivered SNS assets. They are then responsible for initiating a community dispensing plan to get the drugs and vaccines to the hospitals and to the designated Neighborhood Emergency Help Centers and Alternate Treatment Centers to administer to the population. Finally, they are responsible for supplying accurate and timely pandemic information and instructions to the public and reporting the number of cases back to the state.

This requires proper local command and control with Public Health officials working in a unified fashion with both local officials and the area's hospitals and Emergency Medical Services. This requires repetitive training, exercising, and constant evaluations for improvement.

In this respect, the DHHS *Cities Readiness Initiative* (CRI) was created to examine emergency biological preparedness in the cities of the Megaregions where more than 50 percent of the nation's population resides. The CRI project began in 2004 with 21 cities and it expanded to include a total of 72 cities and metropolitan statistical areas with at least one CRI city in every state. The purpose of the CRI was to assist the local Public Health Departments in developing plans to respond to large-scale Biological Warfare event by dispensing antibiotics to the entire population within 48 hours. This useful multipurpose effort spent $27 million over 5-years with an obvious direct applicability for Pandemic Influenza preparedness.[5]

In its review of 2008 State pandemic influenza operating plans, the

DHHS Assistant Secretary for Preparedness and Response (ASPR) found "very few gaps in State-level readiness for antiviral drug distribution." Additionally, ASPR found that States were "doing well" with respect to developing State-level pandemic influenza vaccination plans. This was a glowing report and a review of the various state pandemic plans published on the internet confirms this. However, the CRI review did not assess the local authority preparedness for local vaccine and antiviral drug distribution.

To assess this local Public Health capability, in September of 2009 the DHHS Office of the Inspector General conducted a second series of audits involving 10 selected local public health authorities. The audit was performed by assessing the local planning documents for vaccine and antiviral drug distribution and other preparedness items as based on the formal DHHS pandemic influenza planning guidance.

The results were unexpected as none of the local authorities had any actionable plan for stockpile dispersal into their community. Localities had generally not identified sufficient sources of staff or factored absenteeism into their staffing estimates. They had not addressed most of the vaccine and antiviral drug distribution requirements identified in the DHHS guides. In addition, they were poor at tracking vulnerable populations and priority groups. Failing grades were given for local security for the arriving stockpile items and their storage and dissemination. While all local authorities did conduct at least one exercise related to vaccine and antiviral drug distribution and dispensing, 80% did not create "After Action Reports" and use the "Lessons Learned" to formulate better improvement plans.[6]

The National DHHS Pandemic Influenza Plan assumes a high pre-existing preparedness at all Federal, State, County, and local jurisdictions. However, most federal funding is "stove-piped" to either local emergency management or local public health, but not to both. Funding for nongovernmental or faith-based organizations that could assist a local pandemic response is virtually non-existent. In addition, the federal funding to one jurisdiction is not shared with other jurisdictions and local EMS and local Public Health departments rarely include each other in planning and exercises. *(Note: This has changed a bit with the development of Healthcare Coalitions in all states. Partnerships and collaborative training and exercises is a main objective. It remains to be seen what evolves from this).* Another major problem over the last two decades is that public health nationally has experienced repeated severe budget cuts with a loss of 50,000 health officials.

The failure of local authorities to effectively plan to rapidly distribute stockpile items such as vaccines and anti-viral drugs during a severe Influenza outbreak was a shocking revelation.

In a severe pandemic, vaccines and antiviral agents will initially be strictly rationed. Existing medical facilities will quickly become overwhelmed and as many as 40% of the healthcare workers may become ill or may stay at home. There will be significant shortages of infrastructure personnel and a disruption of essential community services. Existing local mortuary services are likely to become overwhelmed. During such a crisis, any delay is unacceptable when distributing antiviral drugs which may have only a very narrow window for treatment for their effective administration.

The failure of local authorities to plan for the simplest most basic function of rapidly distributing drugs and vaccines to their local community calls into question the entire 2005 federal decision to make the local authorities responsible for the most difficult problems associated with managing a severe Influenza pandemic. However, what other choice is there?

Currently, there are existing efforts underway to upgrade local stockpile distribution using a variety of mass-dispensing methods such as partnerships where public and private organizations assist with dispensing medications to their own pre-identified populations through dispensing sites called "closed" Points of Delivery (PODs).[7,8] However, this will increase the amounts of drugs and vaccine that are required.

The major point to be made is that the local Public Health and Planning Authorities are understaffed and underfunded. This gives some degree of uncertainty as to the effectiveness of the entire National Pandemic Response Plan as it is currently outlined.

There are other areas of a pandemic response that are also troubling, and these will be examined in more detail later. However, at this stage, it appears that a more "bottom up" approach to pandemic preparedness is required for an effective national response. By this we mean that a new concentration needs to be made with respect to Local Authority Public Health and that this be closely tied into the County Public Health Departments within each given State. From this solid foundation, an interlinked solid public health infrastructure can be created up to the national level. Otherwise, it is like trying to construct a building with the foundation placed at the top of the structure.

NOTES FOR CHAPTER 10

[1] CDC. "Strategic National Stockpile (SNS)" webpage. www.cdc.gov/phpr/stockpile/stockpile.htm. Accessed January 31, 2012

[2] https://www.cdc.gov/phpr/stockpile/sustaining.htm

[3] Greenfieldboyce, Nell (2016-06-27). "Inside A Secret Government Warehouse Prepped for Health Catastrophes". NPR.org. Retrieved 2017-06-29.

[4] ASTHO. The Strategic National Stockpile: From Concept to Achievement. August 2010. Available at http://www.astho.org/Programs/Preparedness/Strategic-NationalStockpile/The-Strategic-National-Stockpile--From-Concept-to-Achievement/. Accessed January 31, 2012.

[5] Cities Readiness Initiative CDC https://www.cdc.gov/phpr/readiness/mcm.html

[6] OEI-04-08-00260 Local Pandemic Influenza Preparedness: Vaccine and Antiviral Drug Distribution and Dispensing https://oig.hhs.gov/oei/reports/oei-04-08-00260.pdf

[7] Institute of Medicine (US). Forum on Medical and Public Health Preparedness for Catastrophic Events. Medical Countermeasures Dispensing: Emergency Use Authorization and the Postal Model. Washington, DC. National Academies Press. 2010.

[8] FDA. "Emergency Use Authorizations Questions and Answers" webpage. At www.fda.gov/NewsEvents/PublicHealthFocus/ucm153297.htm. Accessed Jan 31, 2012

11

THE PROBLEM OF THE "VACCINE GAP"

POPULATIONS THAT ARE *PROPERLY* IMMUNIZED against a new Influenza A virus strain by the administration of an effective vaccine, do not suffer serious illness or transmit the virus through their community. They are immune to that strain. Therefore, the hallmark for stopping any serious infectious viral disease outbreak is the ability to rapidly create and manufacture an effective vaccine and to quickly administer it to all populations at risk. This brings up a general question that asks how do flu vaccines prevent the flu?

Influenza vaccines contain an inactivated or "neutered" attenuated strain of the Influenza virus that when injected into the body, stimulate an individual's immune system to produce very specific antibodies in the bloodstream that bind to specific live disease-causing viruses that are causing the infection. It takes several weeks for this process to occur, and with some disease-causing agents, multiple vaccinations may be required. With exception of the Rabies virus, vaccination is not a useful method to treat a viral infection. However, a successful vaccine teaches the body that if it ever sees a virus like the one in the vaccine in the future, it should quickly make antibodies as part of its immune response to deal with the problem. This is called "responding to an antigenic challenge" and the immune system is "trained" by the vaccine to immediately respond by making antibodies within a few hours to a day. In addition, other specialized white blood cells called T-lymphocytes participate in the immune response.

A vaccine, however, is very specific and it only trains the immune system to react to the viral strains that are in the vaccine. At present, there is no universal "Flu" vaccine that teaches the human immune system to recognize all the possible strains of the Influenza A virus found in nature, although scientists are working very hard on this and some early progress has been made.

A well-matched vaccine given quickly to a population is the most important public health measure that can be taken against pandemic Influenza. However, the time required to manufacture a vaccine after the recognition of an outbreak, has always led to too little vaccine manufactured and its globally distribution made too late during each of the last four pandemics.

As an example, in 2009 an ample supply of vaccine for the new H1N1 virus was not available in the United States until after the second pandemic wave had already occurred and subsided. Even after a global production ramp up, there was only 78-million vaccine doses available for the World Health Organization to distribute to 77 developing countries encompassing billions of people.[1]

Unfortunately, with current technology, a new vaccine for a new mutated pandemic Influenza virus strain, cannot be manufactured until an epidemic is already underway. This problem is compounded because the most common technology used for Influenza vaccine production originated in the 1930's using germ-free fertilized chicken eggs. Using this method, there is a 4-6-month delay before a new vaccine can be produced in any effective quantity. Because the new Influenza pandemic will already be underway, this time delay is referred to as the "Pandemic Vaccine Gap." As witnessed during the lethal 1918-pandemic, most Influenza deaths will occur during this period. Even with the relatively minor mutations seen in normal seasonal Influenza, the annual global vaccines usually must be reformulated, and they are based on a "best guess" of which known strains are predicted to circulate during the upcoming influenza season 6-months later.

To address this issue, DHHS has revamped the vaccine production process and has claimed in its 2017 update that it can produce the first initial limited doses of a new vaccine within weeks. Unfortunately, there are things in nature that could be much worse than the 1918 (H1N1 virus) pandemic.

As previously discussed, the H5N1 strain of the Influenza A virus first proved itself lethal to humans in 1997 in Hong Kong. It is now widespread in parts of Southeast Asia and the Middle East, with large agricultural outbreaks in chickens in the United States. This has led to the culling of hundreds of millions of birds in attempts to minimize further mutations of the virus and potential spillover and species jumps into the human population. Although the total number of human deaths from this strain caused by viral spillover has remained low, the H5N1 virus has shown a 50% mortality in humans during micro-outbreaks.

To date, the H5N1 viruses have not been transmitted efficiently by human-to-human contact, and some experts have argued that it is impossible. However, given the potential consequences of a global outbreak of this type, it is crucial to know whether the H5N1 viruses can ever become well-adapted to man. In this respect, scientists have created chimera influenza viruses that have combined the H5 hemagglutinin (H protein) "blueprints" with the remaining "blueprints" from the pandemic 2009 H1N1 influenza virus. This mutant H5-HA/2009 virus has demonstrated an ability to spread between infected and uninfected ferrets (used as an animal model to study the transmission of influenza in humans) in separate cages via respiratory droplets in the air. The ability of H5N1 to recombine with H1N1 or other Influenza strains to create the attributes of a pandemic virus, is extremely worrying.[2]

There is one other significant problem with respect to diminishing the mortality caused by a 1918-type Influenza pandemic, and that is the demonstrated poor effectiveness of current Influenza vaccines in the elderly. Adults aged 65 and over, represent one of the major vulnerable population groups during any Influenza outbreak. Consequently, even during normal seasonal pandemics, the older population are a priority for vaccination, and this has been the situation for the past 40-years.

However, a new Cochrane Systematic Review has brought to light that there is a low effectiveness for Influenza vaccination in this age group. These scientists performed a careful study of previous vaccine trials and determined that the effectiveness of influenza vaccines is modest at best in the elderly. Although this is just an early finding, it shows that additional high-quality trials spanning several flu seasons are urgently required to clarify this potentially serious problem.[3] Another review was made concerning whether vaccinating healthcare workers helps to prevent influenza symptoms and death in people aged over 60, but the results of this study were inconclusive.

To overcome the problems of the "Vaccine Gap," DHHS planners have decided to distribute oral antiviral drugs to select populations to maintain the critical urban infrastructures until a new vaccine can be developed and administered. As we will discuss, there are major problems with this concept as well, most particularly with the drug that has been stockpiled. The effectiveness of the drug (Tamiflu) has been in question for a decade and the stockpile is inadequate to meet the U.S. demand for its entire population. Even if the drug becomes widely available and does prove to be effective in Influenza, it will likely be quickly compromised by a developing drug resistance in the Influenza viral quasi-species. This has already been observed with the seasonal H1N1 Influenza virus.

A WHO Review on the Functioning of the International Health

Regulations (IHR) in Relation to Pandemic H1N1, adopted by the World Health Assembly in May 2011, concluded that the world is ill-prepared for a severe influenza pandemic and that such an event could lead to the death of millions of people.[4] The other conclusion of this useless review, was that there should be another review.

In past Influenza pandemics, groups at increased risk for serious illness and death have differed by age and health status. Specifically, during the 1918 pandemic, healthy young adults were a high-risk group. Because the high-risk groups in the next pandemic are not known, any issued national guidance must be adaptable and responsive to multiple pandemic scenarios.

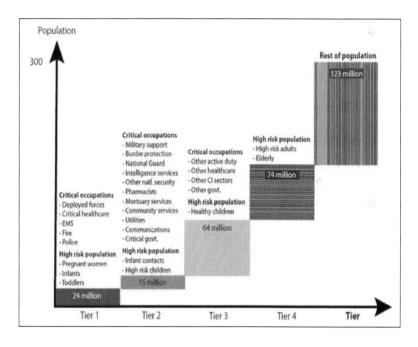

Figure 18. *Tiered Distribution System for Influenza Vaccine.* Public Domain 2008 United States Government Avian and Pandemic Flu Information.

Because there will be only a limited amount of the first new vaccine doses manufactured, the U.S. Government has issued guidelines for who should first receive the first immunizations.

A federal interagency working group has drafted guidance for the administration of the early production of pandemic vaccine with a list of population groups that will be vaccinated in "Tiers," with all groups in an individual Tier vaccinated simultaneously.[5] Tier 1 is considered the most important group. These Tiers are defined in Figure 18.

Within each Tier are target groups collected into 4 broad categories that correspond with the objectives to protect the government and national security, provide health care, maintain critical infrastructure, and finally the general population. Each category contains specific populations based on their occupation or their age and health status. All groups designated for vaccination within a Tier have equal priority for vaccination.

However, it is quickly apparent that both the DHHS and DHS have not properly addressed the vulnerabilities that we have described for the interlinked infrastructures that support the high-density urban regions, or the global just-in-time economy which has neither surge production or distribution capacity for many of the critical products and services.

With respect to vaccine production, even a minor disruption to a single vaccine production reagent, packaging material, or distribution pathway, means that a new vaccine could quickly become unavailable.

Many scientists and public health experts believe that the current federal guidance for vaccine distribution is fatally flawed and that it will not minimize a pandemic-induced infrastructure disruption.[6]

Under the current plan, there will be no antiviral medications or vaccine for weeks, for some 123-million U.S. citizens or about 30% of the American workforce, many of whom ensure that there is electricity, food on the supermarket shelves, gasoline, diesel fuel, spare parts, banking services, mass transportation, and the many other essential services necessary to maintain a high-density urban population. In formulating the federal vaccine distribution plan, DHHS and DHS have failed to construct a priority list of critical products and services, and this may result in a significant increased infrastructure disruption and possibly an increased mortality.

For example, under the current guidance, millions of toddlers will receive pandemic influenza vaccine well before those who provide electricity and transportation. While the need to vaccinate vulnerable populations during a pandemic is logical, and in many previous Influenza pandemics it has been children that contributed to the most spread, the consequences of not protecting the critical infrastructures could be severe. The choices are indeed difficult. For example, would a child with Type 1 diabetes be better off during a pandemic if they receive an Influenza vaccine before those who manufacture and distribute the insulin that is essential for the child's continuing survival if it does not contract Influenza?[6] It will depend on the Influenza strain involved. In a 1918-type pandemic it will be the younger adults that will be hit the hardest and it will be that demographic that would need to receive the first vaccine doses. It may also depend on job classification. An 18-wheel truck driver for a major transportation company might need to receive a dose of the first vaccine over a Harvard-trained lawyer.

This is the situation after some 40-years of government failure to properly address and prepare for the pandemic Influenza problem.

Thus, there is an urgent need for a national prioritization scheme for goods and services to ensure to ensure that these are maintained during a pandemic for the greater good. Better efforts must be made to identify and quantify the personnel essential for maintaining these critical supply chains and infrastructures.

When an Influenza vaccine is in short supply, distributing it quickly and equitably among the different populations and communities remains a significant problem for effective pandemic planning.[7] The distribution of vaccination locations and personnel might not be equal in all state counties and communities.[8] This was observed during the 2009 H1N1 pandemic, when Los Angeles reported unequal vaccine distribution with relatively less vaccine available in areas with higher percentages of uninsured and low-income residents. In this respect, south Los Angeles County received one dose per five people, while West Los Angeles County, which includes Malibu, Santa Monica, and Beverly Hills, received one dose per two people.[9]

To avoid hospital and clinics becoming overcrowded during a severe pandemic, federal response planning suggests a variety of options for local communities to distribute stockpiles of available vaccines from private pharmacies, supermarket chains, private practitioner doctors' offices and other local points of distribution. However, these services are much less likely to be found in lower income neighborhoods and the evidence suggests that during a pandemic, any shortages of influenza vaccine will have a major effect on the socially disadvantaged groups in a community.[10,11] *This is a major problem and it will be specifically discussed later.*

Therefore, vaccine distribution plans may need to include mobile community health centers (staffed by nurses and nurse practitioners) that can travel to low-income areas, along with a variety of community medical and other service providers, as well as use nontraditional sites like soup kitchens, sheltered workshops, and transit points, which already have become popular places for administering the yearly influenza vaccine.[12,13] However, being in proximity to a designated vaccination location, or having a mobile vaccination facility available, does not guarantee that a population will be immunized to the level necessary to develop a "herd immunity."

The term "herd immunity" refers to a means of protecting a whole community from disease by immunizing a critical number of its populace. Just as a herd of cattle or flock of sheep use their sheer numbers to collectively protect any one individual in their community from predators, "herd immunity" protects a community from an infectious disease by the sheer numbers of people immune to the disease. The more members of a human "herd" who are immune to an infectious disease agent, the better protected the whole population will be from an outbreak of that disease. Herd immunity means that not every individual in a community must be vaccinated or have survived an infection for an epidemic or pandemic to stop. The problem occurs when large numbers of people in a community people are unable to get a vaccination because there is no vaccine, they have no money and lack insurance, or because their insurance restricts where they can get preventive care, or simply because they cannot afford to miss work to be vaccinated.[14] The barriers to equitable vaccine distribution require careful local preplanning, even when vaccines are available.

The willingness to be vaccinated also varies. It is especially low among the African American demographic that is disproportionately found the poorer neighborhoods.[15] As will be discussed later, there is both historical and computer modelling data that suggests to maximally reduce the level of Influenza pandemic spread, the poor, low-resource communities should be targeted with the first doses of vaccine because of their high-risk for Influenza infection and their high-risk for secondary transmission to the population of the more affluent areas. More studies on this factor are needed urgently. Without a fast-distributable vaccine or effective antiviral drug, these poor communities will be relegated to the same basic non-pharmaceutical public health measures employed during the 1918 pandemic.

Historically, these measures were not effective in the poor, high-density demographic areas.

NOTES FOR CHAPTER 11

[1] 2011GAO-11-632 Lessons from the H1N1 Pandemic Should Be Incorporated into Future Planning.

[2] Yoshihiro Kawaoka, H5N1: Flu transmission work is urgent. Nature 482, 155 (09 February 2012) doi:10.1038/nature10884, 25 January 2012

[3] Wiley-Blackwell. "Influenza vaccines: Poor evidence for effectiveness in elderly." Science Daily. www.sciencedaily.com/releases/2010/02/100216203146.htm (accessed September 21, 2017).

[4] First Meeting of the Review Committee on the Functioning of the International Health Regulations in Relation to Pandemic (H1N1) 12–14 April 2010, Geneva, Switzerland http://www.who.int/ihr/r_c_meeting_report_1_en.pdf

[5] Guidance on Allocating and Targeting Pandemic Influenza Vaccine DHHS and DHS https://www.cdc.gov/flu/pandemicresources/pdf/allocatingtargetingpandemicvaccine.

[6] M. T. Osterholm, et.al., Comments on the Draft Guidance on Allocating and Targeting Pandemic Influenza Vaccine, December 31, 2007. http://www.cidrap.umn.edu/sites/default/files/public/downloads/hhsvaccpriority.pdf

[7] Zimmerman RK, Tabbarah M, Nowalk MP, Raymund M, Wilson SA, McGaffey A, et al. Impact of the 2004 influenza vaccine shortage on patients from inner city health centers. J Urban Health. 006; 84(3):389–99.

[8] Logan JL. Disparities in influenza immunization among US adults. J Natl Med Assoc. 2009; 101:161–6.

[9] Hennessy-Fiske, M. Los Angeles Times. 2010 Mar 1. H1N1 vaccine was unevenly distributed across L.A. County.

[10] Morland K, Wing S, Roux AD, Poole C. Neighborhood characteristics associated with the location of food stores and food service places. Am J Prev Med. 2002; 22(1):23–9. [PubMed:11777675] 47.

[11] Rangel MC, Shoenbach, VJ, Weigle KA, Hogan VK, Strauss RP, Bangdiwala SI. Racial and ethnic disparities in influenza vaccination among elderly adults. J Gen Intern Med. 2005; 20(5):426–31. [PubMed: 15963166]

[12] CDC. Adult immunization programs in nontraditional settings: quality standards and guidance for program evaluation. MMWR Morb Mortal Wkly Rep. 2000;49:1–39.PubMed

[13] Coady MH, Weiss L, Glidden K, Vlahov D. Rapid vaccine distribution in nontraditional settings: lessons learned from project VIVA. J Community Health Nurs. 2007; 24(2):79– 85.

[14] Blumenshine P, Marks J. et.al. Pandemic influenza planning in the United States from a health disparities perspective. Emerg Infect Dis. 2008; 14(5): 709–15.

[15] Armstrong K, Berlin M, Schwartz JS, Propert K, Ubel PA. Barriers to influenza immunization in a low-income urban population. Am J Prev Med. 2001; 20(1):21–5.

12

THE ANTIVIRAL DRUG "TAMIFLU"

THE MAIN ANTIVIRAL DRUG for Influenza selected for major U.S. stockpiling is called Oseltamivir, (known by its brand name *Tamiflu*). It was the first orally available drug developed for Influenza that could be taken by mouth. The standard adult treatment course is ten-capsules with one taken twice a day for 5-days without missing a single dose. The drug is promoted both as a treatment for infection and a 5-day prevention for infection following a possible exposure to someone suffering from Influenza.

In a previous chapter on the Influenza virus, the neuraminidase protein on the outside of the virus was referred to as the N protein. It has 2 functions. The first of which is to help the virus penetrate the thin layer of mucous that lines the human airways so the Hemagglutinin protein on the outside of the virus can bind to the cells living underneath the mucous layer. The second function of the N protein is to allow the daughter Influenza viruses that have replicated inside the airway cells to bud and exit out of the host cell to cause further infection.

Tamiflu belongs to a new class of drugs called neuraminidase inhibitors. The Tamiflu drug molecules act by binding to the N (neuraminidase) protein to stop it from functioning. Unlike antibiotics that can kill a bacterial invader, Tamiflu does not kill the virus, it just slows down the rate of infection enough so that the body's own immune system has time to mount a proper defense. Therefore, the timing for taking the drug is critical. For normal seasonal Influenza, Tamiflu treatment must start within hours of the first initial symptoms, such as a spiking fever, chills, cough, and body aches. If the drug is taken too late during an infection, there is too much virus being created for the Tamiflu to be effective.

Following the drug's discovery, the giant Swiss pharmaceutical company Roche conducted its own clinical trials to demonstrate Tamiflu's effectiveness. This data was reviewed by the regulatory governing bodies of several nations and in 1999, it was approved for licensing and use in the United States. Consequently, Tamiflu went on sale (by prescription) to the American public to reduce the normal general misery associated with the normal outbreaks of seasonal Influenza.

As already discussed, after the terrorist attacks on the United States on 9/11 the U.S. government rushed to bolster its capability to respond to a wide variety of both man-made and natural disasters. During this process, the worries of many scientists came to light with respect to the growing concern of another natural 1918-type Influenza pandemic. As the G.W. Bush Administration desperately searched for answers to address the decades of neglect in Public Health funding, the drug Tamiflu appeared to provide a quick fix to Influenza pandemic preparedness. The idea was spurred on by the Infectious Diseases Society of America who advocated forming a national stockpile of Tamiflu with enough tablets to treat at least 25% and ideally 40% of the U.S. population. [1] The National Vaccine Advisory Committee and the Advisory Committee on Immunization

Practices called for an even larger 45% drug coverage of the population.

The strategy that the Bush Administration finally settled on was to have a large deployable national stockpile of Tamiflu set aside to keep essential Federal employees and the US military healthy, to ensure the continuity of the Federal Government during a lethal Influenza pandemic. It was envisioned that the stockpile would be augmented by the rapid additional synthesis of more Tamiflu for the rest of the American population.[2] Conceivably, this drug supply would also treat critical population groups like health care workers and the emergency responders such as the fire, EMS, and police forces in the United States. To our knowledge a full scale-rehearsal for this manufacturing was never performed.

When examined closely, the Bush Administration's Response Plan made little common sense. It was designed around the premise that U.S. Health Authorities would have several weeks warning that an Influenza pandemic was developing overseas. This ignored the effects of modern air travel where an individual could be in the middle of an epidemic outbreak in Asia and 24-hours later be in New York City or another high-density metropolitan area.

The plan also failed to address a number of serious problems inherent in a major pandemic response and it seemed to have been designed more as a rushed, quick, stop-gap measure. It ignored the fact that Tamiflu had to be administered quickly within the first hours of developing Influenza symptoms to have a maximum effect, and that it would take several days to disperse the Tamiflu capsules out from the stockpile sites to the target groups selected to receive the medication. Also, there was little data concerning the safety of repeated prophylactic dosing of an individual by administering Tamiflu. There was no mention if the family members of essential federal employees would receive the drug.

Seemingly overnight, Tamiflu was being promoted as being able to significantly reduce hospital admissions, significantly slow the transmission of the virus and decrease the severe pneumonia complications of Influenza. The World Health Organization approved and promoted the concept of national antiviral drug supplies. Consequently, countries around the world rushed to create their own Tamiflu stockpiles. Billions were spent to stockpile Tamiflu and a related drug called Zanamivir (Relenza) that is inhaled through the nose. Most countries could not afford to buy such stockpiles.[3]

The pharmaceutical manufacturer Roche manufactured Tamiflu. In 1999, this company had been criminally indicted for price-fixing vitamins and in the US, and Roche had been fined $500 million for this action. However, the company would soon have the last laugh.[4] With the exclusive license to manufacture Tamiflu held by Roche, the company pursued monopoly pricing that went unchallenged by the Federal government. Countries such as Australia, New Zealand, and some European countries raced to stockpile enough Tamiflu to cover 20% of their population. Some countries spent almost roughly 1% of their annual health budget for this. The United Kingdom spent over half a billion dollars on Tamiflu and the office of the Mayor of London reportedly purchased more than 1 million dollars-worth of this drug for his office and staff.[5]

The United States itself spent over $1.2 billion on antiviral agents and the authorities proudly announced this action and described how it would protect America. During this panic buying, Roche garnered 2005 third-quarter sales that approached $20 billion.[5]

However, all during this process, a few perceptive biomedical scientists were uncertain if Tamiflu was even worth taking at all. During the stockpiling effort, the Cochrane Collaboration was tasked to review and verify Roche's evidence for Tamiflu's efficacy. Although the drug's mechanism of action was well known, some medical scientists wanted to know if it performed as well as the company was claiming. What should have been a routine review became complicated when the Cochrane Group found the company's studies on the drug's effectiveness was unclear. They asked Roche for its full reports and analysis. Roche refused, and it took three-years until the company handed over these reports. In 2014, the definitive final Cochrane review was published. Its major findings included the following points:[6]

1. Roche sponsored all the clinical trials itself. The company reports showed evidence of reporting biases. Roche did not conclusively show that Tamiflu had any effect on reducing the risk of severe disease and the rate of hospitalization during seasonal Influenza outbreaks.

2. Roche's studies were inadequate to determine if Tamiflu could conclusively prevent serious lethal secondary bacterial infections. The FDA had required Roche to print *"Tamiflu has not been shown to prevent Influenza complications"* on the label.

3. The use of Tamiflu did reduce the duration of symptoms by about a day, but only if it was taken at the very first sign of illness. When taken to prevent infection after an exposure, it also seemed to prophylactically reduce the risk of symptomatic influenza in households. The studies were inadequate to determine if Tamiflu decreased the amount of virus that an infected individual disseminated into the immediate environment around them.

4. Tamiflu side-effects included nausea, vomiting, headaches, kidney, and psychiatric effects when it was taken to prevent infection (Influenza prophylaxis). Also, Tamiflu might cause serious heart rhythm problems.

There was more to consider. A later Eurosurveillance study of 85 children in three London schools found that half had experienced side-effects when given the drug as a preventative measure after a classmate was diagnosed with Influenza. Of these, 40% reported gastrointestinal problems including nausea, vomiting, diarrhea and cramps. More shockingly, 18% developed neuropsychiatric side-effects.[7]

At a press briefing in April of 2014, the Cochrane scientists reported that Tamiflu had limited efficacy. One co-author of the report from the University of Oxford, stated that the money for the stockpile *"has been thrown down the drain."* He advised that the United Kingdom should avoid spending another £50 million updating its expiring stockpile.

Shortly after this Cochrane publication, a senior WHO representative made a complete about face in a statement where he emphasized that the WHO *"did not currently recommend pandemic stockpiling of Tamiflu and had no guidelines for its use in seasonal Influenza."*[8] This blatant duplicity went completely unchallenged by the press.

In a contrast, the CDC in the United States still continues to recommend the use of oral Tamiflu as important drug for the treatment of Influenza. This recommendation is claimed to be based on all available data, The CDC criticized both the 2012 and a later 2014 Cochrane report and its 2017 CDC website firmly maintains that Tamiflu treatment when initiated as soon as possible, can have significant clinical and public health benefits during an Influenza pandemic.

In its defense of the drug, the CDC cites a recent meta-analysis of individual participant data that it claims adds to body of evidence showing that Tamiflu can reduce the risk of death in hospitalized Influenza patients. Therefore, the drug should continue to be stockpiled.[9] Yet by its own statements, the CDC is promoting a patently ridiculous position when it also affirms that the drug must be taken early to have any effect. While the CDC has set up an efficient system to deliver prepackaged "Push Packages" of broad-spectrum medical assets to anywhere in the United States within 12-hours, the individual States are still responsible for the distribution of Tamiflu to the local authorities and the local authorities have the responsibility to deliver the drug to their local population. Clearly this process could take several days. How many doses would turn out to be ineffective because it was taken too late?

New Tamiflu Study

In 2017, an expert panel from the European Center for Disease Prevention and Control (ECDC) published its own review. For their analysis, their experts focused on three large systematic reviews and meta-analyses from 2014 and 2015, including one from the Cochrane Collaboration. They also looked at other views and studies.[10]

The final ECDC report reaffirmed that there was clear evidence to support using Tamiflu and other neuraminidase inhibitors to treat and prevent Influenza group A virus infections. The 34-page review agreed that more studies were needed on the outcomes in high-risk groups and that new, more powerful antivirals were urgently needed. It also supported the current CDC guidance and it found that for adults, Tamiflu shortens flulike illness symptoms by about a day. Two of the large reviews it examined showed a statistically significant decrease in patient-reported pneumonia, lower respiratory-tract infections, and hospital admissions. All three of the major reviews that were studied emphasized the importance of starting treatment early (within 48-hours for Tamiflu), and for children treated with the inhaled drug Relenza, within 36 hours. Regarding prophylaxis, they reaffirmed a reduced risk of contracting Influenza after an exposure if Tamiflu treatment was initiated.

The ECDC Report continued by stating that more studies were needed to verify any benefits on severe clinical outcomes and for high risk groups, such as people with asthma, chronic obstructive pulmonary disease, cardiovascular disease, or diabetes. The ECDC found no new evidence to support any changes to already-approved neuraminidase inhibitor recommendations in any of the European Union member states and it affirmed that the use of Tamiflu and other neuraminidase inhibitors is a reasonable public health measure as part of a nation's preparedness planning.

And there the matter stands.

However, when sophisticated statistical methods are needed to demonstrate the actual effectiveness of Tamiflu, it is certainly not the miracle drug it was initially reported to be. Irrespective of the speed of its distribution and effectiveness, the U.S. stockpiles of Tamiflu are acknowledged to be insufficient to treat half of the U.S. population. When fully in place, the National Federal stockpile will contain a total of 50 million doses, with an additional 31 million doses held in State stockpiles.[11] The total US population is roughly 326,691,500. During the 1918 Influenza pandemic, about 28% of Americans became infected. Today that would represent 91,473,620 individuals infected. Using a reasonable 2.5%-3% case fatality rate for the 1918 influenza, this means that between 2,286,841 and 2,744,209 Americans could risk death from the infection over a period of weeks. Although the National Pandemic Response Plan places a heavy emphasis on the use of Tamiflu, the truth is that in a 1918-type outbreak millions of Americans will receive no antiviral drugs at all.

In all reality, the issues of stockpiling and the effectiveness of Tamiflu are probably moot points. This is because the national planners have failed to understand the true nature of RNA viruses, the error-prone replication of their genetic material, and the constant formation of new "quasi-species" of viruses that are very slightly different but still related. This includes the presence or absence of drug resistance in the virus.

Scientists now realize that even a single small change in the N protein (neuraminidase) of the Influenza A virus due to minor mutations in the virus's "blueprints", can create a resistance of the virus to Tamiflu.[12] This suggests that viral drug resistance could spontaneously develop during any Influenza A virus outbreak. This has been repeatedly confirmed during actual outbreaks.

Tamiflu resistance was found in the H1N1 strains of seasonal flu circulating during the 2007–2008 flu season. In 2009, a new influenza A(H1N1) 2009 variant with mildly reduced Tamiflu (and Zanamivir) sensitivity was detected in more than 10% of community specimens in Singapore, and in more than 30% of viral samples from northern Australia.[13] During the 2013–2014 season approximately 1% of the H1N1 viral isolates demonstrated Tamiflu resistance.[14] For the H3N2 virus strain, one study found drug resistance in 18% of the children examined, suggesting that higher and earlier dosing with Tamiflu might be necessary in such populations.[15] This would be likely to create more side effects and further compound drug availability problems. Drug resistance has also been found to develop in the H5N1 Avian influenza and H7N9 Influenza strains during treatment with Tamiflu, and recent data from experiments on mice reaffirms that the customary 5-day course of treatment may not be sufficient for all Influenza strains.[16,17] This again raises the question the actual effectiveness of the National Pandemic Influenza Response Plan as it is written. In 2016, Roche's patents for Tamiflu began to expire and a much lower cost generic version was quickly approved by the FDA.

In summary, there are currently three antiviral neuraminidase inhibitors drugs recommended by the U.S. Centers for Disease Control. These are Oseltamivir (Tamiflu), Zanamivir (Relenza) which must be inhaled, and Peramivir (Rapivab) which must be injected intravenously. The inclusion of Peramivir in the stockpile is curious. The drug cannot be taken by mouth and it has no effect when given intramuscularly. When injected intravenously it has the same mechanism of action as Tamiflu.[18,19] Like Tamiflu, viral resistance can also develop against Peramivir. While it may be suited for individual patients infected with viruses that are resistant to Tamiflu, its requirement for intravenous delivery makes it of little use for managing a large-scale 1918-type pandemic. Yet DHHS apparently provided millions of dollars to assist the drug's manufacturer in bringing it to the market. That money could have desperately been used for other vital problems in pandemic preparedness. Where is the logic for this?

One rational explanation would be that the national antiviral stockpile was designed from the start to primarily ensure the Continuity of Federal Government and some of the infrastructure of the 120 largest American cities. At present, this is most certainly what would happen under existing planning.

However, creating a stockpile based on a single class of antiviral drugs with a common mechanism of action, is a tremendously bad decision. The more total Influenza virus particles that that are infecting, reproducing, and circulating through a community, the greater will be the chance that a quasi-species with a spontaneous drug resistance will develop. It is all about probabilities and how many times the dice are thrown.

SALVAGING THE BASIC NATIONAL PANDEMIC INFLUENZA PLAN

There is, however, hope with respect to the basic strategy of the National Pandemic Response Plan. In this respect, there are multiple compounds that scientists have already developed for use as new, inexpensive Influenza drugs that target less mutable regions of the Influenza A virus.

One target for new antiviral drug development is the Replicase (RNA-dependent RNA polymerase) enzyme of the Influenza A virus. The normal function of this RNA polymerase is so complicated that it can only tolerate few mutations in the blueprints for its construction before it loses its ability to function. This means that it is a highly evolutionarily conserved protein. Hence, unlike the outer proteins of the Influenza virus, the Replicase enzyme has a mainly uniform structure in all the various quasi-species that are viable. This makes it an attractive target for antiviral drugs that can inhibit its function. Even better, this viral enzyme is not found in mammalian cells.

In 2014, scientists at Toyama Chemical in Japan discovered a pyrazine carboxamide molecule that can selectively inhibit the Influenza Replicase enzyme.[20] The molecule underwent clinical trials and was approved for use under the name of Favipiravir (Avigan) in Japan. This remarkable drug shows activity against a wide range of RNA viruses and it has even shown efficacy in an early study of Ebola Virus Disease in West Africa. Consequently, Japan has selected this drug for their national stockpile. Favipiravir appears to selectively inhibit the Influenza RNA polymerase causing it to generate lethal RNA transversion mutations that produce nonviable daughter viruses.[21] Even more important is that the drug can be taken by mouth and it is non-toxic to human cells.

Additionally, a second anti-RNA polymerase drug is currently under development. In 2017, scientists announced the results from a Phase 2b Topaz Pilot Clinical Trial on an experimental drug called Pimodivir (JNJ-63623872).[22] This drug acts to block the PB2 subunit of the influenza RNA polymerase enzyme. Treatment with this experimental drug significantly decreased the amount of Influenza A virus in adult patients infected with acute, uncomplicated seasonal influenza A.

This drug can also be given by mouth and it has not shown any significant safety concerns.

By targeting an alternative part of the viral replication process, both Favipiravir and Pimodivir can successfully treat influenza A virus infections that are resistant or have become resistant to the existing antiviral drugs in the national stockpile. By targeting an Influenza protein that is highly evolutionarily conserved, the chances for the rapid development of viral resistance to these new drugs should be minimized.

A third drug has now been discovered which is an endonuclease-inhibiting compound that is able to block the acid polymerase (PA) enzyme in Influenza A and B viruses. This compound also exhibits low human cell toxicity.[23]

The stockpiling of these new anti-viral drugs and their possible use in combination, adds promising new hope for the Federal strategy of using antiviral agents to transcend the "vaccine gap."

It has taken over a decade and billions of wasted dollars to reach the stage where we may now actually have a few promising drugs to stockpile with enough effectiveness to be useful in a lethal large-scale 1918-type Influenza pandemic. Unfortunately, there are other large problems that must still be overcome.

NOTES FOR CHAPTER 12

[1] Michael Greger. Bird Flu: A Virus of Our Own Hatching. 2006, Lantern Books ISBN 1590560981 (ISBN13: 9781590560983) http://birdflubook.com/

[2] Oxford JS, Novelli P, Sefton A, and Lambkin R. 2002. New millennium antivirals against pandemic and epidemic influenza: the neuraminidase inhibitors. Antiviral Chemistry and Chemotherapy 13:205-17.

[3] Burton B. 2005. Generic drugs only answer to bird flu in Asia. IPS-Inter Press Service, Oct. 27.

[4] U.S. Department of Justice. 1999. F. Hoffmann-La Roche and BASF agree to pay record criminal fines for participating in international vitamin cartel, May 20.

[5] Costello M. 2005. Avian flu fears help sales surge at Roche. The Times, October 19. http://timesonline.co.uk/article/0,,25149-1833185,00.html.

[6] Jefferson T, Heneghan CJ, et.al. (2014). "Neuraminidase inhibitors for preventing and treating influenza in healthy adults and children". Cochrane Database Syst Rev. 4 (4): CD008965. PMID 24718923. doi:10.1002/14651858.CD008965.pub4

[7] A Kitching, A Roche. S Balasegaram, R Heathcock, H Maguire, Eurosurveillance Edition 2009: Volume 14/ Issue 30 http://www.eurosurveillance.org/ViewArticle.aspx?ArticleId=19287

[8] Peter Doshi. Tom Jefferson, Will Tamiflu recommendations change this winter? Has WHO quietly reversed its support for Tamiflu stockpiling? BMJ 2014; 349 doi: https://doi.org/10.1136/bmj.g6742 (Published 27 November 2014)

[9] Stella G Muthuri, Sudhir Venkatesan, et.al. Effectiveness of neuraminidase inhibitors in reducing mortality in patients admitted to hospital with influenza A H1N1 virus infection: The Lancet Respiratory Medicine, Volume 2, No. 5, p395–404, May 2014.

[10] ECDC; 2017. ISBN 978-92-9498-080-9 doi: 10.2900/01723 https://ecdc.europa.eu/sites/portal/files/documents/Scientific-advice-neuraminidaseinhibitors-2017.pdf

[11] Winkenwerder W. Letter to DoD Pandemic Influenza Preparation and Response Planning Guidance, Office of the Assistant Secretary of Defense, September 21, 2004 as cited in Davis M. 2005. The Global Threat of Avian Flu (New York, NY: The New Press, p. 146).

[12] Thorlund, Kristian; Thabane, Lehana, et.al. (2011). "Systematic review of influenza resistance to the neuraminidase inhibitors". BMC Infectious Diseases. 11 (1): 134.

[13] A. C. Hurt., I G Barr, et.al. Increased detection in Australia and Singapore of a Novel Influenza A(H1N1)2009 Variant with Reduced Oseltamivir and Zanamivir

Sensitivity Due to a S247N Neuraminidase Mutation Eurosurveillance, Volume 16, Issue 23, 09 June 2011

[14] CDC Influenza Division Key Points, March 28, 2014" (PDF). CDC. March 28, 2014.

[15] Ward, P; Small, I; Dutkowski, R. et.al. (February 2005). "Oseltamivir (Tamiflu) and its potential for use in the event of an influenza pandemic.". The Journal of antimicrobial chemotherapy.

[16] Yen HL, Monto AS, and Govorkova EA. 2005. Virulence may determine the necessary duration and dosage of oseltamivir treatment for highly pathogenic A/Vietnam/1203/04 influenza virus in mice. Journal of Infectious Diseases 192(4):665-72.

[17] Davis LE. 1979. Species differences as a consideration in drug therapy. Journal of the American Veterinary Medical Association 175(9):1014-5.

[18] Kohno, S.; Shimada, J et.al. (8 August 2011). "Phase III Randomized, Double-Blind Study Comparing Single-Dose Intravenous Peramivir with Oral Oseltamivir in Patients with Seasonal Influenza Virus Infection". Antimicrobial Agents and Chemotherapy. 55 (11): 5267–5276.

[19] BioCryst to File Peramivir NDA Supported by BARDA/HHS Funding". Fierce Biotech. July 11, 2013

[20] Jin, Z; Smith, L. K., et.al. (2013). "The ambiguous base-pairing and high substrate efficiency of T-705 (Favipiravir) towards influenza A virus polymerase". PLoS ONE. 8 (7

[21] Baranovich, T., Govorkova, EA. et.al., "T-705 (favipiravir) induces lethal mutagenesis in influenza A H1N1 viruses in vitro". (2013-04-01). Journal of Virology. 87 (7): 3741–3751.

[22] Pimodivir Alone or in Combination with Oseltamivir Demonstrated a Reduction in Viral Load in Adults with Influenza A - Phase 2b. 5th International Society for Influenza and Respiratory Diseases Antiviral Group (ISIRV-AVG) Conference - Shanghai– June 14, 2017.

[23] J.C. Jones, L. Kreis, E. A. Govorkova. A Novel Endonuclease Inhibitor Exhibits Broad Spectrum Anti-Influenza Virus Activity In Vitro. Antimicrobial Agents and Chemotherapy, April 2018, Vol. 62 Issue 4.

13

THE PROBLEM OF LOCAL AUTHORITY PANDEMIC PREPAREDNESS

NATURAL DISASTERS THAT IMPACT a local region or state, will always require the rapid concentration of emergency resources and assets into a well-defined area. Because of the normally focal nature of the disaster, the surrounding unaffected areas are available to donate their resources to assist in this response.

However, a severe 1918-type Influenza pandemic will have completely different dynamics than other disasters and it may impact almost every community in the United States at roughly the same time. It will affect almost every village, town, city, and county in every state. With modern air and ground transportation systems, it is possible that the first outbreaks would already be underway inside the United States before the severity of the Influenza A strain involved is realized. With all communities affected, there could be little mutual aid available between jurisdictions.

As mentioned, the overall strategy of the National Pandemic Influenza Response Plan seems to be focused on first protecting the federal government and the military and then the state governments, and then the basic infrastructures of the 120 largest cities of the United States. Sufficient quantities of vaccine for the general population will not be ready for weeks and what federal surge medical personnel are available, will be utilized at the federal, military, and state government levels first, with little left over. The smaller cities and towns will essentially be left to their own planning and resources.

The National Pandemic Plan *clearly states* that it is the Local Authorities that are responsible for developing their own community pandemic plans and preparations for overwhelming numbers of Influenza cases. They are responsible for recruiting, training, and managing their own medical surge personnel and the preselection of buildings to use as Alternate Care Sites. They are responsible for making provisions for receiving and distributing antiviral drugs and vaccine doses to their communities, making home care and pandemic information available to their populations, developing a local mortuary surge capability, and making their plans for the continuity of their own local government and first responders.

To foster this process, the Department of Health and Human Services (DHHS) has created general guidance outlines for local authorities to assist them in developing this "self-sufficient" capability. These documents entail how to create a community-based medical surge capability. They show how to conduct local stockpiling and give infection prevention guidance for first responders and guidance for small local businesses and critical infrastructures. Other documents show how to enhance mortuary capability and set up Alternate Care Sites.

In addition, beginning in 2002, DHHS has provided more than $11 billion for programs designed to enhance local authority emergency preparedness for large-scale public health emergencies. DHHS distributed this funding primarily through cooperative agreements under two programs; the *Hospital Preparedness Program* (HPP)[1] and the *Public Health Emergency Preparedness* (PHEP) *Cooperative Agreement.*[2] In addition to providing general emergency preparedness funds, DHHS has provided more millions in supplemental funding specifically for improving Influenza preparedness.[3,4]

Prior to assessing the status of local Public Health capability with respect to their plans for vaccine and antiviral drug distribution, the DHHS Office of the Inspector General conducted an audit to evaluate the medical surge capability of several select Local Authorities. The study focused on local authority coordination; recruitment of medical volunteers; acquisition and management of medical equipment; the development of Alternate Care Facilities; and procedures for altering triage, admission, and patient care. The study looked at 5 States and 10 localities. Considering the amount of federal money supplied to these local communities: the results were outrageously disturbing.[5]

- Fewer than half of the selected localities had started to recruit medical volunteers, and none of the five states had implemented an electronic system to manage them. Only 4 localities had started to recruit, register, and train medical volunteers. However, all 4 had concerns about using volunteers.

- The states were required to have electronic systems to register medical volunteers and verify credentials. None of the five states had fully implemented an electronic system for managing medical volunteers.

- All 10 localities had acquired limited caches of medical equipment; however, many experienced difficulties with inventory tracking the equipment.

- Only three of the five states had implemented electronic

systems to track available hospital beds during an emergency.

- Most of the selected localities were still in the early stages of preselecting Alternate Care Sites using buildings such as schools or convention centers, to alleviate hospital overcrowding. Nine localities had either identified or were in the process of identifying Alternate Care Sites in a pandemic, but few had signed formal agreements.

- None of the localities had plans that included the scope of care and how these sites would be managed, staffed, and supplied.

- During a pandemic, medical care might have to be rationed in a manner that saves the greatest number of lives. Nine localities had not identified guidelines for altering triage, admission, and patient care during a pandemic. Seven of these localities were concerned that they would be legally at risk if they were to alter their standards, and all nine reported that they wanted additional State or Federal guidance.

- All localities had conducted medical surge exercises; however, none consistently documented the "lessons learned." Most of the exercises were discussion-based, rather than operations-based. No locality consistently created "after-action" reports and improvement plans. All the existing documentation that was available for review, showed that localities needed to make improvements within all five of the medical surge components; medical volunteers; medical equipment; Alternate Care Facilities; and procedures for altering triage and patient care.

This lack of community progress in response to federal funding reflects what seems to be a common existing difficulty between city managers and their local public health authorities. Many emergency managers experience frustration in dealing with their Public Health departments. Despite guidance from the CDC and DHHS, many local jurisdictions still lack emergency planning staff capable of developing a rational pandemic response. The poor progress in developing a local medical surge capability also reflects poorly on the city emergency managers who do not seem to appreciate the true seriousness of the pandemic Influenza risk.

One other factor may to be the noticeable increase in the public sector's reliance on making the federal government the answer to many of society's problems. Whether from political, social, or intentional economic design, this increasing government dependency is unrealistic and fraught with potential disaster.

Before the levees in New Orleans collapsed in 2005, U.S. Federal, State, and local authorities had precisely planned how they would respond to a severe Hurricane with a storm surge that overwhelmed existing countermeasures with thousands stranded inside a flooded city. The year before Hurricane Katrina struck, the plan was even practiced in conjunction with FEMA (the Federal Emergency Management Agency).

Yet when this Category 3 hurricane event occurred, the response by local authorities was slow, incompetently coordinated, and only a small fraction of what was needed. Eventually, the U.S. military with its resources, accountability, and its rigid chain of command, had to take over the city's ineffective civilian disaster response.

For local authority guidance, DHHS uses the following guidelines for the impact that a severe Influenza pandemic will pose to a small community in the United States.[6]

- Susceptibility to the virus will be universal.
- Typical incubation period is ~2 days.
- Individuals can transmit infection 1-day before the actual onset of illness.
- Risk of transmission highest during first 2-days of illness.

- Asymptomatic or minimally symptomatic individuals can transmit infection.
- Infected persons will transmit infection to ~2 other people on average.
- 30% of the population will be infected.
- Epidemics will last 6–8 weeks in affected communities.
- Work absenteeism may reach 40% during peaks of community outbreaks.
- Several waves of global pandemic spread may occur with each lasting 2–3 months.
- Children may play a major role in transmission of infection.

These characteristics were constructed from a loose summary of past Influenza pandemics. In 1918, the second wave of infection that came back from Europe to Boston and Philadelphia showed a case fatality rate that rose above 2.5%, compared to the less than 0.1% seen in other influenza pandemics.[7] Today, alarmingly, the current human micro-outbreaks involving the H5N1 and H7N9 Influenza strains has raised fears that a mutated, human-adapted, human-transmissible "quasi-species" could develop with an associated 50% case mortality. With no treatment or immediately available vaccine, local communities could experience an overwhelmed healthcare system within a few days. Without preplanning, the responsibility for healthcare would shift over to untrained families trying to nurse their loved ones at home, with a justified blame on local authorities for their failure to prepare their communities.

Local communities and their managers need to understand the very serious nature of the current pandemic threat and they must prepare rational and constantly rehearsed emergency plans and build a response from the community up to the county level. It is also important for the public to realize that during a national pandemic, the federal government does not have the capability or the capacity to meet the needs of everyone at the same time, and it has never had this ability.[8]

The problems associated with the availability and effectiveness of antiviral drugs and the delay associated with new vaccine production and distribution, make it essential that local authorities try to limit their community Influenza infections to a level that can be handled by their medical surge capability. To some extent, this can be accomplished by very basic public health measures called "*Non-Pharmaceutical Interventions*" or NPI.

In a world of high-technology medicine, these interventions are simple and basic, but they are all that will be left for the roughly 123-million Americans (recently revised to 125-million) that have been left out of the federal top-down planning with no assurance that their local communities will have a rational and functional pandemic Influenza plan.

NOTES FOR CHAPTER 13

[1] Hospital Preparedness Program (HPP)
http://www.phe.gov/preparedness/planning/hpp/pages/default.aspx

[2] Public Health Emergency Preparedness (PHEP) Cooperative Agreement
https://www.cdc.gov/phpr/readiness/phep.htm

[3] "HHS Announces $896.7 Million in Funding to States for Public Health Preparedness and Emergency Response."
http://www.hhs.gov/news/press/2007pres/07/pr20070717c.html.

[4] "HHS Provides More Than $1 Billion to Improve All Hazards Public Health."
Available online at http://www.hhs.gov/news/press/2008pres/06/20080603a.html.
Accessed on March 6, 2009.

[5] HHS Office of Inspector General, Office of Evaluation and Inspections (OEI). State and Local Pandemic Influenza Preparedness: Medical Surge. September 2009. OEI-02-08-00210.https://oig.hhs.gov/oei/reports/oei-02-08-00210.pdf

[6] DHHS Pandemic Influenza Plan; 2017 Update.

[7] Patterson KD, Pyle GF. The geography and mortality of the 1918 influenza pandemic. Bull Hist Med. 1991; 65:4–21.

[8] Testimony of Tara O'Toole, "Protecting the Homeland: Fighting Pandemic Flu from the Front Lines." House Committee on Homeland Security Subcommittee on Emergency Preparedness, Science and Technology, February 8, 2006.

14

NON-PHARMACEUTICAL
INTERVENTIONS (NPI)

WITHOUT AN EFFECTIVE and widely available drug treatment or vaccine, one goal of pandemic preparedness is to slow the spread of a pandemic virus and limit its impact until countermeasures can be widely administered.

The isolation of infected individuals and the use of quarantines is a recorded technique dating as far back as A.D. 541 when the Justinian Plague afflicted the Eastern Roman Empire. Much the same techniques were used during the medieval era during the "Black Death" pandemic of the fourteenth century. For hundreds of years in rural Africa, villages would reverse-quarantine themselves during times of pestilence and not allow outsiders in. Reverse community quarantine also occurred in India during the outbreak of Bubonic Plague in south-central and southwestern India in 1994.

If everyone stayed home with no outside contact at the start of an Influenza pandemic, there would be no further human to human transmission and the pandemic/local epidemic would die out. Unfortunately, in modern society, people must go to and from work or school where they interact with many others. They must shop for food and other necessities which brings them into contact with other population groups outside their immediate circle. These interactions all increase their chance of contact with others that may be in the early stages of infection.

However, there are some simple measures that individuals and communities can use to help "biologically isolate" themselves to some extent from any disease-causing agents in their environment. These community mitigation strategies originated in earlier times and today we call these techniques Non-Pharmaceutical Interventions or NPI.

These NPI are the practical things that can be done during a disease outbreak to avoid infection when there are no drugs or vaccines against an infectious disease. However, one problem with Influenza, is that individuals do not show any obvious signs of infection until several days after they have become infected (Figure 19). During this time the Influenza virus is multiplying in the cells lining the upper respiratory tract and large amounts of live virus is being shed into the environment around the infected individual.

This interval is called the latent or incubation period and most individuals infected with an Influenza A virus strain are infectious for 1 to 2 days before the onset of symptoms. During this "incubation" period, the infected person may feel slightly unwell, but nowhere ill enough to miss work, and they can transmit the virus to others around them.

It is only after several days of infection that individuals start to develop a rising fever and the other classical signs and symptoms of Influenza, and they remain infectious up to 5–7 days after becoming ill.[1]

Of note is the fact that Infants and immunocompromised individuals may shed influenza virus particles for up to 21 days.

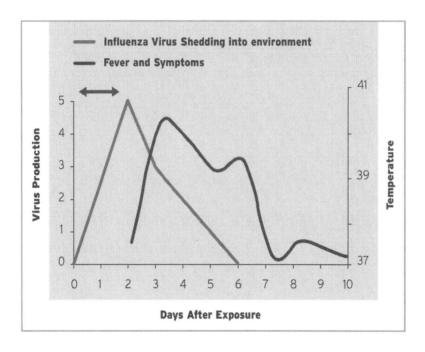

Figure 19. *Influenza viral shedding into the environment occurs before the onset of fever.*[1]

During the 1918 pandemic, the public health authorities of the time understood that Influenza was communicable and transmitted through the air via nasal mucous and coughing. They understood that sputum was infectious, and they issued guidance to prevent droplet infection. Consequently, they promulgated efforts to prevent the infected from sharing air with the uninfected. In the cities, many public institutions were closed, and large public gatherings were banned. Bars and movie theaters were closed. To prevent overcrowding, businesses and factories staggered their opening and closing hours. People were advised to minimize the use of mass transportation. Public funerals were banned in some areas.

The public health authorities also correctly believed that infection could occur by the contamination of the hands and by touching common eating and drinking utensils. Education programs for "respiratory hygiene" were created to teach people about the dangers of coughing, sneezing and the careless disposal of their nasal mucous.

Communities were also taught the value of handwashing before touching the face or eating.[2] Various Public Health Departments also printed public Influenza posters to educate the community how to reduce the spread of infection.

The success of these measures varied with respect to the type of community and its socioeconomic conditions.

One debated public health measure was to close the schools. While possibly of value in small towns and rural areas, these closures were probably less effective in the larger metropolitan areas because of the many chances of infection by other contacts. More restrictive infection control involved a quarantine isolation of the ill. In 1918, these measures required a sacrifice of individual liberty for the societal good and therefore required a strong public health authority. Because of the strain on facilities, only severe cases were to be hospitalized while mild influenza patients were quarantined at home.

INDIVIDUAL NON-PHARMACEUTICAL INTERVENTIONS (NPI)

For individuals, the basic NPI are simple and easy to understand and they provide some degree of reduced personal infection risk, and if adhered to they can lower the infection risk for the entire community. These include; respiratory etiquette, hand hygiene, the routine cleaning of frequently touched surfaces, voluntary home isolation when ill, the voluntary home quarantine of potentially exposed household members, the self-use of face masks in community settings when ill, and the use of individual social distancing measures.[3]

For these to be effective, it is essential that the public be familiar with the spectrum of signs and symptoms of influenza. This includes an initial general malaise, muscle or joint aches, headache, fatigue, followed by cough or chest discomfort, possible sneezing, a sore throat, and a runny, stuffy nose. Sometimes vomiting, and diarrhea occur. Teaching the signs and symptoms of an Influenza infection allows individuals to recognize the infection in themselves and in others. Individuals must also know the correct procedures for taking a body temperature. The ability to recognize a possible early Influenza infection in themselves or others, allows an individual to implement NPI.

Respiratory Etiquette

Respiratory etiquette refers to minimizing the dispersion of droplets contaminated with influenza virus through the air by coughing or sneezing. Individuals should cover their coughs and sneezes, with a tissue and dispose of the tissues safely, while disinfecting their hands immediately afterwards. If a tissue is not available, they should cough or sneeze into their shirt sleeve. Touching a nearby surface or a doorknob and the eyes, nose, and mouth should be avoided until after the hands are washed.

Hand Hygiene

Hand hygiene refers to the practice of performing regular hand washing with soap and water, or with alcohol-based hand sanitizers containing at least 60% ethanol or methyl (rubbing) alcohol. This destroys the outer part of the Influenza virus and reduces the transmission rate between people and surfaces.

Video studies have quantified that people touch their face an average of 3.6-15.7 times per hour.[4] Every time people touch their mouth or nose; they transfer bacteria and viruses between their hands and their face. This "self-inoculation," or transfer of germs from one body part to another, is a primary way that the Influenza virus can spread from sick people to often-touched surfaces, and from these virus-contaminated surfaces to uninfected people's faces.

Rubbing the eyes, nose, or mouth with contaminated hands can place the Influenza virus in contact with the mucous membranes lining the mouth, nose, and eyes, leading to infection, especially in the membranes around the eyes which drain through the nasolacrimal duct into the nose.[5] Numerous studies have demonstrated that increased handwashing reduces self-inoculation via contaminated surfaces.[6]

It is important to remember that Influenza viruses can remain viable on the human hand for roughly 3–5 minutes and infectious on the fingers for up to 30-minutes after contamination.[7,8]

Routine Surface Cleaning

Surface cleaning measures will destroy any influenza viruses on frequently touched surfaces including tables, doorknobs, toys, telephones, work surfaces, night tables, and computer keyboards. Surfaces can be decontaminated with detergent-based cleaners or alcohol-based disinfectants. The routine use of cleaning measures that eliminate viruses from contaminated surfaces will reduce the chance for hand contamination, especially when in the workplace or in the home.[3]

Voluntary Home Isolation

Persons in community settings who show symptoms consistent with influenza and who may be infected, should be separated from others as soon as practical, be sent home, and practice voluntary home isolation. This serves to prevent an ill individual from infecting people outside of their household.

This recommendation is based on studies of previous epidemics in which most Influenza cases could be managed with home care. Individuals with the symptoms of Influenza should stay home until the fever, chills and sweating have abated, and then remain at home for at least another 24-hours (children longer). The individual's temperature should be measured in the absence of taking medication such as Tylenol (Paracetamol) that will lower a fever.

Voluntary Home Quarantine
of Exposed but Non-Symptomatic Family Members

This is called self-quarantine or household quarantine. Household members exposed to symptomatic individuals (with probable Influenza) should stay home for up to 3-days starting from their initial contact with the ill person. This is a community consideration that helps prevent the spread of Influenza from households to schools, workplaces, and other households.

If a household contact becomes ill, then this 3-day temporary quarantine should then become a voluntary home isolation.

Self-use of Face Masks in a Community Setting

Today, disposable surgical, medical, and dental procedure masks are widely used in health care settings to prevent health worker exposure to patient respiratory infections. In 1918, surgical face masks (often handmade) became a widely used intervention during the pandemic with variable reports of their effectiveness. However, reports from that time suggested that face masks did not provide complete protection to healthcare workers in the high viral load environment of the hospital wards.

Since 1918, the topic of wearing face masks for self-protection has undergone much debate, but only recently have definitive experiments been performed with respect to the value of face masks in Influenza. In a study in 2010, some 1,400 volunteers in a university dormitory setting were divided into groups, one wore face mask protection with instructions on its use and one group without any face mask protection. The groups were monitored for 6-weeks after Influenza broke out on the campus. The scientists found a 35 to 51% reduction of infection when compared with the control group, indicating that face masks and hand hygiene may reduce respiratory illnesses in shared living settings and mitigate the impact of an influenza pandemic.[9]

In summary, face masks worn by ill patients may have value by blocking the large-particle respiratory droplets propelled by the sick individual coughing or sneezing. This could have value when ill patients need to go out into a crowded setting or when a family places a mask on an ill family member that they are caring for at home. Face masks that are sized for children are available.

Face masks worn by healthy individuals provide some degree of protection against infection by large particle aerosols generated by coughing and sneezing, but this protection is not complete. This will be discussed further in a separate chapter.

Social Distancing Measures (Individual)

Social distancing refers to practical measures that reduce the face-to-face contact between individuals in a community setting. These include always maintaining a distance of at least 3-feet between individuals to reduce large particle aerosol transmission of the Influenza virus. This applies to everyone, including apparently healthy persons without symptoms. In the event of a very severe pandemic, this minimal distance should be extended out to 6-feet.

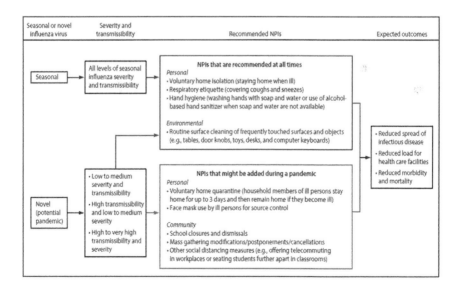

Figure 20. *Phased Addition of NPI Measures to Prevent Community Influenza Spread.*
Source: Centers for Disease Control and Prevention.[10]

Social Distancing Measures (Community)

The U.S. workforce comprises roughly 62.9% of the civilian, noninstitutionalized population over 16 years of age, and DHHS has outlined major guidelines for social distancing techniques for use by businesses and other places of work.[11]

These include telecommuting and the increased use of e-mail and teleconferences, or staggered shifts to minimize the number of office staff at any one time. However, the practicality of these measures in the Megaregions and large cities that are mass-transit-dependent remain problematical.[12]

Other social distancing measures can be implemented in a wide range of community settings including educational facilities and other public places where people gather. These community NPIs might include the temporary closure of child-care facilities and schools. Public health authorities might also recommend the cancellation of mass gatherings, the closure of parks, religious institutions, theaters, and sports arenas during a pandemic.

Even though the evidence base for the effectiveness of some of these measures is limited and there is limited empirical evidence supporting the implementation of any individual measure alone, there is some evidence for the effectiveness of using multiple social distancing measures to slow an Influenza outbreak (Figure 20).

THE EFFECTIVENESS OF NPI

The NPI that were used during the 1918 pandemic were much the same as would be recommended today, although different cities undertook different interventions in their attempts to reduce Influenza transmission.

Historically, the *early* introduction of NPIs appears to be a key factor in reducing person-to-person viral transmission. One study found that the cities that established early NPI in 1918 had less mortality than those that did not. The utilization of multiple interventions appears to have been more effective than the use of a single intervention.[13] Also important was the ability of the population to maintain their NPI measures. When intervention use fell off, viral spread appeared to increase.[14]

Retrospective studies have examined the death rate in the second 1918 pandemic wave in Philadelphia and have compared this with the death rate in St. Louis where the city health authorities proactively closed schools early and quickly prohibited public gatherings in places like theaters, churches, and restaurants.[13,15]

In this respect, Figure 21 shows the excess mortality over 1913-1917 baseline in Philadelphia and St. Louis from September 8 to December 28, 1918. It illustrates that the excess death rate in Philadelphia was 5-times greater than St. Louis.

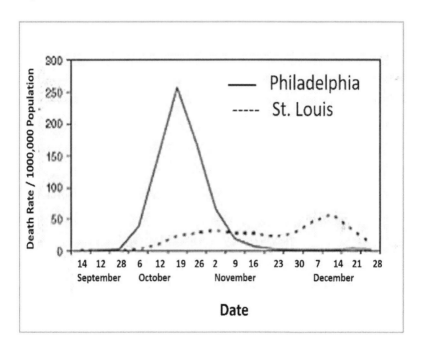

Figure 21. *1918 Pandemic Death Rates in Philadelphia and St. Louis.*
Source: Collins SD, Frost WH, Gover M, Sydenstricker: Mortality from influenza and pneumonia in the 50 largest cities in the United States. First Edition Washington: U.S. Government Printing Office. 1930.

The resulting burden of this on Philadelphia's hospitals, mortuaries, and the economy has previously been described. There, the introduction of NPI was left too late to have any effect until the resulting high levels of mortality eventually reduced individual personal contact rates out of fear. What is interesting is that although the percentage of cases reported on a daily basis were far fewer in St. Louis, the pandemic wave in that city lasted almost twice as long as that seen in Philadelphia. *This is precisely the goal for the modern use of NPI.* It is to spread out a pandemic's impact on the surge medical resources so that they are not completely overwhelmed, and to buy time until a drug treatment and vaccine program can be implemented.

The ability of the public to comply with NPI was a concern in 1918, and it remains a concern today. This underscores the need to develop adequate individual and community NPI education programs that are effective in modifying behavioral patterns. This is especially true with respect to the members of the poor, low resource, high-density communities in the 120 largest cities of the U.S.

This reinforces the concept that any intervention outside of the rapid administration of orally effective antiviral drugs or a mass vaccination of the public with an effective vaccine, will not completely halt an Influenza pandemic.

NOTES FOR CHAPTER 14

[1] Carrat, F. Valleron, A., et.al. Time-Lines of Infection and Disease in Human Influenza: A Review of Volunteer Challenge Studies (2008). Am. J. Epidemiology, 167 (7), 775-785 DOI: 10.1093/aje/kwm375

[2] Influenza, Report of a Special Committee of the American Public Health Association., JAMA. 1918;71(25):2068-2073. doi:10.1001/jama.1918.26020510014010b

[3] MMWR / April 21, 2017 / Vol. 66 / No. 1 US Department of Health and Human Services / Centers for Disease Control and Prevention. https://www.cdc.gov/mmwr/volumes/66/rr/pdfs/rr6601.pdf

[4] Nicas, M. A study quantifying the hand-to-face contact rate and its potential application to predicting respiratory tract infection. Journal of Occupational and Environmental Hygiene. June 2008; 5(6):347-52.

[5] Macias, A. Controlling the novel A (H1N1) influenza virus: don't touch your face! Journal of Hospital Infection. 2009: 73, 280-291. August 20, 2009.

[6] Levy JW, Simmerman, JM, et al. Increased hand washing reduces influenza virus surface contamination in Bangkok households, 2009–2010. Influenza Other Respir. Viruses 2014; 8:13–6. 59.

[7] Bean B, Balfour HH Jr, er.al. Survival of influenza viruses on environmental surfaces. J Infect Dis 1982; 146:47–51. https://doi.org/10.1093/infdis/146.1.47 60.

[8] Thomas Y, Kaiser Lm. Survival of influenza virus on human fingers. Clin Microbiol Infect 2014;20: O58–64. https://doi.org/10.1111/1469-0691.12324

[9] T. L. Daniels, T.R. Talbo, Unmasking the Confusion of Respiratory Protection to Prevent Influenza-Like Illness in Crowded Community Settings., JID 2010:201 (15 February). DOI: 10.1086/650395

[10] https://www.cdc.gov/mmwr/volumes/66/rr/rr6601a1.htm#T8_down. Accessed 9/22/18.

[11] Source: US Bureau of Labor Statistics. The employment situation—September 2016. Washington, DC: US Department of Labor; 2016.

[12] https://stacks.cdc.gov/view/cdc/44313

[13] Morse, S.S. "Pandemic Influenza: Studying the Lessons of History." PNAS vol. 104, no. 18, 2007, pp. 7313–7314., doi:10.1073/pnas.0702659104.

[14] Hatchett, R.J., Mecher, C.E., and Lipsitch, M., Public health interventions and epidemic intensity during the 1918 influenza pandemic, PNAS, vol. 104 no. 18, 7582–7587, doi: 10.1073/pnas.0610941104http://www.pnas.org/content/104/18/7582.full.pdf

---

[15] Martin C. J. Ferguson, N.M., et.al. The effect of public health measures on the 1918 influenza pandemic in U.S cities, PNAS May 1, 2007, vol. 104, no. 1., 7588–7593.

15

THE CONCEPT OF HOME MEDICAL CARE

To AVOID HOSPITAL OVERCROWDING and minimize the demand for limited surge medical personnel, as well as reduce Influenza transmission rates, the current DHHS doctrine is for local communities to care for their ill family members at home whenever possible. However, to safely do this without becoming infected themselves, home caregivers need some basic knowledge as well as some training, and practice.

It is therefore useful to outline just what would be involved in caring for a family member suffering from a lethal strain of Influenza. The reader can then judge for themselves if a simple Public Health poster would give them enough information to safely care for an infected loved one without becoming infected themselves. Again, it must be emphasized that Influenza strains may differ in their infectivity and ability to survive in the environment. For lethal strains with no vaccine or treatment it is best to err on the side of caution.

One excellent basic reference for this has been written by Michael Greger, and the book is titled *"Bird Flu: A Virus of Our Own Hatching."* 2006, Lantern Books ISBN 1590560981. The author has conducted an exhaustive literature research on Avian Influenza and has concluded that the on-going massive growth of the poultry industry may be a factor in the trafficking of Influenza strains between different species. His book also contains a number of useful suggestions for the homecare of ill family members. As a public service he has made his book freely accessible on the internet at http://www.birdflubook.org/a.php?id=34 (Access July 2019).

Another useful publication is "Good Home Treatment of Influenza" by Dr. G.C. Woodson.[3] This author has also made his work available on the internet. These and some of the internet-available documents from the CDC and DHHS, can be used to create a small home library useful to help manage a family member with seasonal Influenza at home. The measures that are outlined in these publications are standard and have extremely useful information applicable for normal seasonal Influenza. We reference some of these in this chapter.

However, based on current research we believe that for a 1918-type Influenza strain, the caregiver should wear full-face protection with the eyes completely covered. This will be discussed in the next chapter.

THE CLINICAL COURSE OF HUMAN INFLUENZA INFECTION

The signs and symptoms of influenza are easy to recognize, but it is first necessary to rule out the "Common Cold" as a cause of the symptoms. The common cold is a localized, sniffing, runny nose, sore throat, full-sinus type of infection. The primary target for the many different viruses that cause the "Common Cold" are the mucous membranes that line the inside of the nose.

As the infection progresses, the erectile tissue of the nasal turbinates (the ridges deep inside the nose) become engorged with blood. Outside of the genitalia, this is the only other erectile tissue in the human body.

This turbinate swelling is evident by the changes in the tone of the sufferer's voice when they try to talk. In contrast, while a cold sufferer may have a fever for a few days it is neither marked nor severe. In addition, while a cough, headache, and chest discomfort can accompany a "cold," this is normally mild and self-limiting.

The initial signs and symptoms of Influenza initially resemble those of a cold, but then it quickly runs a much different clinical course. In the airways, the Influenza virus infects the membranes lining the trachea that passes down from the throat and into the chest where it branches into two main bronchi with one going to each lung. There, the virus begins to attack and kill the cells of the mucous membranes that line the airways. The victim develops a moderate to very-high fever with a sore throat and a dry, hacking cough.

When the Influenza virus enters the blood stream, it triggers a rapid immune response with the release of a shower of inflammation-causing chemicals into the blood. It is these inflammatory chemicals that cause the symptoms of severe muscle and body aches, shaking chills, and headaches accompanied by profound fatigue.

The classical symptoms of Influenza appear suddenly from one to four days after exposure to the virus and infected patients can secrete virus into the environment for an average of 24-hours before they run a fever. As the infection progresses the victim feels miserable, the high temperature, coughing and sneezing continue, but normally within two to three days, the worst symptoms quickly subside. However, the dry cough and profound fatigue may linger for several more weeks afterwards. Children with Influenza develop the same symptoms as adults with a high fever. Occasionally they may also vomit with the fever.

The most common complications of Influenza are due to the damage the virus causes to the mucous membranes lining the airways. This damage reduces the ability of the airway to secrete mucous to trap bacteria and viruses in the inspired air and sweep it out of the airways as sputum. This reduced ability makes influenza patients very prone to secondary bacterial respiratory tract infections.

CARING FOR A PERSON WITH INFLUENZA

It is important to recognize the first signs of influenza and the victim should be isolated in bed in a private room with sunlight and good ventilation, preferably with outside air. This helps decrease the amount of virus in the room after the patient coughs or sneezes, and the ultraviolet rays in sunlight inactivate the virus. If the windows can be opened for outside circulation that is all the better. Ideally, they should have their own bathroom to use.

The individual should also remain in bed rest as much as possible. In 1918, some victims developed an inflammation in their heart muscle (myocarditis).

Influenza victims will have a significant fever and although this may be uncomfortable, this fever is part of the immune response. There are some indications that an elevated body temperature may inhibit the replication of some strains of influenza virus, and this may have a beneficial effect on the course of infection. In addition, many of the biochemical reactions involved in an immune response operate more efficiently at a raised body temperature. Lowering a fever by using the combination of a tablet of Tylenol and a tablet of Motrin may make a patient feel better, but it may slightly undermine the immune system as it tries to fight off a viral infection. The exception is in children that are five years or less years in age, where Tylenol syrup can be given to lower the fever to prevent febrile convulsions.

At no time, should any child less than 12-years of age be given aspirin for a fever because of the risk of a rare but serious side-effect known as *Reye's Syndrome.* [1] This is a rapidly progressive inflammation of the brain with liver damage and vomiting, personality changes, confusion, seizures, and an eventual loss of consciousness. The mortality rate of Reye's syndrome is 20-40% and the survivors usually have suffered some degree of brain damage. The biochemical mechanism involved in this syndrome is uncertain, but it usually starts shortly after recovery from a viral infection and 90% of the cases are associated with the use of aspirin in children. As an alternate, a cool cloth on the forehead and a tepid sponge bath can make a child with a fever feel better without the risk.

As an alternate, a cool cloth on the forehead and a tepid sponge bath can make a child with a fever feel better without the risk. When the fever is high an individual may also feel chills, feel very cold, and want more blankets. They should be allowed to adjust these themselves to their own comfort level.

Of more concern is a condition known as a *febrile convulsion*. This is the sudden epileptic seizure in a child with a temperature usually above 38 °C (100.4 °F). It is most common in children between the ages of 6 months and 5 years. It usually lasts less than five minutes and the child is completely back to normal within an hour of the event.

Parents should remain calm, note the start time of the seizure, and call an ambulance if the seizure lasts longer than 5 minutes. The child should be positioned on their side to prevent choking and to rule out encephalitis or meningitis, quickly assessed by a doctor.

Helpful supplies to have include a thermometer, Tylenol, an anti-inflammatory tablet, or capsule, as well as Zinc cough drops, a cough syrup, and a variety of warm and cold drinks including water, fruit juices, soda. Light foods and soups are ideal. [2]

The household needs to have a supply of personal protective equipment, ideally with disposable examination gloves purchased from a pharmacy. Reusable dishwashing gloves are a possibility if disposable gloves are not available, but the gloves must be decontaminated. Bottles of methyl alcohol (rubbing alcohol for surface and glove disinfection) and a supply of disposable face masks for the patient and care giver to wear are essential if the victim is actively coughing and sneezing. It must be kept in mind that the face mask will not fully protect against infection. This will be discussed in more detail in a later chapter.

The actual nursing of an individual with influenza at home is rather simple. The first goal is to keep the patient as comfortable as possible while keeping them isolated to prevent the infection of other family members. The second goal is to observe the patient for the early development of any of the serious complications that can occur in Influenza. The sick person should be allowed to drink as much fluids as possible to replace the body fluid lost by sweating.[2,3]

Fluids are more important than food in the first few days when the fever is highest. It is essential to keep the patient well hydrated by drinking at least one full cup of fluid every hour while awake. This may help to loosen mucus secretions and help the patient cough.

If a patient is not eating, a simple but adequate oral rehydration electrolyte solution can be made by mixing the following:[2,3]

- 1-quart (or liter) drinking water
- 1 "pinch" of table salt
- 1 level tablespoon of sugar
    Mix well to make approximately one quart (or liter)

The level tablespoon of sugar will help the fluid absorb from the gut. If available, add a ½ cup of orange or lemon juice to provide potassium to the mixture if the patient has been vomiting.

As mentioned, most people with Influenza will recover in several days to a week, but some will develop moderate to severe complications from the tissue damage caused by the viral infection. Some groups are more at risk for developing complications than others.

COMPLICATIONS IN ADULTS

Average CDC statistics indicate that about 5% to 20 % of the U.S. population contract Influenza every year. Seasonal Influenza can vary in its severity depending on the strain of Influenza that is involved, and an average of 200,000 people are hospitalized for flu-related complications each year. Estimates of normal seasonal Influenza-associated deaths in the United States are variable and range from 3,000 to 49,000 fatalities depending on the virus strain. Roughly 90% of these deaths occur in patients above the age of 65 years.[2] Globally, between a quarter to half a million people die from the complications of Influenza each year.

Complications can appear with infection by any of the wild Influenza viruses that infect man including the H1N1, H1N2, and H3N2 strains. These are currently the only known strains to freely circulate among humans.

Usually, the groups most at risk for developing complications are children below 5-years of age, individuals above 65 years of age, and people with a weakened immune system. Pregnant women and individuals with chronic diseases of the heart and lungs are also at a high risk for complications, and an infection can affect insulin use in people with diabetes. It must be remembered that during the 1918 pandemic, there was a reversal of this age group demographics and it was the physically fit young adults that suffered the worst mortality rates from Influenza.

Individuals with asthma in all age groups are at a special risk because an Influenza infection may worsen their asthma and their chronic airway changes make them prone to developing a bacterial bronchitis.[2,4] Finally, the caregivers of influenza patients are at risk because without using proper procedures they will be exposed to prolonged high levels of the Influenza virus when they nurse patients.

The complications of Influenza typically appear after the main symptoms of viral infection are subsiding and the fever is diminishing. The return of a fever is often an early sign that a secondary bacterial infection has started to colonize the damaged airways. When nursing an Influenza patient at home it is necessary to recognize any developing complications early so that professional medical care can be quickly initiated. Any delay can be serious.

The two most common complications of Influenza A infection are Acute Bronchitis and a much more serious condition called Pneumonia.

ACUTE BRONCHITIS

Bronchitis is common in Influenza. It is caused by the virus damaging the cells lining the bronchi (large and medium-sized airways) in the lungs. The most common symptom of is an initial "dry" hacking cough. Other symptoms include coughing up yellowish mucus. This color is due to the dead white blood cells that have been fighting the infection as part of the body's natural defenses. Other signs and symptoms are wheezing, shortness of breath, fever, and chest discomfort. The infection may last from a few days to a week and it may require a proper medical examination and antibiotics to clear the bacterial infection. Sometimes the cough may persist for several weeks afterward.

PNEUMONIA

Pneumonia is the most common, serious, complication of influenza and it is associated with a mortality rate of 10-20%. The highest-risk patients are those over 65-years of age, together with children below the age of five years. The delayed onset of pneumonia is normally due to a bacterial infection that has penetrated deeply into the lung to affect the actual air sacks (alveoli). The alveoli perform a gas exchange by bringing oxygen into the body and eliminating carbon dioxide. It is a very serious condition. The more virulent strains of the Influenza virus such as H5N1, can directly attack the deep airways of the lung with secondary bacteria that invade the spaces between the alveoli. As part of the body's defense, white blood cells attempt to kill the bacteria. These white cells release chemical messengers called cytokines and pyrogens, which cause a further general activation of the immune system. This leads to the fever, chills, and fatigue common in bacterial pneumonia.

The patient's white blood cells fighting the infection and fluid leaking from the surrounding blood vessels, start to fill the lung tissue and the patient may have difficulty maintaining the levels of oxygen in their blood. Mixed infections with both the Influenza virus and bacteria may occur in up to 45% of Influenza infections in children and in 15% of infections in adults. The common symptoms of pneumonia include:

- Lethargy and weakness
- Headache
- Joint and muscle pain
- Fever of 102°F or more

- Chills
- Cough with yellow sputum production
- Shortness of breath with chest pain (may be sharp and worse on inspiration),

A secondary bacterial pneumonia can usually be treated with antibiotics if recognized early. However, antibiotics are only effective against bacteria. They have no effect on the Influenza virus itself. In the elderly or people with other lung problems, recovery may take up to several months. In patients that require intensive care for lung complications, the mortality may reach 30–50% even with normal seasonal Influenza strains.

ADDITIONAL SEVERE COMPLICATIONS OF INFLUENZA INFECTION

Other serious complications of Influenza may occur if large amounts of the virus spread into the blood stream. This depends on the specific strain of the Influenza virus and it was observed during the second wave of 1918 pandemic.

In 1918, doctors observed on autopsy that the most serious cases of the disease showed tissue damage and inflammation in the wall of the heart (myocarditis), in the brain (encephalitis), in the membranes surrounding the brain (meningitis), and in the skeletal muscles (rhabdomyolysis). The widespread inflammation in the body caused by the 1918-strain resulted in what is today termed the *Systemic Inflammatory Syndrome*. This can quickly lead to Multiple Organ Dysfunction and damage with respiratory failure, together with kidney and liver damage. This condition is more commonly known as "septic shock" and much of the tissue damage is caused by the patient's own over-active immune response.[5] There are numerous Influenza cases described where previously healthy individuals died within hours from respiratory failure due to this process.

Influenza like many other viral infections can cause serious complications in pregnancy such as premature delivery before 37-weeks or stillbirth. As previously mentioned, Diabetics may show an increased demand for insulin. The presence of any neurological signs and symptoms such as confusion or seizures, obviously requires immediate medical attention. Individuals providing home care must be aware of the basic signs and symptoms of these complications and they need to seek medical assistance at the earliest appearance of any signs.

To recap, medical help should be called for any Influenza patient that starts to exhibit a fever of 100° F or higher for 3 or more days or starts to feel better and then develops a new fever or sore throat. Rapid medical care should also be sought for any Influenza patient who develops shortness of breath or wheezing, or who is coughing up small flecks of blood mixed with mucous.

Urgent medical care is also required for any patient that suddenly begins to have chest discomfort or trouble with their balance, speech, walking, or becomes confused.

SAFELY NURSING AN INFLUENZA PATIENT

If no complications develop, an influenza patient is normally infectious for roughly a week and they are most infectious during the first 3-4 days. However, small children may excrete live virus for up to 21 days.[2] It is essential during this time for the caregiver to avoid becoming infected themselves. This is a major challenge and it was a significant factor during the 1918-pandemic, especially in the overcrowded hospitals and in the homes of the poor, overcrowded, low-resource communities. In 1918, entire families became infected to the point where all the family members were incapacitated and unable to look after each other. When nursing an Influenza patient, there are certain basic protective equipment and practices that must be used when entering and leaving an infected patient's room.

Hand "Hygiene"

Hand hygiene is an essential element of what are termed Universal Standard Precautions. The term includes handwashing with either plain or antiseptic-containing soap and water, or the use of alcohol-based products (gels and foams). Why this is effective is because the Influenza virus has a fatty covering around its outer protein structure that is acquired when the virus buds out of its host cell as a new daughter virus. This makes it especially susceptible to detergents and alcohol-based sanitizers. These detergents, ethanol, or methyl alcohol (rubbing alcohol) will quickly dissolve this fatty envelope. Studies suggest that products containing between 60% and 80% alcohol are more effective at quickly destroying the virus because of their solvent action.

Frequent hand washing by both the patient and the caregiver alike, is an important Non-Pharmaceutical Intervention (NPI) and supplies for performing hand hygiene should be both inside the patient's room as well as immediately outside the room. The caregiver should disinfect their hands before touching their eyes, nose, or mouth and after every bathroom visit. While alcohol-based sanitizers can be found in any supermarket or drugstore, during an Influenza pandemic these are likely to be in short supply. Also, alcohol-based hand sanitizers can lose their potency with time. Fortunately, a cheap, effective substitute can be made at home.[2]

Simple Preparation of an Alcohol Sanitizer

- 4 cups of 70% methyl (rubbing alcohol) (1 quart)
- 4 teaspoons of glycerin (can be purchased at supermarkets)

This solution makes an effective hand sanitizer and the 70% rubbing alcohol alone can be used to wipe surfaces to kill the Influenza virus. While methyl alcohol (rubbing alcohol) is highly toxic if ingested, little of it will absorb through the adult skin. Hand and wrist jewelry and watches should never be worn inside a patient's room.[2] The caregiver must wash their hands before and after caring for an ill family member and avoid touching their face until their hands have been disinfected.

When providing homecare, visitors to the home should be limited and they should avoid all direct contact with the infected patient for the first week of illness. Family members should be checked often for the symptoms of influenza and if present they should also be separated into their own room. The caregiver should ensure that the patient adheres to respiratory hygiene, cough etiquette, and hand hygiene throughout the duration of their illness. They should cover their nose and mouth when coughing or sneezing. If they use paper tissues, these should be placed into a lined wastepaper basket. Obviously, this is going to be difficult when dealing with small sick children.

The caretaker must take all infection precautions when disposing of the heavily virus-contaminated tissues, soiled bedding, towels, and patient clothing. However, the risk of disease transmission is negligible if they are handled, transported, and laundered in a safe manner. This involves not shaking the items and avoiding direct contact of one's body, ungloved hands, and personal clothing with the soiled items being handled. These soiled items should be placed into a single plastic garbage bag and washed immediately with the hands well-disinfected after placing the clothing into a washing machine. A combination of hot water and the detergents used in modern washing machines is sufficient to destroy the Influenza virus on clothing and bedding. The door handles of the washing machine must also be disinfected with alcohol sanitizer. After laundering, the clean items should be bagged and kept outside the patient's room until use.

Hot water and dish soap is sufficient to sanitize the plates, cups, and eating utensils used by the patient. Alternately, paper dishes and disposable eating utensils can be used by the patient. Thermometers should be cleaned with hand sanitizer before and after use and kept in the patient's room.

PERSONAL PROTECTIVE EQUIPMENT (PPE)

This refers to the variety of barriers and respirators that can be used in combination to protect the caregiver's mucous membranes, airways, skin, and clothing from direct contact with infectious agents. The selection of PPE is based on the nature of the caregiver's patient interaction and infected children will normally require a maximum use of precautions.

Gloves

"Gloves' are used to prevent contamination of the hands when they come into contact with infected surfaces or body fluids and they should be worn always inside an infected patient's room. Besides protection, this serves as a reminder for the caregiver not to touch their own face. The gloves manufactured for general healthcare purposes are subject to FDA standards and they are made from a variety of materials. They are nonsterile, disposable, come in sizes, and are made of a variety of materials such as vinyl or nitrile for routine patient care. However, the user needs to be shown and then practice how to remove the gloves without touching the outside of the glove.

Disposable gloves should be worn before entering a patient's room. When finished in the patient's room, the door handle to the room should be disinfected with hand sanitizer then the outside of the gloves disinfected and removed using proper technique and disposed of in the patient's room. After leaving the room, a supply of hand sanitizer located outside the room should be used to disinfect the bare hands again.

A plastic or disposable apron

If caring for a child, the healthcare giver should wear a plastic apron when in the patient's room.[2] Donning both an apron and gloves upon room entry will address any unintentional contact with contaminated environmental surfaces. If this is done, the front of the apron should be wiped with disinfectant before removal and it is left in the room. When redonning it, the apron should be sanitized again before putting it on.

Masks

The main mode of influenza virus transmission is by coughed and exhaled respiratory droplets of virus-laden secretions. Conversational speech alone can produce thousands of these tiny droplets which extend about 3-feet out into the person's immediate environment. Infection can occur if one of these droplets happens to land on the surface of the caregiver's face, eye, or mouth, or if a provider's hand becomes contaminated when they touch an infected surface and they then rub their eyes.

Masks can be worn by the Influenza patient to minimize their secretions into the air. However, this may not be tolerated in children.[2] With respect to healthcare providers, basic federal guidance indicates that masks should be worn in healthcare settings. Although this was referring to hospitals, it is reasonable when nursing an Influenza patient at home. The actual effectiveness of this will be discussed later.

There are two general types of masks. The first is the common "surgical mask" that can be purchased from a pharmacy. These are typically made of paper. The patient should use these to minimize the infectious droplets they cough and sneeze into the environment around them. If the patient is coughing and sneezing, the mask should ideally be changed for a fresh one every 4-6 hours. The masks from a patient will contain active Influenza virus and the mask is therefore highly infectious. It should be disposed of in a bag in the patient's room. If handled by the caregiver, it is important to remove the mask carefully for disposal and that they disinfect their gloves immediately after handling it.

The second type of mask is more efficient and should be used by the caretakers themselves. It is called an N-95 mask. The "N" denotes it has been certified by NIOSH, the U.S. National Institute for Occupational Safety and Health. The numerals 95 refer to the fact that if properly worn, the mask can filter out 95% of the aerosol particles within the critical 1 to 5-micron droplet size range and larger. The N-95 masks are more expensive, but the CDC is now recommending these for healthcare providers.

In hospitals, the N-95 masks are fit tested to an individual to ensure they are suitable for the healthcare provider's head. In a homecare setting this is impractical. Therefore, a strip of duct tape can be placed around the edges of the mask before entering a patient's room. Removing the mask should be in the order of; apron, mask, and the gloves last, with disinfection of the outside of the gloves after each step. None of the masks that have been described will protect the eyes and for some influenza strains this is an important fact.

Like alcohol and examination gloves, masks should be stockpiled before a pandemic is underway. This is because unfortunately, most of the masks are made overseas which renders this item vulnerable to infrastructure disruption, although the HHS 2017 update states that U.S. continental production has now been upgraded for the N-95 mask.

Shoes

A pair of cheap slippers that can be donned and removed without touching them by hand should be left in the patient's room, put on after entry through the door and removed at the door before leaving.

Surface Disinfection

Frequent cleaning and disinfecting surfaces in patient-care areas are essential, especially those surfaces closest to the patient that will certainly be contaminated (bedside tables, potties or bedpans, doorknobs, sinks, bedside tables, dressers, and any chairs near the patient). The frequency of cleaning may change based on the patient's level of hygiene and the degree of illness.[2]

If a common bathroom is shared with the rest of the family, it should be disinfected after each use by the patient if possible and there is a good reason for this. Infected birds are known to shed the Influenza A viruses in their saliva, nasal secretions, and feces. Humans also secrete infectious Influenza virus in their stool as well. Live Influenza virus has been isolated from the diarrhea of a child dying from the H5N1 Influenza virus, as well in individuals suffering from seasonal Influenza.[6] This raises the possibility that the Influenza virus could be spread from human to human via a fecal-oral route as well.

There is also a concern about the inhalation of microscopic fecal droplets aerosolized by toilet flushing. Experiments with fluorescent dye-stained water have demonstrated that not only are toilet seats significantly contaminated, but a plume of aerosolized toilet water is generated by flushing. This invisible large-particle aerosol rises 3-4 feet around the bowl. Good bathroom hygiene should include lowering the toilet lid before flushing and disinfecting all the surfaces in a bathroom after a patient with influenza uses it.[2]

As a rule, a care giver should avoid any unnecessary touching of surfaces in a patient's room to avoid both the contamination of their gloves and the transmission of Influenza virus from their contaminated gloves to other surfaces. The popular so called *"3-second rule"* for food dropped on the floor, is a complete myth. The contamination occurs instantly.

With respect to small particle viral aerosols, the RNA viruses show a decreased viability under the conditions of high atmospheric humidity, oxygen, and exposure to the ultraviolet radiation in sunlight. If it is possible, the patient's room air should be directed to the outside to reduce the concentration of 1 to 5-micron particle aerosols which can remain suspended in the room for several hours.

Use of Ultraviolet Light for Viral Disinfection

This brings us to the question of using ultraviolet lights for disinfection. This is a disinfection method that uses short-wavelength Ultraviolet (UV-C) light to kill viruses by causing dimer-damage to their genetic material. Its effectiveness depends on the length of time the Influenza virus is exposed to UV, the intensity and wavelength of the UV radiation, and the presence of dust particles that can protect the virus from UV exposure.

For humans, skin and eye exposure to UV light can cause damage. Consequently, this is a lot more difficult than simply hanging UV "party" lamps around the house. Small, commercially available UV air purification systems provide the safest, most effective method and these can be purchased as free-standing units with shielded UV lamps that use a fan to force air past the UV light. The UV wavelength for disinfection is most typically generated by a mercury-vapor lamp with a strong emission line at 254 nanometers. This is within the range of wavelengths that demonstrate a strong viral disinfection effect.

There are advantages to having this in an Influenza patient's room.

However, they are expensive (around $300) and numerous models of variable effectiveness are on the market. During our design of the floating laboratory outlined in Chapter 30, we found an excellent review site for these devices on the internet (https://www.damagecontrol-911.com/buyers-guide-top-quiet-uv-air-purifiers/).

The guidelines outlined in this chapter are an upgrade from what is recommended in federal homecare guidance for Influenza. Now a historical document, the advice given to homecare providers in 2009, was inadequate for a severe Influenza pandemic with a virus that is associated with a high mortality.[7]

In this light, there appears to be a serious disconnect between the federal advice that is being given to homecare providers and the Influenza guidelines being issued to hospitals.[8] In addition, the CDC website is poorly designed and difficult to navigate to find information pertaining to current home care recommendations for severe Influenza. This precludes easy access by the general public to the national guidelines on this important matter.

There is the appearance that for several decades now, the federal health agencies have been issuing advice to the public simply as they go along, without making careful studies of up-to-date scientific literature and assessing the effectiveness of what they are promoting. This is reflected by their constant issuing of new interim guidelines that contradict their earlier federal guidelines for even the simplest matters such as wearing protective masks. Time and again, these guidelines fail to err on the side of caution. This is important when dealing with a lethal viral agent with no vaccine or effective drug treatment.

This seems to be a persistent problem that was very noticeable when the first infection control guidelines were issued by the DHHS/CDC during the 2014 Ebola outbreak. One of the absurd statements made by leading infectious disease authorities at the CDC and the National

Institute of Allergy and Infectious Diseases, was that "double-gloving" was not necessary when managing Ebola patients, and that a single layer of surgical gloves was sufficient. This repeated statement was ludicrous, as double gloving is a standard procedure used for many well-known infectious diseases such as hepatitis. This only served to further erode the public trust and cause concern. There is a repeating pattern here.

In summary, the federal pandemic doctrine is shifting towards an emphasis that the home care of influenza patients will be an important solution to minimize hospital overcrowding and the medical surge requirement necessary during a severe Influenza pandemic. However, when dealing with a lethal Influenza strain, there is more to safely doing this than simply giving bed rest, food, and fluids to a patient and the early detection of Influenza complications.

It is essential for the caregiver and the rest of the family to ensure that they avoid contracting the infection themselves. As previously mentioned, during the 1918-event, entire families quickly became co-infected to the point of their incapacitation. Therefore, it is essential that home caregivers take every practical precautionary measure that is possible. These techniques must be learned and practiced before a severe pandemic occurs, or entire families will run the risk of infection which will further add to the problem of the pandemic response.

THE CONCEPT OF A NURSE TRIAGE LINE

During a severe pandemic, the public needs timely and accurate information about when and where to seek care. Emergency rooms, clinics, and medical offices will be crowded. If effective antiviral drugs are available, any delay in seeking treatment may be accompanied by a delay in initiating antiviral drug therapy and a missed "window" for treatment.

Although there are medical/legal considerations, one of the concepts being considered for improving information flow and improving home care is called the Nurse Triage Line. The rationale for this is that when a pandemic expands to the point that medical care is shifted away from individuals and more towards groups; an experienced Registered

Nurse's "*Scope of Practice*" might be expanded under certain guidelines. This is somewhat like the Philadelphia Filbert 100 "Hot Line" used during the 1918 pandemic. This concept has a more modern precedent.

During the 2009 H1N1 outbreak and fearing the worst because of the WHO pandemic level announcement, the highly competent Minnesota health authorities established what was called the Minnesota-Nurse Triage Line.[9] In this respect, the Minnesota Department of Health quickly partnered with 8 state health plans and two hospital systems, to establish a common protocol and a toll-free number. The purpose of this number was for citizens to call-in so that duty nurses could offer antiviral prescriptions to the callers per a standard protocol and orders approved by a State-licensed physician. The Department of Health also created an additional Nurse Triage Line for the uninsured, and for those whose health plans were not participating in the Triage Line concept.

From Oct 2009 through to March 2010, over 27,300 calls were received where nurses performed a survey evaluation and issued prescriptions. Using this method, an estimated 11,000 unneeded health care facility visits were avoided. This served to decrease public confusion by providing accurate information and assistance, minimize any misinformation and rumors about the pandemic and it helped to reduce the spread of Influenza by reducing the number of ill individuals gathering in the waiting rooms of health care facilities.

It also helped the state healthcare system meet the needs of the uninsured or underinsured patients, along with those who did not have easy access to health care. Conceivably, in a severe pandemic it could reduce the medical surge requirement on a local healthcare system and help to ensure that other priority medical needs outside of Influenza, to continue to be met.

With modifications, an extension of this obviously successful Minnesota program could have an effect with respect to helping individuals participate in the home care of an ill family member. The Telephone Triage nurse could help the patient or family define the nature of their problem and if they should be seen by a physician, and what health education the family may need for home care.

An assessment is now underway concerning any existing laws that might impact the ability to set up effective Nurse Triage Lines. This involves a 50-state assessment with respect to allowing Registered Nurses to give medical triage advice over the phone, their ability to prescribe medications under strict protocol over phone, and their ability to provide triage and prescriptions across state lines based on the standards of nursing practice set by the American Nursing Association and the National Council of State Boards of Nursing. If this is established, a further physician-directed expansion of the concept could start to achieve some of the capability of the original Filbert-100 multiple call-line system used in Philadelphia in 1918.

If a single physician is available to work with the nurses that are operating multiple call lines, this functional collaboration can expand the capability of the call lines to better assess and attempt to diagnose the nature and urgency of an existing problem in home care, or with a call-back, may even be able to monitor the problem and assess the effectiveness of antiviral treatment or a resolution of the problem.

Using critical thinking and clinical judgment, a physician-directed call center should be able to decide if a home visit by a small home-visit health team is required to develop a more individualized plan of care. Such small dedicated visiting health teams could act as a force multiplier for the medical response. The CDC is currently working with the states and public health partners to develop an approach to Nurse Triage Lines as a national model with guidance for use during a severe pandemic scenario.

A coordinated network of pandemic Nurse Triage Lines would provide another very critical function, and that is to collect community data on Influenza case numbers and their severity, while the pandemic is still unfolding. If a dedicated national information/GIS system can be linked into the call-line system and updated by manual input as the nurses take their calls, this could generate real-time data which would be vital for state and national planners.

A GIS system (geographic information system) is computer

software designed to capture, store, manipulate, analyze, and present geographic data. The concept of a GIS dates as far back as 1854 when Dr. John Snow determined the source of a cholera outbreak in London by marking points on a map depicting where the cholera victims lived.[10] Such a system would aid a local pandemic response by graphically depicting where in their communities the worst influenza outbreaks are occurring. In addition, modern software packages provide an ever-increasing set of analytical tools to use on GIS databases and their data displays. This will be discussed later on in this book,

In summary, the U.S. government has spent billions of dollars on its pandemic response plan, but it has underestimated the capability of local authorities to make rational, tested, end-user preparations. At the same time, it has failed to acknowledge the decay of the healthcare system that has allowed this to happen.

Realizing that most local authorities are not capable of managing the medical surge required in a severe Influenza pandemic, the bulk of the problem is now shifted further down the chain to the individual families of a community. The concept of Home Care is promoting that families with no medical background, now nurse their own moderately ill family members at home without contracting the infection themselves. The family is also expected to suddenly acquire an ability to make an early diagnosis of when their ill family members are developing a severe complication that requires urgent professional medical attention.

However, with the addition of Nurse Triage Lines, this approach does gain some plausibility and the concept of home care is backed by previous Influenza pandemic data. However, it fails to consider what is currently happening in nature with respect to the Influenza virus itself.

As human habitation-density is changing and the domestic poultry industry continues to expand, the natural constraints and selection pressures on the Influenza virus can be expected to change.[2] It is entirely possible that a new strain may emerge with a high human to human transmissibility and a 40% or greater mortality that extends to all population age-groups.

In this respect, pandemic planners are living in the past, not erring on the side of caution, or looking towards the future. There is little or no Influenza home-care training for the general population taking place and a severe pandemic outbreak is not the time to try and rush such community preparedness efforts into play.

Most high schools require some type of general health classes and the pandemic problem and NPI could be added to the curriculum for little cost.

Notes for Chapter 15

[1] Pugliese, A; Beltramo, T; Torre, D (October 2008). "Reye's and Reye's-like syndromes.". Cell biochemistry and function. 26 (7): 741–6. PMID 18711704. doi:10.1002/cbf.1465.

[2] Michael Greger. Bird Flu: A Virus of Our Own Hatching. 2006, Lantern Books ISBN 1590560981 (ISBN13: 9781590560983) http://birdflubook.com/

[3] G C Woodson, "Good Home Treatment of Influenza". drgcwoodson.com/wpcontent/uploads/2017/10/Good-Home-Treatment-of-Influenza.pdf).

[4] Asthma and Influenza. https://www.cdc.gov/flu/asthma/index.htm.

[5] CDC sepsis, https://www.cdc.gov/sepsis/index.html

[6] Chan M, Lee N, Chan P, et al. Seasonal Influenza A Virus in Feces of Hospitalized Adults. Emerging Infectious Diseases. 2011; 17(11):2038-2042. doi:10.3201/eid1711.110205

[7] Home Care Guidance. https://www.cdc.gov/h1n1flu/homecare/caregivertips.htm

[8] Feb 15, 2017 Update Guideline for Isolation Precautions in Healthcare Settingshttps://www.cdc.gov/infectioncontrol/pdf/guidelines/isolation-guidelines.pdf

[9] A.B. Spaulding, D, Radi, H. Macleod, A,S. DeVries, et.al., Design and Implementation of a Statewide Influenza Nurse Triage Line in Response to Pandemic H1N1 Influenza. Public Health Rep. 2012 Sep-Oct; 127(5): 532–540. doi: 10.1177/003335491212700509

[10] Snow, John (1849). On the Mode of Communication of Cholera (PDF). London: John Churchill. www.ph.ucla.edu/epi/snow/publichealth118_387_394_2004.pdf 9. Geographical Information System https://www.nationalgeographic.org/encyclopedia/geographic-information-system-gis

16

CURRENT DHHS/CDC INFLUENZA PROTECTION GUIDELINES ARE STILL INADEQUATE

BEFORE ANY FURTHER DISCUSSIONS concerning home care or pandemic preparedness and the bolstering of medical surge capability, it is necessary to carefully review how Influenza is transmitted from animals to humans, and from humans to humans.

The study of the medical effects of any virus requires closely examining infected human cases and infected human tissue cultures in the laboratory. Unfortunately, in many cases, it is also necessary to develop a laboratory animal model of the infection. Animals like humans, show different susceptibilities to different viruses. Therefore, it is necessary to search for an animal species that can be infected by the virus being studied.

Usually, the selection of special laboratory mice and rats fulfill this role. These animals are easy to keep and study, and they can show where a virus will replicate in a mammalian body. They can also help us understand how well various vaccines and antiviral drugs work. Such experiments are conducted with utmost consideration and follow strict protocols for how the animals are housed and fed, as well as their compassionate care. Occasionally, an animal species is found where the virus being studied causes signs and symptoms that very closely match what is observed when humans are infected with the virus. This then becomes the preferred animal model for the disease.

For Influenza, a small mammal called the ferret serves as the model for human infection. These highly intelligent animals make delightful, interesting pets, and they have greatly advanced our knowledge of Influenza transmission. Ferrets and humans share similar lung structures and function, and human and avian influenza viruses exhibit similar patterns of binding to the sialic acids (the receptor for influenza viruses), which are distributed throughout the respiratory tract in both species. Ferrets show the same clinical signs as humans when experimentally infected in the laboratory, including a nasal discharge and sneezing. Like humans, they run a fever starting a day after infection. Human and avian influenza viruses replicate well in the respiratory tract of ferrets without prior adaptation, and the spread of the virus through the body after infection with High-Pathogenic Avian Influenza viruses is like that seen in the human cases that have been described.

Ferrets have demonstrated Influenza virus spread by direct contact (i.e. by housing an infected and an uninfected ferret together) or by the spread of respiratory droplets in the absence of direct contact (i.e. separating infected and uninfected ferrets with a perforated wall that only allows an air exchange.[1]

The H1N1 virus that caused the great 1918 pandemic was by itself highly dangerous, but as discussed previously, some of the mortality associated with this event was due to a secondary bacterial pneumonia that developed after the Influenza virus had damaged the respiratory tract. Ferrets show this same pattern, corroborating the historical human data showing that cases of pneumonia are increased during some pandemic influenza outbreaks.

Based on ferret and human data, it is acknowledged that the Influenza virus may be transmitted to humans in three ways: by direct contact with infected individuals; by contact with contaminated objects and then touching the face, eyes, or mouth (doorknobs, elevator buttons, work surfaces, dust, children's toys, light switches, etc.); and finally, by the inhalation of virus laden aerosols. The relative importance of each one of these during a human pandemic spread is ill defined, but in a healthcare setting, all routes of infection must be guarded against.

Numerous scientists have emphasized that droplet transmission is an important mode by which influenza virus infection is acquired and there is over 50-years of data on the behavior of small particle aerosols and the viability of infectious viruses in such aerosols. Yet the previous 2006 DHHS Pandemic Influenza Plan, recommended the use of simple surgical masks as part of the personal protective equipment (PPE) for routine patient care. This recommendation was wrong inside a healthcare setting with an environment of dehumidified air, low ambient ultraviolet light, and high concentrations of virus in the environment.[2,3,4,5,6,7] It took until 2017 for the DHHS to update its Pandemic Plan to fully recommend and stockpile high-efficiency particulate air (HEPA) filtered N95 masks for which they use the term "respirators".

The new interim guidance document says the use of N-95 "respirators" (designed to stop 95% of small airborne particles) is *prudent* for medical workers providing direct care for patients with confirmed or suspected pandemic flu and is recommended in caring for those with secondary pneumonia. It also says respirator use is "prudent" for support workers in direct contact with patients. The 2017 pandemic plan also advises healthcare facilities to expect and plan for shortages of N-95 respirators and similar protective equipment in the event of a pandemic. This is because the majority of these are now made overseas with a lengthy supply chain vulnerable to pandemic disruption.

These new recommendations reflect an increased concern about the possibility of airborne transmission of flu viruses. Yet the DHHS 2017 update says the CDC has found no new scientific evidence on this question. DHHS says the new guidance "augments and supersedes" previous advice. While it discusses the use of N-95 HEPA (High Efficiency Particulate Air) respirators for other direct care activities involving patients with confirmed or suspected pandemic influenza, it provides little guidance about the home health care activities that it promotes during a pandemic.

There is a disconnect here. If it is prudent for healthcare workers to be wearing N-95 respirators, then that should be the baseline for protection for anyone in contact with an influenza patient. This should include home caregivers.

Irrespective, repeated experimental data now shows that even the current 2017 DHHS guidelines are inadequate for complete protection against Influenza infection in healthcare setting featuring a low humidity, controlled environmental condition. This is because a patient's coughing and sneezing can produce both large and small particle aerosols. If this aerosol has droplets in the 1 to 5-micron mass-median-diameter size-range it will have the same physical behavior as a gas. Consequently, infected mucous droplets in this size range can remain suspended in the air and some strains of the influenza virus can remain viable and infectious for at least 2-hours in a floating aerosol.[8,9]

It has been known for some time that a variety of respiratory viruses (including Influenza A virus strains), can cause documented human eye infections.[10,11] While rare, sporadic reports of eye-related symptoms following H5N1 and the 2009 H1N1 Influenza strains have been documented. The dangerous Influenza A viruses of the H7 subtype have resulted in over 100 cases of human infection since 2002, and these frequently cause eye inflammation in infected individuals along with severe respiratory disease and death.[12] Eye exposure as a route for Influenza virus entry into the body has been confirmed by documented accidental laboratory exposures (e.g., by liquid Influenza virus tissue culture fluid being splashed or infected ferrets sneezing into a scientist's face and eyes) and occupational exposures (e.g., by direct ocular exposure to infected poultry or eye abrasions from contaminated dust during chicken culling operations).

A large body of evidence now makes it clear that the human eye is a target for the entry of some Influenza A virus strains into the human respiratory tract. In the eye, both the transparent clear part of the eye (the cornea), the inner lining of the eyelids, and the white part of the eye (the conjunctival epithelial cells) contain the sialic acids molecules that serve as the receptors for the H protein of the Influenza virus.[12,13] When the human eye contacts a suspended large and small small-particle Influenza-laden aerosols from an infected patient's cough or sneeze, a surface tension effect can draw the viral particles to the moist epithelial cells on the ocular surface where they adhere. Once adherent, the nasolacrimal drainage system of the eye, will drain the attached viruses from the surface of the eye through the tear ducts and into the inside cavity of the nose within 30-minutes. Surprisingly, even the deeper structures of the human eye have been shown to support Influenza virus replication.

Experiments reveal that ocular-only exposure to virus-containing aerosols constitutes a valid exposure route for a potentially fatal respiratory infection, even for viruses that do not demonstrate an ocular viral tropism. Ferrets inoculated solely by the ocular aerosol route with avian (H7N7, H7N9) or human (H1N1, H3N2) strains were able to transmit these Influenza viruses to uninfected animals by direct-contact or respiratory-droplets. This underscores the public health implications of human ocular exposure in clinical or occupational health care settings. These experiments have shown that eye exposure alone to Influenza A virus strains are sufficient to cause a lethal infection in the surrogate ferret model.

Therefore, respiratory protection alone will not fully protect against influenza virus exposure, infection, and severe disease.

Under Federal Respiratory Protection Standards 29 CFR
1910.134 and Personal Protective Equipment Standard 29
CFR 1910.132, any medical surge capability must also focus on
the safety of the medical surge providers and staff.

The demonstrated vulnerability of the human eye as a point of infection with some strains of the Influenza Group A virus, indicates that without recommending full eye covering, the current 2017 DHHS/CDC guidelines being promoted for healthcare workers are inadequate to afford complete 100% protection during a global Influenza pandemic, Therefore its recommendations might not be in compliance with Federal law. In addition, the DHHS guidelines being given to home caregivers are also inadequate to prevent infection,

As was seen in the 2014 Ebola debacle in the United States, it is essential for DHHS and the Public Health authorities to keep up to date with the latest peer-reviewed research before making national guidelines. Apparently, this is being done very slowly for Influenza.

In a global Influenza pandemic, U.S. healthcare workers must be assured that the protective measures and personal protective equipment that they use, will prevent them from contracting the disease. The infection of even a few volunteer workers with Influenza could have a domino effect on the rest of the volunteer workforce and an existing surge personnel capability could vanish overnight because of illness and fear of infection.[14]

Adding eye goggles to the protective ensemble would be one solution, but this would require additional training in decontamination when doffing PPE. This is because the outer surface of the goggles should be considered to be contaminated with live Influenza virus. Therefore ideally, full airway protection requires not only HEPA filtered air, but also full-face protection and this must be combined with alcohol-based wipe disinfection of both the protection device and the hands after use.

In this respect, a significant number of full-face respirators are manufactured by a variety of companies. Their cost range is between $120 to $420. However, they require a precise donning and doffing procedure, and some may require submersion for complete decontamination. Some models are bulky, heavy, and require fit testing to ensure a good face seal. Some require OSHA-mandated respiratory medical clearance for institutional use.

Hence, there is an urgent need for an affordable, simple, negative pressure, air purifying respirator that is lightweight, easy to don and doff, and able to reliably achieve a face-seal without qualitative fit testing. Searching the internet for concept ideas, we came across a design called the "*social gas mask*".[15] We were immediately attracted to the design and in Figure 22, we have made suggested improvements for use of this basic concept by both healthcare workers and by the minimally-trained general public during a severe 1918-type Influenza pandemic.

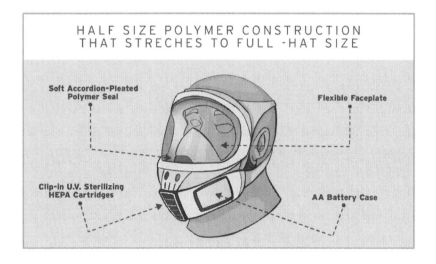

Figure 22. *Integral Pandemic Respirator.*

Such a design would be comfortable, low profile, and compatible with wearing corrective eyeglasses or contact lenses. Because this could be used by the public, a suitable modified design would feature dual self-sterilizing filter units based on low-voltage U.V. LEDs embedded into the inside of an insertable, replaceable HEPA filter cartridge.

These inexpensive 3-volt Ultraviolet (UV) Light Emitting Diodes (LED) would supply a wavelength sufficient to create nucleic acid dimer formation to sterilize any viral agent trapped in the HEPA material of the filter cartridge. Minimal training could ensure that the wearer properly decontaminates both the respirator and their hands when doffing.

The most critical component of this respirator concept would be the novel use of a soft polymer "pleated accordion cup" which would act to seal the HEPA filters to the mouth and nose using only the mild outside pressure provided by the chin extension and the top polymer retaining band. Such a product could be extremely useful during the projected "Vaccine Gap" between an initial severe Influenza outbreak and general vaccine availability for the public. A "just-in-time" manufacturing capability could be pre-arranged as part of the Strategic National Stockpile. It is likely that such a reusable "Integral Pandemic Respirator" could be mass produced for the same price as a single course of generic Tamiflu ($155.86). Unlike Tamiflu, the respirator can be used for long periods of time (days) and if hermetically sealed packaging is used in conjunction with oxygen absorbing packets, it could feature an extended shelf life.

THE PROBLEM OF CIRCULATING BANKNOTES

The successful control of any viral disease outbreak requires knowledge of the different circumstances or agents that could promote its transmission among hosts. In this respect, there is one final aspect of general pandemic preparedness that must be addressed. This concerns the survival of the Influenza virus on common circulating banknotes.

In a series of experiments, banknotes were experimentally contaminated with representative influenza virus subtypes at various concentrations, and the virus survival time was tested after different periods. Influenza A viruses tested by cell culture methods, survived up to 3-days when they were inoculated at high concentrations. The same inoculum in the presence of respiratory mucus showed a striking increase in survival time (up to 17-days) in the laboratory.[16] When the nasopharyngeal secretions of naturally infected children were used, the Influenza virus survived on banknotes for at least 48-hours in one-third of the cases.

The unexpected stability of the Influenza virus in this non-biological environment suggests that this possibility for environmental contamination should be considered in the setting of pandemic preparedness. Banknotes might be a significant factor in Influenza transmission, but our research indicates that no federal agency has yet addressed this concern. This potential mode for transmission might be negated by the simple exposure of banknotes to sunlight, by dunking in methanol, or by impregnating bank notes with an inorganic antiviral substance at the time of their manufacture.

NOTES FOR CHAPTER 16

[1] T. Sutton, et.al. Airborne Transmission of Highly Pathogenic H7N1 Influenza Virus in Ferrets J. Virol. June 2014 vol. 88 no. 12 6623-6635. Posted online 2 April 2014, doi:10.1128/JVI.02765-13

[2] Moser, M. R., T. R. Bender, H. S. Margolis, G. R. Noble, A. P. Kendal, and D. G. Ritter. 1979. Outbreak of influenza aboard a commercial airliner. Am. J. Epidemiol. 110:1-6.

[3] Raymond Tellier, Perspective; Emerg. Inf. Dis. Volume 12, Number 11, November 2006. Samira Mubareka, et.al., Transmission of Influenza Virus via Aerosols and Fomites in the Guinea Pig Model J Infect Dis (2009) 199 (6): 858-865. 15 March 2009.

[4] Yao. M. Zhang, X. et.al. The Occurrence and Transmission Characteristics of Airborne H9N2 Avian Influenza Virus. Beri Munch Tieraztl Wochensehr Zoll. Mar-April; 124 (3-4) 136-41.

[5] Noti JD, et al. Detection of infectious influenza virus in cough aerosols generated in a simulated patient examination room. Clin Infect Dis 2012 Jun; 54(11):1569-1577.

[6] Cowling BJ. Airborne transmission of influenza: implication for control in healthcare and community settings. (Editorial) Clin Infect Dis. 2012 Jun;54(11):1578-80. doi: 10.1093/cid/cis240. PMID: 22460979

[7] N. Nikitin, O. Karpova, et.al., Influenza Virus Aerosols in the Air and Their Infectiousness. Advances in Virology. Volume 2014 (2014), Article ID 859090, http://dx.doi.org/10.1155/2014/859090

[8] J.R.Brown, et.al. Influenza virus survival in aerosols and estimates of viable virus loss resulting from aerosolization and air-samplingJournal of Hospital Infection. Volume 91, Issue 3, November 2015, Pages 278-281 https://doi.org/10.1016/j.jhin.2015.08.004

[9] J. Belser, et.al. Ocular Tropism of Respiratory Viruses Microbiol. Mol. Biol. Rev. March 2013 vol. 77 no. 1 144-156. doi: 10.1128/MMBR.00058-12

[10] J. Belser, D. Wadford, Terrence M. Tumpey, Ocular Infection of Mice with Influenza A (H7) Viruses: a Site of Primary Replication and Spread to the Respiratory Tract, J. Virol. July 2009 vol. 83 no. 14 7075-7084. posted online 20 May 2009, doi: 10.1128/JVI.0053509

[11] J. Belser, Hui Zeng, T. Tumpey, et.al. Ocular Tropism of Influenza A Viruses: Identification of H7 Subtype-Specific Host Responses in Human Respiratory and Ocular Cells. J. Virol. October 2011 vol. 85 no. 19 10117-10125. posted online 20 July 2011, doi: 10.1128/JVI.05101-11

[12] J. Belser, Terrence Tumpey, et.al. Pathogenesis, Transmissibility, and Ocular Tropism of a Highly Pathogenic Avian Influenza A (H7N3) Virus Associated with

Human Conjunctivitis. J. Virol. May 2013 vol. 87 no. 10 5746-5754 Accepted manuscript posted online 13 March 2013, doi: 10.1128/JVI.00154-13

[13] J, Belser, et.al. Influenza Virus Infectivity and Virulence following Ocular-Only Aerosol Inoculation of Ferrets. J. Virol. September 2014 vol. 88 no. 17 9647-9654posted online June 2014, doi: 10.1128/JVI.01067

[14] Rossow, C., W. Fales, et.al. Healthcare Providers: Will They Come to Work During an Influenza Pandemic? Disaster Management and Human Health Risk III, WIT Transactions on the Built Environment, Vol 133, 2013, ISSN: 1743-3509, ISBN: 978-1-84564-738.

[15] The Social Gas Mask; Designer: Zlil Lazarovich http://www.yankodesign.com/2014/07/11/the-social-gas-mask/

[16] Y. Thomas, G. Vogel, L. Kaiser., Survival of Influenza Virus on Banknotes Appl. Environ. Microbiol. May 2008 vol. 74 no. 10 3002-3007. posted online 21 March 2008, doi: 10.1128/AEM.00076-08

17

THE PROBLEM OF MEDICAL SURGE CAPABILITY

WE HAVE ALREADY DISCUSSED the problems with just-in-time medical inventories and the possible pandemic-induced disruption of the materials needed to keep hospitals functioning. To recap, very little of these supplies are manufactured in the United States. In addition, some 80% of U.S. drugs are manufactured by offshore suppliers which may be affected by illness and absenteeism. The federal solution to this problem was to create the National Strategic Stockpile of rapid deployable medical surge supplies. We have already discussed the existing problems with respect to the rapid distribution of time-critical items such as antiviral drugs to local community populations. However, having adequate supplies is only one factor in pandemic preparedness.

Medical Surge Capacity refers to the measurable ability of hospitals and Emergency Medical Services, to manage a sudden, dramatic increase in the number of patients seeking medical care. The concept of medical surge is a cornerstone of preparedness and it is dependent on a well-functioning incident management system, the ability to garner extra bed space for patient care, and the ability to muster extra doctors, nurses, and staff. The presence of highly contagious patients will further complicate a medical surge requirement.

HOSPITAL BEDS

Considering registered hospitals, psychiatric hospitals, long-term care, and federal government hospitals, there are currently a total of 5,564 hospitals with 897,961 hospital beds in the United States. This is for a total U.S. population of around 320 million people.[1] In 2000, the World Health Organization determined that the U.S. had a Medical Surge Immediate Bed Availability of 36 beds per 10,000 population. By 2006, that number had dropped to 33 per 10,000; and by 2012, the number was only 30 beds per 10,000.[2] This is almost a 17% erosion of surge capacity in the form of free hospital beds in the U.S.

Although Congress has allocated approximately $5 Billion since the inception of the National Hospital Preparedness Program, most this money has been spent on equipment and material. The ugly truth is that the U.S. healthcare system is moving farther away from meeting the need for the medical surge capacity required for pandemic readiness. In a severe pandemic, the demand for hospital beds will greatly exceed capacity and capabilities.

So where can the projected ~10 million Influenza cases requiring hospitalization go for medical care as their currently well-resourced megaregions quickly become overwhelmed? The situation is serious and the U.S. Department of Health and Human Services (DHHS) has now recommended that hospitals and healthcare providers develop plans to manage a serious influenza pandemic (such as the ones that occurred in 1957 and 1968), and a second plan for a more catastrophic 1918-type pandemic.

To aid this process, the DHHS Office of the Assistant Secretary for Preparedness and Response (ASPR) has developed a 2017-*2022 Health Care Preparedness and Response Capabilities* document that outlines what the national healthcare system should do to prepare for a major surge requirement. This guidance outlines a priority improvement of four capabilities to ensure Healthcare organizations deliver timely, efficient care to their patients even when the demand for services exceeds available supply.[3]

In 2016, an additional $616 million was allocated to 62 jurisdictions for this. However, DHHS does not seem to acknowledge the problems that local authorities will face in responding to a pandemic. These are numerous, and they include the following:[4]

1. The U.S. Healthcare system is uncoordinated, fragmented, and a largely private system.
2. One-third of U.S. hospitals are operating at a deficit.
3. There are severe manpower shortages, especially in nursing, with a recently estimated need for ~100,000 nurses (or ~8% of the nursing workforce).
4. Approximately 48% of emergency departments operate at capacity or at over-capacity.
5. Nationwide, the number of hospitals, emergency departments, and intensive care unit beds has been constantly decreasing.

All hospitals currently have emergency surge plans to expand their capacity for beds, emergency rooms, and critical care. Anywhere from 15 to 25% of a hospital's bed capacity can be made available by the early release of patients (surge discharge) and the cancellation of elective admissions. In addition, many hospitals have procedures to use the hospital corridors for overflow.[5,6] In an emergency, an additional 5 to 20% of a hospital's bed capacity could also be made available by transferring stable patients needing ward-type care (not needing oxygen and mechanical ventilation) to non-hospital facilities (Alternate Care Sites).

Conceivably, in a severe pandemic these measures could free up an extra 100,000 hospital beds throughout the nation. However, hospital staff and healthcare personnel will have illness and absenteeism issues themselves, and all levels of a Hospital will be impacted by a medical surge requirement, not just patient care. This includes the Hospital Food Services, Housekeeping, Laundry, Clerical Support, and Billing.[6] The mathematics of reduced staffing plus a large increase in the number of patients will not have a good outcome for any hospital.

THE USE OF ALTERNATE CARE SITES

As we have emphasized, a severe 1918-type Influenza pandemic will be a sustained widespread event occurring through large swaths of the United States and the rest of the world. It is important for all local communities to realize that unlike hurricanes or other large-scale natural disasters, outside help from surrounding areas may not be available.

Many cities and towns will be trying to cope with the Influenza outbreak in their own area. The National Guard will be assisting their own states and the Megaregion medical centers will most likely not be able to provide relief to their referral basin local hospitals. Although touted as a great collaboration in the updated 2017 DHHS Pandemic Plan, the so-called *Health Care Coalitions* (HCCs) do not seem to have produced or influenced anything to date with respect to pandemic preparedness. This concept may be problematical if a large severe U.S. pandemic breaks out simultaneously in multiple states. This will be discussed further later on in this book.

The need for medical equipment and hospital beds will be dictated by the particular virulence and contagiousness of the pandemic Influenza strain involved. Current modeling suggests that a mild Influenza pandemic would stress local healthcare systems but with basic surge efforts, the Intensive Care and non-Intensive Care adult cases could be managed adequately in most settings.

However, a moderate to severe pandemic with 35% attack rate, would likely overwhelm existing resources during the first 12-weeks of the outbreak. Maximum hospital bed capacity and Intensive Care beds and available mechanical ventilators would be exceeded during the first 2-3 weeks, with a peak Intensive Care bed requirement that is 785% of the current total U.S. capacity and non-Intensive Care beds that would exceed available national capacity by an astounding 214%.[7]

Even under normal daily circumstances, the hospital Emergency Rooms nationwide are increasingly being used as a patient holding area until a bed on the wards becomes vacant. This problem will be magnified during a pandemic, and it is vital that the hospital Emergency Rooms are not used for temporary patient holding.[8] It is essential that the Emergency Rooms remain open and uncrowded to be functional, and the hospitals themselves must remain able to admit serious non-influenza cases. How can this be achieved?

This problem is not new and in the past, facilities called Alternate Care Sites were set up to respond to large-scale medical emergencies such as the 1950's Polio epidemic. In this book we use the terms Acute Care Center, Alternate Care Sites, Acute Treatment Center, and Isolation /Treatment Center interchangeably. A recent third-world example of Alternate Care Sites was seen in West Africa during the 2014 Ebola outbreak. During this event, the hospitals in several regional African countries became quickly overwhelmed. In response, Médecins Sans Frontières (Doctors Without Borders), quickly worked to establish a series of tent-based Ebola Isolation and Treatment Centers in an attempt to address the medical surge requirements in the worst affected areas.

THE FEDERAL MEDICAL STATIONS

To help address the problem of hospital bed availability and assist select hospitals with performing a surge discharge, the Federal Strategic National Stockpile is a holding site for what are termed Federal Medical Stations (FMS). These are essentially rapidly deployable Alternate Care Sites. These were established in response to Homeland Security Presidential Directive 10 and developed by DHHS as a federal-level asset to address the nation's shortfall in all-hazard mass casualty care (Figure 23).[9,10]

Each FMS is a transportable, general medical center that can be quickly set up in suitable location such as a vacated High-School, to temporarily house and care for large numbers of patients that require low-grade hospitalization or have special health needs or chronic health conditions. Each FMS package has beds, supplies, and medicine to treat 250 people for up to three days and can care for all age populations. This requires local authority pre-planning and pre-identification of potential locations and Memorandums of Understanding, based on specific selection criteria and in coordination with DHHS regional emergency coordinators.

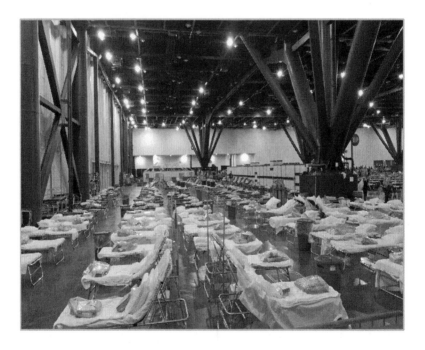

Figure 23. *A 250-bed FMS set up inside a suitable building of opportunity.*

A 250-bed FMS set includes administrative, food service, housekeeping, basic medical and quarantine supplies, basic personal protective equipment, medical/surgical items, and pharmacy medications to treat acute exacerbations of chronic conditions. It requires a minimum of 40,000 square feet of enclosed, climate-controlled space, with parking and loading ramps, food preparation area, waste disposal, laundry capability in the area, security, refrigeration and controlled substance storage, bathrooms and showers, and medical staff from the local community.

While the FMS addresses the supplies for an Alternate Care Site, in most cases, the local medical personnel will have to operate the facility themselves. This may require up to 150 staff of all types.

Each FMS package also deploys with several federal technical specialists having specific knowledge of the Strategic Stockpile and supply operations. This assistance team can also request additional material if needed.

DHHS is planning the acquisition of 138 FMS deployable units totaling 34,500 beds. This will require some 9000 local health care personnel to operate. The eventual goal is to expand the concept to 36,000 beds. However, the serious problem of meeting the local staffing requirement remains. During a severe global pandemic, where are the surge medical personnel necessary to operate these temporary FMS and other Alternate Care Sites going to come from?

THE FEDERAL MEDICAL SURGE CAPABILITY

During the progression of a severe pandemic, the concept of individual care will be shifted over to a population-based system to provide the best outcome for the greatest number of people. However, some form of individual medical care must remain available to prevent a "secondary surge" caused by the deterioration of older people with chronic conditions. All of this will require a significant increase in the number of doctors, nurses, and ancillary medical personnel. Again, this is not a new problem.

From its earliest history, the United States has recognized the need for a national medical surge capability. In 1793, the infrastructure of Philadelphia collapsed due to a horrendous outbreak of Yellow Fever. At the time, this city was the seat of the United States government and federal authorities evacuated the area to prevent contracting the infection.

In 1798, in response to this and other viral epidemic outbreaks such as Dengue, the government created several hospitals specifically designed to treat infected sailors arriving at U.S. ports. Under the banner of a Marine Hospital Fund, these medical facilities provided a surveillance function against the arrival of epidemic diseases into the United States. This early beginning would gradually evolve into our modern National Public Health Service.

Today, the federal government has three principle resources that it can deploy in an emergency medical surge capacity. These are;

- The Commissioned Corps of the U.S. Public Health Service
- The National Disaster Medical System (trained and licensed medical volunteers)
- The Medical Reserve Corps (local community volunteers with federal guidance).

The Commissioned Corps of the US Public Health Service

The United States Public Health Service Commissioned Corps (PHSCC), is the federal uniformed service of the U.S. Public Health Service, and it is one of the uniformed services of the United States.[10] It consists only of commissioned officers and its members hold ranks equivalent to those of U.S. Naval Officers. They wear the same naval uniforms with a special Commissioned Corps insignia. The PHSCC is led by the Surgeon General, who holds the rank of Vice Admiral under the Department of Health and Human Services.

The Commissioned Corps numbers over 6,700 officers in 11 professional categories with multiple specialties. It maintains a Rapid Deployment Force of 525 multidisciplinary staff organized into 5 pre-identified teams. In times of a national disaster, it can provide a rapid medical surge capacity at shelters, casualty collection points, Federal Medical Stations, or other Alternate Treatment Centers.

The Commissioned Corps can also be militarized as a branch of the U.S. Armed Forces by an act of Congress, or by an Executive Order by the President. At present, it can surge up to 2000 assisting medical personnel and still retain a residual response capability.[11] Until recently, these deployment forces were traditionally augmented by the Inactive Reserve Corps (IRC). The IRC was composed of some 10,000 inactive Public Health Commissioned Corps officers who would voluntarily come onto active duty for medical and public health emergencies. These personnel proved to be invaluable during emergency response missions that required a broad medical/public health surge capacity in hardship underserved areas. They played important roles in incidents such as Hurricanes Katrina, Rita, and Wilma. It was the Inactive Reserve Public Health Commissioned Corps which helped make this surge of medical providers a success.

Sadly, this inactive reserve capability no longer exists. For reasons that are unclear, in 2010, the *Health Care Affordability Care Act* (ACA) established a new organization called the *Ready Reserve Corps* to serve as the new surge capability for the US Public Health Service subject to an active duty call by the Surgeon General.[12] As part of this major transformation, the *Affordable Care Act* abolished the Inactive Reserve Corps. Consequently, the commissions of 10,000 IRC officers were withdrawn and this medical surge capability was lost. The standards for appointment into this new Ready Reserve Corps appear to be still under review.

The National Disaster Medical System

The National Disaster Medical System (NDMS) is a federally coordinated healthcare system in partnership between the U.S. Departments of Health and Human Services (DHHS), Homeland Security (DHS), Defense (DoD), and Veterans Affairs (VA). The purpose of the NDMS is to support State and local authorities following disasters and emergencies by supplementing their medical response capability. NDMS is also designed to support the military and the Department of Veterans Affairs health care system with respect to a surge capability should it be required.[13,14,15]

Some common missions for NDMS have included augmenting the hospitals in a defined disaster area to reduce the case load of its emergency department, providing veterinary services to federal working animals during Special Events, and supporting the National Transportation Safety Board with fatality management services following a major transportation disaster. The NDMS is composed of several types of operational teams who perform specific functions during a disaster event.[16,17]

With respect to a medical surge capability the NDMS has two resources that could possibly be applicable in a developing Influenza pandemic:

1. Disaster Mortuary Operational Response Teams (DMORT): These teams work under local authorities to recover, identify, and process the deceased. DHHS also maintains several Disaster Portable Morgue Units (DPMU). There are 10 DMORT teams organized into 10 regions, each with a Regional Coordinator. The DMORT teams work under local civilian authorities at a disaster site and their professional licenses are recognized by all states. However, with only ~10 teams available, it is uncertain what significant role these would play in a severe Influenza pandemic with a projected 1-2 million civilian deaths.

2. Disaster Medical Assistance Teams (DMAT): These mobile medical surge personnel are designed to provide acute care, triage, initial resuscitation and stabilization, advanced life support and preparation of sick or injured for evacuation. The DMAT teams are designed to be mobile within 6-hours of notification and can arrive at a disaster site within 48-hours. These team can sustain operations for 72-hours without external support and remain on-site for up to several weeks.

Originally, the NDMS had 9,000+ licensed health and medical personnel organized into ~107 response teams. These provided a significant volunteer civilian medical surge capability. Team members were required to maintain their certifications and licensures, and most were typically affiliated with a medical center or health department. Upon activation, these personnel were reclassified as intermittent federal employees.

NDMS was originally under the U.S. Public Health Service in the DHHS. In 2003, this was changed and the new Department of Homeland

Security (DHS) was granted authority over the NDMS. After Hurricane Katrina, amidst allegations of mismanagement, the NDMS was reorganized back under DHHS in 2007 under the *Pandemic and All Hazards Preparedness Act* (Public Law 109-417). The effect this confusion and shuffling had on moral, medical readiness and response, was compounded by the fact that NDMS management staffing was reduced from 144 down to 57 personnel in the transition to DHS and then back to DHHS.[15,17]

From what can be ascertained, there are currently only ~80 NDMS response teams of which only 55 are Disaster Medical Assistance Teams. While there are definite uses for these DMAT teams in a severe pandemic, (transporting patients, conducting mass vaccinations, assisting with isolation and quarantine, and assisting with surge capacity including critical care), none of these teams are prepared for a pandemic. They do not have an endogenous Strategic Influenza Response Plan and there is insufficient management staffing at the NDMS headquarters.[15,17]

With respect to working in a potential highly infectious environment such as an Alternate Treatment Center, the DMAT members lack both specific infectious disease training as well as personal protective equipment at the team level. As far as can be discerned, there is no specific planning on how the DMAT teams would be deployed and utilized in an Influenza pandemic.

The NDMS operates under the assumption that its volunteer teams will be 100% available for a response. However, in a severe pandemic this is an unreasonable assumption for several reasons. The hospitals, public health departments, or medical systems with which the NMDS civilian medical professionals are affiliated, may not allow their participation within the NDMS system during a pandemic. The primary reason for this refusal would be the anticipated exponential increase in patients and the reduced health care workforce in their own communities. In addition, there is not sufficient medical personnel available to formulate and deploy these NDMS teams to the extent that they have been promoted in the past.[15,17]

While the NDMS is certainly of use during localized medical

disasters such as hurricanes, the problem of not being released for a pandemic emergency, the apparent continuing process of low morale, a loss of personnel, leadership changes, reduced funding, and the low number of operational teams, makes it unlikely it could provide any significant national medical surge capability in a pandemic response.

The failure to mention the assets of the NDMS in the 2017 Update of the DHHS Pandemic Influenza Plan, indicates that the NDMS is not a priority organization in a pandemic response.[18] The emphasis now seems to be placed on Healthcare Coalitions and state and local health departments, as the federal government continues to place the fundamental responsibility for pandemic preparedness directly on the states and local communities.[19]

Medical Reserve Corps

The concept of using volunteers to address the emergency needs after a disaster is probably as old as civilization. For decades now, the American Red Cross has successfully provided temporary support to communities that have suffered natural disasters. The concept of using volunteer physicians and nurses to provide medical care has been demonstrated successfully for many large-scale disasters, including international relief efforts such as the response to the Asian tsunamis in 2005, and after numerous hurricanes and other natural disasters.

A relatively new concept, however, is that of identifying, recruiting, and sustaining doctors and nurses and associated ancillary medical personnel as "volunteers-in-waiting" for emergency service. This is both for their own local communities and for other distant communities that have suffered a disaster.

In this respect, the Medical Reserve Corps (MRC), was originally established as a 2-year demonstration project within the Office of the Surgeon General (OSG). The purpose of this was to demonstrate a national ability to create auxiliary teams of local medical and public health professionals who would voluntarily contribute their expertise during times of community need, and occasionally for specific projects.[20,21] The concept was to have a pre-identified reserve force of volunteer physicians, nurses, epidemiologists, and other workers that could also insert into a federal or state disaster response, or address broader public health needs.[22,23]

The OSG initiated the MRC by using a small grants program that was in operation from 2002-2006. During the first 2-years of the demonstration project, 42 units were funded for start-up in 2002, and 124 units were funded in 2003. This was typically with a federal grant of $50,000 annually provided directly to each MRC unit's local sponsoring organization (i.e., local health department, university medical school, or hospital).

In 2006, the MRC partnered with the National Association of County and City Health Officials (NACCHO) to help promote and expand the program and increase its number of volunteers. This capacity expansion effort reportedly increased the stated number of units to 982 throughout the US and its Territories.[21] In 2013, the Office of the Assistant Secretary for Preparedness and Response (ASPR) in the Department of Health and Human Services took over the responsibility for the entire MRC program.

The MRC system is reportedly made up of 192,861 volunteers from a variety of medical and healthcare professions, as well as a substantial number of non-medical individuals. The original size of each MRC unit varied greatly from a few individual volunteers to over 1000, depending on the location. Almost half of the units serve populations of less than 100,000 in their area.[21] Volunteers are from a variety of professions and disciplines, with roughly one-third consisting of non-public health or non-medical personnel such as logistics specialists, chaplains, interpreters, legal advisors, office workers and others.[22,23]

On average, registered nurses make up 27 % of volunteers, EMT's 9 %, licensed practical nurses/licensed vocational nurses 5 %, and physicians 4%. Other medical and healthcare personnel make up 11 % of volunteers, with mental health and substance abuse professionals, nurse practitioners, pharmacists, and veterinarians providing approximately 2 % each of all MRC volunteers.[24]

The MRC organizational framework is less structured than other federal medical assets. Governed under the DHHS with leadership authority ultimately under the DHHS Office of the Assistant Secretary of Preparedness and Response, the organizational structure consists of a headquarters operation and 10 regional liaisons. In addition, each state and territory has a State Coordinator responsible for maintaining the data, operations, overall communications, and coordination of the units within their area.[24]

A 2015 survey conducted by the National Association of County and City Health Officials (NACCHO), demonstrated that the MRC conducted activities in numerous programmatic areas.[21] Under public health activities, the top 5 were listed as: community outreach events (e.g. health fairs), seasonal flu vaccination programs, health education, staffing medical/first aid booths for marathons or 5k races, and health clinic support/staffing. As mentioned, some units specialize in one type of activity while others may take part in general activities, depending on the expertise of their members. During Hurricane Katrina in New Orleans, MRC units from several other states were brought into the area as part of the federal response plan where they performed a variety of roles supporting the medical needs of the victims and the disaster workers as well.[24,25,26]

MRC VOLUNTEER TRAINING AND PERSONNEL RETENTION

There is a heavily emphasis on training as a primary MRC mission component and although 71% of MRC units have a training plan in place for their volunteers, most units have no funds to spend on training and exercises.

In a survey assessment, NACCHO has stated that roughly 49% of those units responding to the survey were made of up non-medical volunteers. Almost all training outside of first aid, basic CPR (cardiopulmonary resuscitation) or citizen preparedness, is through FEMA's (Federal Emergency Management Agency) Independent Study curriculum.[27] These FEMA courses are without cost and they provide a basic knowledge of disaster management and the Incident Command

System. Depending on the focus of a given MRC unit, other more specialized training may address topics such as basic universal precautions (wearing protective gloves).

However, the planning/training philosophy for many units appears to be one of conducting specific just-in-time training if it becomes necessary. This will not be sufficient for a rapidly moving lethal pandemic.

MRC Funding Problems

Most of MRC funding comes from the DHHS Office of the Assistant Secretary for Preparedness and Response (ASPR) through their Capacity Building Award (CBA) and Challenge Awards program. Other funding comes through the CDC Public Health Preparedness Grant Program and Hospital Preparedness Program. With a few exceptions, units are funded to a maximum of $5000 per award with larger units receiving up to $10,000 per award.[28,29] Although the funding for MRC units has never been substantial, for the past several years funding has been steadily decreasing.

Interviews with MRC Members

When activated, the MRC is composed of committed and dedicated volunteers. For the MRC unit interviewed, its last full activation was for Hurricane Katrina where it helped staff Red Cross shelters and medical stations. Nurses were the primary expertise that was utilized. This MRC unit was sponsored by an academic institution and it received no internal funding at all.

After Katrina, member retention fell, and the unit interviewed was never again properly staffed and could never maintain any real operational capacity. Volunteer numbers fell dramatically and if a catastrophic event would have occurred, the unit would have had to be rebuilt using volunteers that were less trained. By 2013, the unit had only 20 or 30 active members that could be counted as reliable.

Although the MRC was designed to provide both a medical surge capacity as well as participate in community health activities, the public health aspect has never been given the same priority. Also, the number of MRC volunteers as stated on the MRC website is possibly misleading and the data needed to accurately analyze the MRC's true capacities and capabilities is not readily accessible. The MRC unit that was interviewed has not been operational since 2013-2014, yet in 2017, the data listed for the website had the unit listed as having 900 volunteers. Maintaining of different databases collecting similar volunteer information data may have led to a double and triple counting of volunteers. To improve this, the MRC website was recently upgraded in September 2017 to now show more current data for some specific MRC units.

Several challenges exist for the MRC to remain operational and adequate funding continues to be an issue for most units. During the national flurry of pandemic planning in 2005, the MRC was somewhat incorporated into the community planning process. However, in hindsight the expectations for the MRC to support any long-term staffing needs of hospitals, shelters, and alternative care sites during a pandemic seem to have been overstated.

PROBLEMS WITH VOLUNTEERS IN A PANDEMIC

In the wake of the terrorist attacks of 9/11, the lack of a coordinating structure to manage the multitude of self-deployed medical volunteers responding to this incident, provided a rationale for the creation of the Medical Reserve Corps. However, as over a decade and a half of hurricanes have demonstrated, volunteer participation of these medical volunteers may be variable.

A study of the MRC program found six factors that could influence an individual's decision to join or remain a MRC member. These included; the time commitment required, the professionalism of an MRC unit and its management, the availability of MRC-sponsored training or education sessions with Continuing Medical Education credits, concerns regarding the safety of family members during a disaster, and finally the professional liability protection afforded for work performed during MRC operations.[30]

The MRC is not trained to deal with a highly infectious pandemic situation, but rather other types of national disasters. In an infectious pandemic, studies have shown there will be other issues concerning the willingness of both volunteers and professional healthcare personnel to report for duty. The perception of the biological risks associated with a pandemic, safety concerns for the worker's own family, safety concerns for duties requiring direct patient contact, a lack of adequate infection control training and experience, and the quarantine or infectious death of a fellow colleague, will all have a negative impact on the availability of medical personnel.[31]

With respect to medical professionals, several studies indicate there is a wide disparity in the exact number who would be willing to work under severe influenza pandemic conditions.[32] These studies included several worker categories encompassing physicians, nurses, EMS providers, and others, The willingness to respond to a pandemic ranged from as low as 23 percent to as high as 93 percent.

When considering planning for a pandemic, a consensus figure is that only 1 in 4 healthcare workers will be willing to work during a severe Influenza pandemic. If that figure is adjusted for illness-related absenteeism of healthcare professionals, the estimation could go as low as 15%. This is a significant problem which only adds to the difficulty in providing a medical surge capacity.

With respect to volunteer personnel, the reasons for not reporting for duty include transportation problems, child and elderly care, pet care obligations, as well as personal health problems. Most were willing to report during snowstorm, mass casualty accidents, and environmental disasters. They were least willing to report to the more technical disasters such as an infectious disease outbreak, an event involving radiation, and a toxic chemical event.

THE SURGE CAPACITY FORCE

The DHS *Surge Capacity Force* (SCF) is an attempt to augment the federal workforce in response to a catastrophic disaster.[33] The program is managed by FEMA and the SCF is composed of federal employees from DHS and other agencies. Volunteers are required to already be full-time federal employees from any federal agency, have sexual anti-harassment training within the last 365 days, have their supervisor's approval, and have completed online Independent Study courses and exams through the FEMA Emergency Management Institute. These courses include a safety orientation, an introduction to the Incident Command System (ICS), the National Incident Management System (NIMS), and the National Response Framework (NRF).

Established by the Post-Katrina Emergency Management Reform Act of 2006 (Public Law 109-295) the Surge Capacity Force has been activated several times. The first was in 2012 in support of Hurricane Sandy where some 1,100 Federal employees deployed to New York and New Jersey to supplement the FEMA disaster workforce. In 2017 it was activated in response to hurricanes Harvey, Irma, and Maria and for the wildfires in California. More than 2,740 individuals from eight DHS components were deployed and the SCF was expanded to agencies outside DHS for the first time, increasing SCF personnel by more than 1,300 employees. In March 2019, the SCF was activated for the immigrant crisis on the Southern U.S. Border. These volunteers receive no medical training and for a variety of reasons, most probably will be of limited or no practical use during a severe pandemic event.

LOCAL AUTHORITIES MUST IMPROVE THEIR PANDEMIC PREPAREDNESS THEMSELVES

The success of any federal disaster plan lies with the local authorities that govern our towns and cities. The federal government has clearly outlined what it sees as its responsibility in a pandemic, and it has clearly outlined what the local authorities will be responsible for. Yet outside of a few exceptional cities, there has been little effective local preparedness efforts to date.

As outlined in Chapter Thirteen, most localities have not put in an effort to recruit medical volunteers, verify their credentials, implement an electronic system to register and manage them, and train them. Equipment inventories are not being consistently maintained and formal agreements are lacking for the selection of Alternate Care Sites along with local authority guidelines for their staffing and operation. Improvements are needed within all five of the medical surge components; *medical volunteers, medical equipment, Alternate Care Facilities, procedures for triage, and procedures for altering mass patient care.*[34] The states have also been delinquent with respect to covering localities for any legal risk entailed if they were to alter their standards during a pandemic.

This lack of community progress in response to federal funding reflects the existing difficulty between city managers and their local public health authorities. Despite federal guidance and funding, many local jurisdictions lack the necessary emergency planning staff to develop a rational pandemic response. This poor progress reflects on the city managers who do not seem to appreciate the true seriousness of the pandemic Influenza risk. The Federal Pandemic Influenza Plan will not work without the local authorities having a well-constructed and periodically rehearsed medical surge capability.

Another major problem is financial. In this respect, there currently are no authorized funding programs to provide grants, benefits, and incentives to help minimize the financial impact on community service programs when disaster-caused needs exceed the capabilities of their current program funding and resources. In addition, there are no real incentives to build a local authority mass-care capability and there are no grants available for local agencies and for voluntary community-based and faith-based organizations through existing FEMA programs.

In summary, if deployed to assist in a severe 1918-type pandemic Influenza response, it is likely that the Commissioned Public Health Service will be primarily tasked to support Continuity of Government efforts and the National Medical Disaster System will support the Veteran's Administration. The Medical Reserve Corps is at present, largely untrained and unequipped to participate in a pandemic response in a meaningful way. Consequently, the NDMS in its current size and structure will likely not be a factor in a national civilian medical surge response.

Stated again, in a severe Influenza pandemic, the local authorities will be responsible for organizing their own medical surge capability and pandemic procedures in alignment with their own local resources and planning. Most local authorities in the United States remain unprepared for a severe 1918-type pandemic event.

Notes for Chapter 17

[1] American Hospital Association, AHA Hospital Statistics, American Hospital Association, Chicago, IL, 2017; Accessed at http://www.aha.org/research/rc/stat-studies/fastfacts.shtml

[2] World Health Organization (WHO), Epidemic and pandemic alert and response. Available at: http://www.who.int/csr/en/ Accessed 18 June 2017.

[3] U.S. Public Health Service, Public Health Preparedness and Response, National Snapshot 2017, Atlanta, Ga, April 2017, 51 pgs., https://www.cdc.gov/phpr/whyitmatters/00_docs/2017_PublicHealthPreparednessSnapshot_508.pdfAccessed on 18 June 2017.

[4] Ten Eyck R., Ability of regional hospitals to meet projected avian flu pandemic surge capacity requirements. Prehospital Disast Med 2008; 23:103-112.

[5] U.S. Department of Health & Human Services, Hospital Available Beds for Emergencies and Disasters: A Sustainable Bed Availability Reporting System (Final Report), Report Under Contract #HHSA2902006000201, AHRQ Publication No. 09-0058-EF, April 2009.

[6] Kaji, A. et al. Surge capacity for Healthcare systems, a conceptual framework. Academic Emergency Med 2006; 13:1157-9

[7] Sobieraj, JA et.al. Modeling hospital response to mild and severe influenza pandemic scenarios under normal and expanded capacities. Mil Med. 2007 May;172(5):486-90.

[8] Siegel JD, Pandemic influenza planning in Texas: the pediatric perspective. Tex. Med., Oct 2007 pp 48-53.

[9] HHS, ASPR FMS Concept of Operation, 2014 http://www.kdheks.gov/cphp/download/cacs_template/FMS_Fact_Sheet.pdf

[10] U.S. Public Health Service Commissioned Corps". U.S. Department of Health and Human Services. Retrieved 24 June 2008.

[11] Reese, CA. The National Disaster Medical System. American Association of Nurse Anesthetists. AANA Journal. December 1989/ Vol. 57/No. 6 493.

[12] Knouss, RF, "National Disaster Medical System", Pub Health Rep, 2001;116 (suppl 2):49–52

[13] HHS Concept of Operations for ESF #8 phe.gov

[14] National Disaster Medical System. Federal Coordinating Center (FCC) Guide. April 2014.

[15] Delaney, John. The National Disaster Medical System's Reliance on Civilian-Based Medical Response Teams in a Pandemic is Unsound. Homeland Security Affairs 3, Article 1 (June 2007). https://www.hsaj.org/articles/146

[16] US Department of Health and Human Services, Pandemic influenza plan: 2017 update. Washington, DC. 2017.

[17] United States. (2005). HHS pandemic influenza plan. Washington, D.C.: U.S. Dept. of Health and Human Services.

[18] Medical Reserve Corps webpage. https://www.medicalreservecorps.gov/HomePage.

[19] Accessed September 17, 2017. Frasca DR. The Medical Reserve Corps as part of the federal medical and public health response in disaster settings. Biosecur Bioterror. 2010 Sep;8(3):265 71. doi: 10.1089/bsp.2010.0006.

[20] Gotzer DL, Rinchiuso A, Rekow ED, Triola MM, Psoter WJ. The Medical Reserve Corps. An opportunity for dentists to serve. N Y State Dent J. 2006 Jan;72(1):60-1.

[21] National Association of County and City Health Officials. The 2015 Network Profile of the Medical Reserve Corps. Connecting with communities, The MRC: A network of dedicated volunteers. October 2015. http://archived.naccho.org/topics/emergency/MRC/upload/TTCNACCHO-MRC-2015v1-20.pdf.

[22] Watson M, Selck F, Rambhia K, et.al. Medical Reserve Corps volunteers in disasters: a Survey of their roles, experiences, and challenges. Biosecur Bioterror 2014;12(2):85-93.

[23] Ibid. 2015 NACCHO Report.

[24] United States. The Federal Response to Hurricane Katrina: Lessons Learned. Washington, D.C: White House, 2006.

[25] Young D. Medical Reserve Corps pharmacists assist evacuees. Am J Health Syst Pharm. 2006 Feb 15;63(4):296, 299-300, 302.

[26] Hoard M, Middleton G. Medical Reserve Corps: Lessons learned in supporting community health and emergency response. J Bus Cont Emer Plan. 2008 Jan;2(2):172-8.

[27] FEMA, Emergency Management Institute. Independent Study Program. https://training.fema.gov/is/. Accessed September 16, 2017.

[28] Qureshi K, Gershon RM, Conde F. Factors that influence Medical Reserve Corps recruitment. Prehosp Disaster Med. 2008 May-Jun;23(3): s27-34.

[29] MRC PROGRAM REVIEW

[30] Rossow, C., L. Ivanitskaya, L. Fulton, W. Fales. Healthcare Providers: Will They Come to Work During an Influenza Pandemic? Disaster Management and Human

Health Risk III, WIT Transactions on the Built Environment, Vol 133, WIT Press, 2013, ISSN: 1743-3509, ISBN: 978-1-84564-738.

[31] Martin, SD. Predictors of Nurses Intentions to Work During the 2009 Influenza A (H1N1) Pandemic. American Journal of Nursing: December 2013 - Volume 113, 12

[32] Qureshi, K, Gershon, RRM, Sherman, MF, et al. Health care workers' ability and willingness to report to duty during catastrophic disasters. Journal of Urban Health: Bulletin of the New York Academy of Medicine. 2005; 82 (3): 378-88.

[33] Aoyagi et al. (2015) Healthcare worker willingness to work during an influenza pandemic: a systematic review and meta-analysis. Influenza and Other Respiratory Viruses 9(3), 120

[34] HHS Office of Inspector General, Office of Evaluation and Inspections (OEI). State and Local Pandemic Influenza Preparedness: Medical Surge. September 2009. OEI-02-08 00210. https://oig.hhs.gov/oei/reports/oei-02-08-00210.pdf

18

THE ROLE OF THE DEPARTMENT OF DEFENSE (DoD) IN A SEVERE PANDEMIC

OVER THE PAST SEVERAL DECADES, the utilization of military assets and resources has been slowly inserted into the national strategy for responding to major disasters. *The Robert T. Stafford Disaster Relief and Emergency Assistance Act* is the primary legal authority for Federal participation in a civilian disaster response. Federal assistance may be in the form of financial assistance, direct provision of goods and services, technical assistance, and manpower augmentation. The DoD is designated as a support agency for all emergency support functions and can cooperate in several pre-planned responses.

The *Defense Support of Civil Authorities* (DSCA) is the process by which United States military assets and personnel can be used to assist in missions normally carried out by civil authorities. These missions have included: responses to natural and man-made disasters, special events, and other domestic activities.[1] Examples of the use of the DSCA was the military response to Hurricane Katrina, Harvey, and Irma and it is the overarching guidance of how the United States military can be requested by a federal agency and the procedures that govern the military during its civilian assistance deployment.

Title 10 of the United States Code outlines the role of Armed Forces and provides the legal basis for the roles, missions, and organization of the United States Department of Defense and each of the services. With a few specific exceptions, the US military are forbidden from engaging in law enforcement activity by the Posse Comitatus Act. This is now part of Title 18 of the United States Code. However, the limitations of the Posse Comitatus Act can be waved in specific instances and it does not apply to the National Guard.

It must also be noted that to date, the previous civilian disasters that required military support were all local or regional events. This is a much different scenario than a serious Influenza pandemic which will rapidly affect the entire country.

An analysis of the tasks assigned by the National Strategy for Pandemic Influenza Implementation Plan indicates that DoD's role during a pandemic would be to augment disease surveillance, assist with a surge laboratory diagnostic capability, transport select response teams with vaccines, medical equipment, supplies, diagnostic devices, and pharmaceuticals. In addition, it could provide base and installation support to federal, state, local, and tribal agencies as well as help control movement into and out of areas or across borders. Current DOD plans do not anticipate a federal mobilization of the National Guard or Reserves to respond to a flu pandemic, although these forces may be used for an individual state response.[2]

As stated in the Department of Defense Implementation Plan for

Pandemic Influenza, DoD's priority will be to ensure sufficient personnel, equipment, facilities, materials, and pharmaceuticals, *to protect and treat US forces and dependents, civilian military contractors, and beneficiaries to preserve DoD's worldwide military readiness.* It may also be tasked with assisting partner nations through military-to-military assistance.[3]

However, there is one other possible role for the U.S. Military in pandemic preparedness that will be discussed in a later chapter. This involves direct assistance to the poor, low-resource, high-density urban areas which to date, have largely been left out of specific national and state pandemic planning efforts.

As a final note, the coordinating authority for the U.S. Armed Forces in civilian disasters is the *Joint Task Force Civil Support* (JTF-CS), headquartered at Fort Eustis, Va., which now operates under the authority of the U.S. Northern Command (NORTHCOM). The JTF-CS is an active duty joint headquarters whose primary mission is to provide command and control for DoD forces responding to a catastrophic event on U.S. soil.

When approved by the Secretary of Defense and directed by the commander of USNORTHCOM, the JTF-CS can deploy to a specific civilian disaster site to provide command and control of the assembly and disposition of the required U.S. military forces that will provide civil authority support. The proviso is that this support cannot impair the ability of the U.S. Armed Forces to conduct its primary military mission. It is critical to understand that the military is always in a supporting role and never in the lead. In addition, along with the national and state governments, the military will have a priority access to the first antiviral drugs and vaccine during a pandemic.

CONTINUITY OF GOVERNMENT

The U.S. Federal Government is poised to protect itself through the Continuity of Government (COG) and Enduring Constitutional Government (ECG) programs and laws. While much of the planning behind these programs was originally designed to minimize the disorder in the aftermath of a nuclear attack, it has been expanded to include a broad range of circumstances and threat scenarios and is DoD supported.

Presidential Decision Directives (or PDDs) are a form of an executive order issued by the President of the United States with the advice and consent of the National Security Council. National Security Presidential Directive-51 (NSPD-51) / Homeland Security Presidential Directive 20 (HSPD-20), National Continuity Policy, specifies certain requirements for continuity plan development, including the requirement that all Federal executive branch departments and agencies develop an integrated, overlapping continuity capability. Federal Continuity Directive FCD 1 serves as a guidance to State governments for COG and Continuity of Operations (COOP) planning.

DoD policy guidelines currently specify that if extra military personnel are required to respond to a national pandemic, the services are to use the Military Reserve units first, leaving the National Guard forces available to meet their state-based missions.[4]

MAINTAINING SOCIETAL STABILITY DURING A SEVERE PANDEMIC

Martial law is a condition initiated when the government or civilian authorities fail to function effectively (e.g., maintain order and security, or provide essential services). It refers to the imposition of temporary direct military control over the normal civilian functions of government in response to a national emergency.

In the United States, the concept of martial law is closely associated with the right of habeas corpus, which is the right to a hearing on lawful imprisonment. This provides a form of supervision over law enforcement by the judiciary. The ability to suspend habeas corpus is related to the imposition of martial law. Article 1, Section 9 of the US Constitution states, *"The Privilege of the Writ of Habeas Corpus shall not be suspended, unless when in Cases of Rebellion or Invasion, the public safety may require it."*[5]

The declaration of martial law is limited by several court decisions. While the concept of martial law is complex, there are other extreme examples of a catastrophic pandemic response that may intersect with state and federal laws. For example, there is a lack of clarity on the federal and state roles and responsibilities in the areas of state border closures and influenza vaccine distribution. Confusing or conflicting messages from the many bureaucracies at all levels of government, could inhibit the coordinated control of a pandemic response. For example, some State Emergency Operations Plans may incorrectly recommend that the Governor close their borders during a pandemic, which would have a great impact on the national highway system and hinder the delivery of essential goods and services.

THE NATIONAL GUARD

The National Guard has a long historical pedigree and its concept is descendent from the colonial-era state militias. National Guard personnel would almost certainly be involved in state efforts to respond to a serious pandemic under the control of their Governor. As part of a state response, the Governor could order state National Guard personnel to full-time duty under state law. This is referred to as "state active duty." In this capacity, the state National Guard would assist civil authorities in a wide variety of tasks, and they are not subject to Posse Comitatus (i.e., they can perform law enforcement functions).

Title 32 of the United States Code outlines the role of the United States National Guard which can operate across both State and Federal responses, in the form of State Active Duty (SAD), Full-Time National Guard Duty (Title 32), and Active Duty (Title 10).[6]

DEDICATED NATIONAL GUARD
CONSEQUENCE MANAGEMENT RESOURCES

Since the first World Trade Center bombing in 1993, the DoD has worked to effectively respond to a major Chemical, Biological, Radiological, Nuclear, Explosive (CBRNE) incident in the United States. Initially, the Presidential Decision Directive 39 approved the creation of the Army National Guard's Weapons of Mass Destruction Civil

Support Teams (WMD-CSTs). These 22-person teams, postured in every State and Territory, can respond to a CBRNE incident within three-hours, identify CBRNE materials, assess the consequences of a CBRNE incident, and advise civil authorities on appropriate response measures.

By the late nineties, it became obvious that a catastrophic CBNRE incident would require a more comprehensive response from the DoD. Thus, the Nunn-Lugar-Domenici Amendment 4349 was eventually introduced, creating an additional response element called the Chemical, Biological, Radiological, and Nuclear Enhanced Response Force Packages (CERFPs). These CERFPs can locate and extract victims from a contaminated environment, perform mass patient decontamination, and provide medical treatment to stabilize patients for evacuation. Each of the nation's 17 CERFPs are comprised of approximately 186 members of the Army National Guard and can respond to an incident within six-hours.

In 2010, the National Defense Appropriations Act gave the DoD an even greater role in CBRN response, authorizing the formation of National Guard Homeland Response Forces (HRFs). There are currently 10 HRFs co-located in each of the ten FEMA regions throughout the United States. Each HRF consists of approximately 566 Army National Guard Soldiers and Airmen, and can perform all the functions of a CERFP, plus provide additional security and command and control capabilities. The HRFs can respond to a catastrophic incident within 12-hours.

Because of their specialized training, these forces would have a definite use in a pandemic response. Additional forces may be assigned by NORTHCOM to conduct approved missions in the form of Joint Task Forces or in the form of a very specialized asset called the Defense CBRN Response Force.

THE DEFENSE CBRN RESPONSE FORCE (DCRF)

On 1 October 2008, the 3rd Infantry Division's 1st Brigade Combat Team was assigned to U.S. Northern Command, marking the first time that an active combat unit has been given a dedicated assignment to the

Pentagon's Northern Command (NORTHCOM). In 2009, this unit was termed the CBRNE Consequence Management Response Force, and it was quickly molded into an on-call federal response asset designed to provide domestic support following a catastrophic terrorist attack.[7]

This active duty unit has now been expanded and renamed the Defense CBRN Response Force (DCRF). It is designed to directly assist state and local civil authorities in the consequence management of a catastrophic Chemical, Biological, Nuclear, Radiological, or Explosive (CBRNE) incident. This includes events such as a biological attack on a major metropolitan area, a Chernobyl-type nuclear accident, or a Bhopal-type large area chemical release that causes thousands of casualties.

In 2013, this unit was reorganized into two sections; an active duty DCRF comprised of 5,200 personnel from all four services capable of a response within 24-48 hours; and two Command and Control CBRN Response Elements (C2CRE). An Army Reserve Major General commands one C2CRE, and a National Guard Major General commands the other. Each C2CRE consists of 1500 personnel that are a mix of Active, Reserve, and National Guard soldiers.

In a catastrophic event, these Title 10 active duty military forces can integrate with the previously described Title 32 National Guard organizations working in support of their respective State Governors. This includes the 57 Civil Support Teams, the 17 Chemical, Biological, Radiological, Nuclear and High Yield Explosive Enhanced Response Force Packages, and the 10 FEMA-associated Homeland Response Forces.

*All together, these units make up the DoD's **Defense CBRN Response Enterprise (CRE)** consisting of approximately 18,000 soldiers assigned to respond to a catastrophic domestic incident with NORTHCOM in overall command and control.*

NOTES FOR CHAPTER 18

[1] Joint Chiefs of Staff, Joint Publication 3-28, 14 September 2007; Defense Support of Civil Authorities. https://fas.org/irp/doddir/dod/jp3-28.pdf

[2] Office of the Assistant Secretary of Defense, Homeland Defense, Department of Defense Implementation Plan for Pandemic Influenza, Washington, DC. http://fhp.osd.mil/aiWatchboard/pdf/DoD_PI_Implementation_Plan_August_2 006_Pub lic_Release.pdf.

[3] David S.C. Chu, Memorandum "Mobilization of Reserve Component Medical Support Personnel Supporting the Local Medical Infrastructure during an Influenza Pandemic,"

[4] Washington, DC, November 18, 2008, p. 1, http://fhp.osd.mil/aiWatchboard/pdf/RC_MED_PI_Policy (1108).pdf.

[5] G. Edward White (2012). Law in American History: Volume 1: From the Colonial Years Through the Civil War. Oxford University Press. p. 442. ISBN 978-0-19-972314-0

[6] CRS Report RL30802, Reserve Component Personnel Issues: Questions and Answers, by Lawrence Kapp, pp. 17-20.

[7] Consequence Management-Operational Principles for Managing the Consequence of a Catastrophic Incident Involving CBRNE. 2013 ISBN-10: 1481990829. ISBN-13: 978-1481990820

SECTION

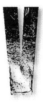

ADDITIONAL MAJOR PROBLEMS
IN PANDEMIC PREPAREDNESS

19

PANDEMIC WARNING LEVELS
AND MODERN AIR TRAVEL

THE DEFINITION OF EPIDEMIC is an infectious disease that spreads to many people in one specific geographic area. The term *pandemic* is much different. A pandemic is an epidemic that is not limited to one specific geographic region, but instead it has spread to many populations in many countries around the globe.

In 1999, the World Health Organization (WHO) defined six-stages of a developing pandemic with suggested measures for countries to take at each stage. This six-stage classification starts with an Influenza virus that is only infecting animals. Then, the virus occasionally spills over to cause a few scattered infections in humans who have been exposed to a high concentration of the virus. This process can go on for months or even years until eventually, some of the viral "quasi-species" acquire the ability to be efficiently transmitted directly from person-to-person. The virus has now become adapted to use humans as its new host, and it now has the potential to spread as a worldwide pandemic.[1]

- In WHO **Pandemic Level 1**, none of the Influenza viruses that have been detected to be circulating in nature have been reported to cause human infections.
- In **Pandemic Level 2**, an animal influenza virus that is circulating among domesticated or wild animals is discovered to have caused at least one infection in humans, usually due to a spillover event (described in Chapter Three).
- In **Pandemic Level 3**, an animal or a human/animal hybrid Influenza virus has caused multiple sporadic individual cases or small clusters of cases in people, but it has not yet acquired the ability for efficient human-to-human transmission.

The world is currently already at Pandemic Level 3

- In Pandemic **Level 4**, a verified human-to-human transmission of an animal or hybrid human/animal Influenza virus has occurred, that has led to a sustained "community-level outbreak". This is an indication that the virus has improved its ability for human-to-human transmission, and it marks a significant shift in the risk for a pandemic.
- In **Pandemic Level 5**, there is now a documented human-to-human spread of the virus in at least two separate areas as reported by the WHO network of 120 National Influenza Centers in 90 different countries.
- In **Pandemic Level 6**, there are community level outbreaks occurring in more than one country. This phase indicates that a global pandemic is now well under way.

The WHO uses these 6 pandemic levels, to indicate what type of a global response is necessary at the time. It does not describe how lethal the virus is to humans or how many people have contracted the infection. Instead, it relates to where the outbreaks are located and how the virus is spreading from one area to another. It also considers how novel the viral strain is, because humans may have little or no previous immunity against a new Influenza strain.

With respect to the global response that is necessary, Phases 1–3 correlate with planning for medical surge requirements and other response activities. Phases 4–6 signal the need for activation of the actual pandemic response and mitigation efforts.

However, there were problems with this Pandemic Alert System. As previously mentioned, a new H1N1 swine Influenza outbreak occurred unexpectedly in Mexico in 2009. When genetic sequences of the new virus were found to be similar with already known pandemic viruses, the outbreak was considered a pandemic threat. As the new epidemic progressed through the various Pandemic Level criteria, the WHO declared a Level-5 and finally a Pandemic Level-6. The virus did indeed spread around the world, but it caused an infection and mortality equivocal to normal seasonal Influenza outbreaks of moderate severity. Most patients experienced mild symptoms with a rapid and full recovery.

Consequently, there were complaints from some member states that the WHO had triggered unnecessary fear which had caused them to prepare for a pandemic of high severity. Other complaints argued that the WHO phases should reflect the severity of the disease, not just its geographic spread.

In response, the WHO revised its warning system and in 2013, it released a new 4-phase alert system to replace the 6-phase classification.[2]

- **Interpandemic,** The period between pandemics.
- **Alert:** A new virus subtype has been identified and increased surveillance is warranted.
- **Pandemic:** Global spread of a new virus based on virologic and clinical data.

- **Transition:** The global risk drops, with a step-down in global actions and response.

The WHO considers the world is currently at the *"Alert"* Pandemic Level when it comes to both the H5N1 and H7N1 bird flu viruses, compared to *"Level Three"* in the old system.

Current U.S. planning assumes that there will be a warning period of at least several weeks for a developing pandemic. This time is essential for pandemic preparedness. However, other factors may ensure that there is little warning and that a global pandemic may already be underway by the time a severe pandemic is declared. This has happened with every major Influenza Pandemic for the last 100 years and the new WHO Pandemic Warning System appears to be nothing more than bureaucratic paper shuffling.

THE PROBLEM OF MODERN GLOBAL AIR TRAVEL

The world has become smaller in terms of communications and the ability of humans to travel quickly around the globe. Consequently, the speed of pandemic spread has increased and the possibility for adequate pandemic warning has decreased. Today, modern air travel can disseminate an infectious disease agent around the globe within hours. This was typified by the 2002 outbreak of the Severe Acute Respiratory Syndrome (SARS).[3] From 1970 onwards, the number of global air travelers has increased by more than 800% and industry forecasts project a growth rate of 5-7.5% per year with an increase in the connectivity of most global regions.

Pandemics have always spread through human travel. Historically this was by ship, horse, and caravan. By the late 1800's this was superseded by the railroads which had become a new method for long-range travel and an important modem for disease spread.

The first pandemic to occur in this era of increased global connectivity was the 1889 Influenza pandemic which began in Russia. By 1918, steamships could make a transatlantic crossing in 5-6 days and the catastrophic 1918 Influenza pandemic was thus amplified by the vast ship and rail movements of troops during the First World War. It was India's rail system that spread the disease explosively through that nation.

Today, millions of passengers fly on commercial aircraft every day. Traveling from New York to England by air takes only 6-8 hours, and a non-stop trip from New York to Sydney can be made in 22-hours.

There have been four major Influenza pandemics since commercial air travel became available. The first was in 1957 which began in Asia but spread globally within six-months. This was before the Boeing 707 jet airliner came into commercial service in 1958. In 2009, the "swine" flu pandemic took only 3-months to widely spread and the initial number of cases in a region was significantly correlated with the number of air travelers arriving from Mexico where the pandemic started.[4]

A variety of computer models have been used to study the spread of diseases within high-density communities; the most classical being the famous Rvachev model.[5] More recent computer models have been upgraded to assess the impact of modern air travel on Influenza spread. One of these is the *AIR Pandemic Flu Model* which has been used to assess pandemic effects, both with and without the use of public health mitigation techniques and the use of different travel patterns.[6,7]

Using the AIR Pandemic Model, scientists have determined that the major cities for pandemic importation, (measured by the number of days until the first pandemic case arrives via air travel) is New York as the number one city, followed by Dubai which serves as a hub between Europe and Asia, followed by San Francisco. Other cities in order of importance were found to be Washington, D.C., London, Los Angeles, Houston, Paris, Atlanta, and Miami.

These studies show that global air travel patterns can have a major impact on the pattern of pandemic spread. For example, Brazil and Mexico have now become Latin America's two largest markets for air travel. Consequently, the 2015 spread of the Zika virus from the Pacific Ring islands to Brazil is a case in point.[8] The Mideast is another developing hub driven mainly by flights to and from Dubai and the 236%

increase in air traffic to and from the Middle East since 2000. This was a public health worry during the Middle East Respiratory Syndrome (MERS) outbreak in 2012.[9]

THE QUESTION OF PANDEMIC TRAVEL RESTRICTIONS

Acknowledging that modern-day air travel can have a large effect on pandemic spread, the question becomes, would air travel restrictions help mitigate a Pandemic? History has shown that Island countries can limit pandemic importation by initiating reverse-quarantine and isolating themselves. However, this is impractical in the highly globalized areas of the world.

Scientists are trying to study what effect travel restrictions might have and if this could be a reliable method to decrease the rate of pandemic spread. The goal is to slow the spread of a pandemic to provide more time to initiate pandemic preparedness efforts such as NPI, antiviral drug distribution, and new vaccine development. In this respect, scientists have used the AIR model to examine the effect of travel restrictions on Influenza spread. The model's findings indicate that early travel restrictions might indeed be beneficial, but the travel ban had to be over 99% effective to delay the pandemic peak by anything more than 2-3 weeks.

Hong Kong represents a critical port in Asia and as such, it receives arrivals from 44 other countries via air, sea, and land. Scientists have used what is known as an SEIR computer model together with 2009 H1N1 influenza pandemic data to examine the effect of regulating air, sea, and land transport to this city during an Influenza pandemic. They also modeled the use of a hypothetical antiviral drug together with hospital isolation strategies to compare the effectiveness of these control measures.[10]

With respect to air travel, the scientists found that a ban on the main air routes connecting Hong Kong to an influenza source area with a 99% effective air travel restriction, could delay the peak of an epidemic by up to two weeks. Hypothetical antiviral drugs and hospital isolation were found to be more effective on reducing the infection rates than air travel restrictions, but a combined strategy (with 99% restriction on all transport into and out of the city) consistently deferred the peak of the simulated epidemic. The researchers concluded that air travel restrictions should be a priority for consideration when a new influenza pandemic begins overseas.

In contrast, scientists at the Centre for Infections, Health Protection Agency in the United Kingdom, also performed mathematical modelling using the data on how Influenza spread during the pandemic outbreak in 1968-1969.[11] Using this model, they concluded that restrictions on air travel would achieve very little. Once a major outbreak was under way, banning flights from affected cities would be effective at significantly delaying worldwide spread only if all travel between cities could be stopped almost as soon as an outbreak was detected in each city.

To date, travel restrictions have yet to gain widespread acceptance and this is still the subject of much debate.

NOTES FOR CHAPTER 19

[1] WHO Pandemic Phase Descriptions
https://web.archive.org/web/20110910112007/http://www.who.int/csr/disease/i
nfluenza/GIPA3AideMemoire.pdf

[2] Pandemic Influenza Risk Management WHO Interim Guidance
http://www.who.int/influenza/preparedness/pandemic/GIP_PandemicInfluenzaR
iskMana gementInterimGuidance_Jun2013.pdf?ua=1

[3] Smith, R. D. (2006). "Responding to global infectious disease outbreaks, Lessons from
SARS on the role of risk perception, communication and management". Social
Science and Medicine. 63 (12): 3113–3123.

[4] Khan, K., J. Arino, W. Hu, F. Calderon, M. Macdonald, J. Liauw, A. Chan, and M.
Gardam 2009, "Spread of a novel influenza A (H1N1) virus via global airline
transportation." New England Journal of Medicine 361, 212-214.

[5] Rvachev, L., and I. M. Longini Jr 1985, "A mathematical model for the global spread of
influenza," Mathematical Biosciences 75,3-22.

[6] Ferguson, N. M., D. A. T. Cummings, C. Fraser, J. C. Cajka, P. C. Cooley, and D. S.
Burke 2006, "Strategies for mitigating an influenza pandemic," Nature, 442, 448-
452.

[7] Madhav, N. (Edited by M. Markey) 2013, "Modeling a Modern-Day Spanish Flu
Pandemic." AIR Currents (February 21, 2013). Available at:
http://www.airworldwide.com/Publications/AIR-Currents/2013/Modeling-a-
Modern-Day-Spanish-FluPandemic/

[8] Sikka; V. Chattu, Vijay Kumar, Raaj K.; et al. (February 11, 2016). "The emergence of
zika virus as a global health security threat: A review and a consensus statement of
the INDUSEM Joint Working Group (JWG)". Journal of Global Infectious
Diseases. 8 (1): 3–15. ISSN 0974-8245. PMC 4785754 . PMID 27013839.
doi:10.4103/0974-777X.176140

[9] De Groot RJ; et al. (15 May 2013). "Middle East Respiratory Syndrome Coronavirus
(MERSCoV): Announcement of the Coronavirus Study Group". Journal of
Virology. 87 (14): 7790–2. PMC 3700179 PMID 23678167.
doi:10.1128/JVI.01244-13.

[10] Reference: Chong KC and Chung Zee BC. Modeling the impact of air, sea, and land
travel restrictions supplemented by other interventions on the emergence of a new
influenza pandemic virus. BMC Infectious Diseases 2012, 12:309
doi:10.1186/1471-2334-12-309 154

[11] Cooper BS, Pitman RJ, Edmunds WJ, Gay NJ (2006) Delaying the international
spread of pandemic influenza. PLoS Med 3(6): e212.
http://dx.doi.org/10.1371/journal.pmed.003021

20

IN A SEVERE PANDEMIC, WILL THE GOVERNMENT AND NATIONAL MEDIA TELL THE TRUTH?

POLITICIANS IN THE U.S. GOVERNMENT have a long history of lying to the American public and the reasons for this are multifold. During wartime, it may be to protect the security of soldiers on the battlefield, and this can be understood and forgiven. However, there are cases where the lies told are to make the government look better in the public eye, or to hide its apparently ever-increasing abject incompetence. Occasionally the government makes a well-meaning but ignorant mistake. Also, sometimes the lies are well-intentioned due to a reluctance of the authorities to generate undue panic among the American population.

This seems to be a reoccurring phenomenon and when the lies have involved matters concerning public health, these actions have only tended to make things worse. At the same time, the national media may unpredictably either follow the federal government's lead and maintain a charade, or it may turn around and attack the government's stance on a public health matter. Sometimes incredibly, it may try to do both.

Throughout the 1918 Influenza pandemic, the reaction of the federal and state governments was one of denial with a constant reaffirmation that there was no cause for alarm. When the second deadly wave of the 1918 pandemic arrived, the government's combination of rigid control and dangerous disregard for the truth was maintained to avoid damaging the war effort. Officials and the newspapers continued to insist that it was only ordinary Influenza and they assured the public that the worst of the outbreak was over. Soldiers continued to be loaded onto troop transports under high-density, with mass Influenza outbreaks occurring onboard as the ships sailed to Europe. Instead of being challenged, the National Press was in full cooperation with the government's propaganda and it continued to assist in the pandemic cover up. This was to the degree that until recently, the third deadliest plague in recorded human history was almost forgotten. To inform the public, it took thousands of hours of painstaking effort by pioneering literary researchers, to piece together the fragmented history of the 1918 Pandemic. We have heavily referenced two of these works in this book.[1,2] However, there are many others that tell the story all the way down to the small community and personal level.

In Philadelphia in 1918, the Public Health Commissioner finally closed all schools, theaters, and other public gathering places even as one newspaper in the city reported that the closure order was not a public health measure and that there was no cause for alarm. But as people heard these reassurances, they could see some of their neighbors, friends, and family becoming ill with some dying horrible deaths. They knew that the event was not due to a normal outbreak of the "Flu."

It was this disconnect between the constant reassurances from the authorities and what the population was observing with their own eyes, that destroyed all government credibility. While the pandemic itself generated fear, the false reassurances given by both the government and the media destroyed public trust and turned this natural fear into abject terror. People stopped helping one another, Philadelphia's volunteer pool disappeared, and people would not go near the sick. This was in face of the numerous reports of families where every member was ill, and their children were starving because there was no one to give them food.

What was made clear from the 1918-event, was that when handling a public health crisis, it is crucial for the authorities to maintain their credibility with the American population. However, beginning with the 1979 Level-Five nuclear incident at the Three-Mile Island Complex in Pennsylvania and the partial meltdown of its Reactor Number 2, the tendency for political lies and media disinformation seems to have become the rule of norm. This was especially evident following the World Trade Center attacks on September 11 in 2001.

2001 WORLD TRADE CENTER ATTACKS

For several months after the 9/11 attack, dust from the destroyed buildings in New York City filled the air downwind from the wreckage with 10-million tons of building materials and toxic fumes generated by materials burning at temperatures above 1,000 degrees Celsius. The event crushed and incinerated thousands of computers and miles of electrical cable along with insulating material from the heating and cooling ducts. This material was spewed into the air as aerosols and toxic gases that contained more than 2,500 contaminants including hundreds of tons of asbestos. The levels of a DNA damaging chemical called dioxin measured in the air near the ruins, showed the highest ambient levels of this chemical ever recorded anywhere in the world.[3]

The toxic World Trade Center cloud extended from lower Manhattan across the East River into Brooklyn and beyond. It also contained heavy metals such as lead, and the chemicals called polychlorinated biphenyls (PCBs) used in electrical transformers. PCBs are extremely toxic when burned at a high temperature. This was in addition to the microscopic particles of silica and glass fibers that lodged in the lungs of anyone who breathed the fumes.[3]

Above all else, the Environmental Protection Agency (EPA) is tasked with ensuring clean air quality, and the highly toxic nature of the cloud was well known to EPA scientists at the time of the tower's collapse. Indeed, it was known by any undergraduate student that ever took a basic toxicology course, and it was well known to the "so-called" medical experts that constantly appeared on television to demonstrate their "profound" knowledge on a variety of medical matters.

Yet on September 13, 2001, Christie Whitman (Administrator of the EPA and former Governor of New Jersey) said, "*The EPA is greatly relieved to have learned that there appears to be no significant levels of asbestos dust in the air in New York City.*"

She added: "*We will continue to monitor closely.*" Five days later, she announced: "*I am glad to reassure the people of New York and Washington, D.C., that their air is safe to breathe.*" Statements by Mayor Rudy Giuliani in the first month after the attacks, also confirmed that the air quality was safe and acceptable.

In reality, the EPA knowingly misspoke about the air quality in the weeks after 9/11. Ignoring the safety of thousands of residents and workers, the Bush administration had pressured the EPA to remove cautionary information about the air at Ground Zero and it never enforced the existing federal laws requiring the wearing of respirators.

Repeated warnings from some scientists were continually ignored and in response, the press remained mute on the subject, completely failing in their code and their proclaimed responsibility to inform the American public. At any time, the national media could have brought prominent toxicologists into their news coverage. Such pressure from the national media would have ensured that proper protective gear was worn by the workers at the site. They failed to do this, and the press are just as culpable as the Bush administration for thousands of worker injuries and the premature deaths that are now underway.

It was later learned that the New York State Department of Environmental Conservation had conducted a study of the World Trade

Center site, but it refused to release the results of its study, saying they were part of a criminal investigation.[4] A later review also found numerous key differences between the draft and final versions of a series of public EPA statements. A recommendation that homes and businesses near ground zero be cleaned by professionals was replaced by a request that citizens follow orders from NYC officials. Statements on the excessive amounts of asbestos in the area were altered by officials to drastically minimize the dangers it posed.[5]

There was no doubt that personnel working at the collapse site were receiving toxic exposures to a variety of hazardous chemicals. Dogs in the area began suffering premature deaths and other ailments and human monitoring over the course of the first year after the disaster showed long-term loss of lung capacity in the firefighters.

In its own report, the EPA's Inspector General concluded in 2003 that 25% of the dust samples the EPA collected in the first week after the attack, showed asbestos levels that were "a significant health risk," The EPA OIG report also noted that "Competing considerations, such as national security concerns and the desire to reopen Wall Street, also played a role in EPA's air quality statements."[6]

In a later incompetent or intentionally deceiving analysis published in 2007 by the EPA, their scientists concluded that the air around Ground Zero was harmless to the civilians living and working in the areas around the collapse site. In its report, the EPA deemed any increased risk of cancer from PCBs in the air during the immediate aftermath of 9/11 as "insignificant".[7]

Only several years later, when it became apparent that there were indeed health effects associated with the smoke and dust at the collapse site, did the national media now suddenly become involved. EPA scientist Dr. Cate Jenkins was brought on television on September 8, 2006, where she bluntly stated that agency officials lied about the air quality in the weeks following September 11, 2001. She said that the EPA knew about the toxicity of the air, and that dust included asbestos and disturbingly high Poly-Aromatic Hydrocarbon levels and that some of the dust was "*as caustic and alkaline as Drano* (drain cleaner)."[8]

Ground Zero Illnesses

The end-result has been a 70% illness rate among the 9-11 rescue and recovery workers and respiratory illnesses grew by more than 200% in the year and a half after the September 11 attacks. Workers who inhaled Ground Zero air essentially lost 12-years of lung function and this was progressive with some victims developing pulmonary fibrosis and end-stage lung disease.

The National Institute for Occupational Safety and Health (NIOSH), is the United States federal agency responsible for the prevention of all work-related injury and illness. This Institute was established specifically to ensure safe working conditions in the United States by gathering information and conducting scientific research. In a 2011 report, NIOSH experts made the conclusion that there was no firm evidence of any association between air exposures at the World Trade Center site and cancer occurrence in the responders and survivors. Siting an impressive but mind-numbing number of references and appendices, this "armchair" study conducted no original field research itself. Yet NIOSH and the World Trade Center Health Program determined that there was "insufficient evidence" to add cancer to the List of World Trade Center related health conditions.[9]

However, in the largest cancer study of 9-11 firefighters ever conducted, outside scientists and health experts conducted an original peer-reviewed study that compared the cancer incidence rates in the World Trade Center-exposed firefighters, with the cancer incidence in non-exposed firefighters. This research was published a few months after the release of the NIOSH report, and it found that New York City firefighters exposed to the 9/11 World Trade Center disaster site were at least 19% more likely to develop cancer in the seven-years following the disaster as their non-exposed colleagues, and up to 10 % more likely to develop cancers of all types than typical American men in the general U.S. population.[10]

On December 10, 2007, civilian legal proceedings began on the question of the responsibility of government officials. Former EPA Director Whitman was among the defendants for saying that the Manhattan air was safe to breath in the aftermath of the attacks. Later the United States Court of Appeals for the Second Circuit ruled that Whitman could not be held liable because she had based her information on contradictory information and statements from President G.W. Bush. The U.S. Department of Justice argued that holding the EPA liable would establish a risky legal precedent.

2014-2015 EBOLA CRISIS

The tendency for the senior members of government to lie and be backed up by the head of various federal agencies was again witnessed during the abject failure of the government to generate an effective response to the 2014 West Africa Ebola event. Despite the billions of dollars spent on biological defense over the last two decades, the response to the outbreak of Ebola in the United States was badly designed and poorly implemented. Either in their effort to minimize public concern, incompetence, or under direct instructions from superiors, some leading U.S, health authorities made far over-reaching statements that were not supported by scientific research.

During the crisis, U.S. health officials repeatedly emphasized that fever is a reliable sign of individuals with Ebola becoming infectious to others around them. Consequently, as a defense against the spread of the virus, the U.S. Government ordered that passengers arriving from West Africa at five U.S. airports be checked for fever. As such, a brief fever screening was conducted on the more than 1,000 air passengers that were arriving each week in the United States from West Africa.

However, in late 2000, scientists reported that although fever is the most common symptom of Ebola virus infection, this only occurred in 85% of the cases. Another study on 24 confirmed cases of Ebola, found fever in only 88% of cases. A later large study in West Africa during the outbreak looked at 3,343 confirmed cases of Ebola. Sponsored by the WHO and published by the New England Journal of Medicine, the study found that 87.1% of cases of early Ebola infections exhibited fever-but 12.9% did not. In the study, fever was defined as a body temperature of 38 degrees Celsius (100.4° Fahrenheit).[11]

Therefore, the absence of fever was not a reliable indication that an individual was free from Ebola infection, and the lack of fever should not have been used to assess the level of infectiousness of an infected case to others. Although a small number of scientists spoke out, the federal assumption about the frequency of fever in Ebola patients was never challenged by the media.

Another inaccurate statement was that an airborne transmission of the Ebola virus could not occur. While it is presumed that the Ebola virus infects through the skin, or with contact with mucous membranes, the only two routes of exposure that have been extensively experimentally verified in animal models, are by direct injection, droplet exposure, and aerosol inhalation. While classical epidemiologic evidence indicates that aerosol exposure is not an important means of virus transmission in human-to-human epidemics of Ebola in African villages, infective Ebola virus particles are present in the oral fluid of infected patients, and experimental studies have verified that Ebola infection can be effectively transmitted by airborne droplet and oral or conjunctival contact in monkey and other animal models.[12,13,14,15,16]

The government readily acknowledged that droplet transmission of the Ebola virus can occur. These droplets would of course be *spread through the air* and small particle aerosol droplet transmission has been demonstrated in animal models. The government intentionally used word-semantics when it assured the public that aerosol transmission could not occur.

Other questions about the virus remain to be answered, especially because research has showed abundant viral proteins and Ebola viral particles in the skin of Ebola patients reaffirming the role of contact transmission in EVD. However, the timing of when live viral particles appear in the skin has not been well defined during early infection. While epidemiological studies suggest this is not a factor for early human-to-human viral transmission, further studies need to be done.[17,18,19]

The Management of Ebola Patients

The Ebola virus is classified as a Biosafety Level-4 (BSL-4) infection and is required to be contained and handled in a BSL-4 laboratory environment. Realizing the dangers and uncertainties associated with this viral disease, a previous generation of physicians and scientists acted to establish a special U.S. Army military team designed to aeromedically transport patients infected with dangerous viruses to a specialized BSL-4 medical isolation treatment facility in the United States.[20,21,22,23] During the Obama military sequestrations of 2010, this Army unit was decommissioned and this unified capability was lost. Under CDC recommendations, health care professionals became relegated to managing EVD patients under less safe BSL-3 conditions as has previously been done with African outbreaks.

The response of the CDC to the management of the first Ebola case in Texas was to promote inadequate and inexcusable guidelines that did not provide adequate health worker protection. Proper science along with previous experience and caution, were ignored. Sending an Ebola patient to a normal hospital with inexperienced staff is not a substitute for proper protective equipment, negative-pressure isolation rooms, and proper and well-practiced decontamination procedures. Neither are "tear sheets" instructing air travelers from epidemic areas to check their temperature.

During the Ebola crisis, passengers arriving in the United States from Liberia, Sierra Leone, and Guinea, were handed a flier instructing them to "call a doctor" if they should feel ill. This ignored the fact that it is impossible today to get any doctor on the phone, and if you did make contact, you would be told to go to the nearest emergency room.

The common-sense approach for "information fliers" would have been to include a toll-free number for returning passengers that would contact a special centralized office, which would then dispatch a designated ambulance with prepared personnel to take the patient to a hospital. The hospital would be warned that a possible Ebola patient was on the way and the individual would be brought in by avoiding the main emergency room entrance. Local public health authorities would be waiting to perform rapid testing using the already existing multimillion-dollar Laboratory Response Network or LRN. Established in 1999 and continuously upgraded, the LRN is a collaborative effort within the federal government which involves the Association of Public Health Laboratories and the CDC.[24]

The carelessness of the U.S. Ebola response was unfathomable and repeated statements by the CDC Director at the time "*That any hospital can care for Ebola patients*" has been heavily criticized.[25]

Pandemic Journalism

Pandemics provide many challenges to news organizations, and it appears to be difficult for news organizations get their reporters quickly knowledgeable not only about a rare virus outbreak, but almost any topic that requires some understanding of science. The supposed "journalistic code" requires a reporter to be independent and they are required to triple check their sources and avoid the use of anonymous sources.

Without having a working background knowledge of the subject, reporters are forced to use independent "experts" which sometimes are just as clueless as the reporters. All this makes it difficult for reporters to point out errors to the public. In addition, the modern news media seems to have become so desperate for ratings that everything is 'breaking news' or a 'crisis.' The quality of news and journalistic standards have dropped to the state that the news channels and newspapers often have a cheap tabloid quality to their coverage with little fact checking and contextual framing of their news items. Occasionally the facts that are exaggerated to such a degree, that they might as well be complete fabrications. In some cases, they actually are fabrications such as the reporting of the Amerithrax situation by senior correspondent Brian Ross at ABC News and Nicholas Kirstof of the New York Times. Yet, no disciplinary actions against these reporters were ever taken by these news outlets, which only further encourages such activity.

Every branch of the U.S. Government employs a team of media experts to influence the media and place their branch in the most favorable light. This should incentivize reporters to be more careful in fact checking and to use multiple sourcing of their stories to ensure that they are not being used for propaganda towards a political agenda. But very few news organizations invest any time in doing so.

In a severe pandemic, it is critical for the press to remain impartial and accurate. Communities will be desperate as the event unfolds and there is nothing better for cable news networks and online news sites than to focus on the latest rumors about an outbreak of a deadly disease. People search channels to get the latest updates, and then log on to social media and discussion forums to discuss conspiracy theories and rumors that eventually become wrongly turned into fact. News reports can easily become sensationalized to the point where the financial markets react negatively.

In the confusion of a severe pandemic, many communities may be challenged by contradictory guidance, such as in Connecticut in October 1918, when communities received precisely opposite recommendations from federal and state health officials on closing schools, theaters, and other places of public gathering.[26]

The risk of such contradictory guidance can only be decreased if accurate information is given to the public by both the government and the press.

At present, it has become almost axiomatic that when the U.S. government repeatedly tells its citizens that there is no cause for alarm or worry, no danger of an epidemic, or that effective plans are in place, then it is the time to start preparing for the worst.[27]

With respect to an answer for the question, "Can the government and the national media be trusted to accurately report the facts during a major Influenza pandemic?" Historically, the answer seems to be no.

NOTES FOR CHAPTER 20

[1] Crosby, Alfred W. America's Forgotten Pandemic: The Influenza of 1918. New York: Cambridge University Press, 1989.

[2] Barry, John M. The Great Influenza: The Epic Story of the Deadliest Plague in History. New York: Viking, 2004.

[3] Biello, D., What Was in the World Trade Center Plume? Scientific American. September 7, 2011 https://www.scientificamerican.com/article/what-was-in-the-world-tradecenter-plume/

[4] Juan Gonzalez, "Fallout: The Hidden Consequences of 9/11", In These Times, September 10, 2002 http://www.alternet.org/911oneyearlater/14073/

[5] Laurie Garrett (August 23, 2003). "EPA Misled Public on 9/11 Pollution". Newsday. Archived from the original, November20,2006. https://web.archive.org/web/20061120200307/http://www.commondreams.org/headlines03/0823-03.htm

[6] EPA OIG Evaluation Report. EPA's Response to the World Trade Center Collapse: Challenges, Successes, and Areas for Improvement. Report No. 2003-P-00012. August 21, 2003. https://www.epa.gov/sites/production/files/201510/documents/wtc_report_20030821.pdf

[7] Lorber, M., Gibb, L., Grant, J.P., et.al. Assessment of Inhalational Exposures and Potential Health Risks to the General Population That Resulted from the Collapse of the World Trade Center Towers. Risk Analysis. Blackwell Publishing, Malden, MA, 27(5):1203-1221, (2007). https://cfpub.epa.gov/ncea/risk/recordisplay.cfm?deid=127846#Download

[8] Insider: EPA Lied About WTC Air". CBS News. September 8, 2006. https://www.cbsnews.com/news/insider-epa-lied-about-wtc-air/

[9] First Periodic Review of Department of Health and Human Services, CDC, NIOSH; Scientific and Medical Evidence Related to Cancer for the World Trade Center Health Program. DHHS (NIOSH) Publication Number 2011–197 July 2011. https://www.cdc.gov/niosh/docs/2011197/pdfs/2011-197.pdf

[10] Rachel Zeig-Owens, Mayris P Webber, et.al. Early assessment of cancer outcomes in New York City firefighters after the 9/11 attacks: an observational cohort study. Volume 378, No. 9794, p898–905, 3 September 2011 DOI: http://dx.doi.org/10.1016/S01406736(11)60989-6

[11] WHO Ebola Response Team, Ebola Virus Disease in West Africa-The First 9 Months of the Epidemic and Forward Projections. New Eng Journal of Med; 371:1481-1495 October 16, 2014.

[12] Formenty P, Leroy EM, Epelboin A, et al. Detection of Ebola virus in oral fluid specimens during outbreaks of Ebola virus hemorrhagic fever in the Republic of Congo. Clin Infect Dis 2006; 42:1521-1526.

[13] Jaax NK, Davis KJ, Geisbert TJ, et al. Lethal experimental infection of rhesus monkeys with Ebola-Zaire (Mayinga) virus by the oral and conjunctival route of exposure. Arch Pathol Lab Med 1996; 120:140-155.

[14] Twenhafel NA, Shaia CI, Bunton TE, et al. Experimental aerosolized guinea pig-adapted Zaire ebolavirus (variant: Mayinga) causes lethal pneumonia in guinea pigs. Vet Pathol 2014 May 14.

[15] Zumbrun EE, Bloomfield HA, et al. Development of a murine model for aerosolized Ebolavirus infection using a panel of recombinant inbred mice. Viruses 2012; 4:258-275.

[16] Kobinger GP, Neufeld J, et al. Replication, pathogenicity, shedding, and transmission of Zaire ebolavirus in pigs. J Infect Dis 2011; 204:200-208.

[17] Bausch DG, Towner JS, Dowell SF, et al. Assessment of the risk of Ebola virus transmission from bodily fluids and fomites. J Infect Dis 2007;196(Suppl 2): S142-S147.

[18] Zaki SR, Shieh WJ, Greer PW, et al. A novel immunohistochemical assay for the detection of Ebola virus in skin: implications for diagnosis, spread, and surveillance of Ebola hemorrhagic fever. Commission de Lutte contre les Epidémies à Kikwit. J Infect Dis 1999; 179 (Suppl 1) : S36-S47.

[19] Delta's CEO is wrong about Ebola. https://qz.com/282345/deltas-ceo-is-wrong-aboutebola/

[20] Clayton AJ. Containment aircraft isolator. Aviat Space Environ Med, 1979;50:1067-1072.

[21] Christopher GW, Eitzen EM Jr. Air evacuation under high-level biosafety containment: the aeromedical isolation team. Emerg Infect Dis 1999; 5:241–246.

[22] Marklund LA. Patient care in a biological safety level-4 (BSL-4) environment. Crit Care Nurs Clin N Am 2003; 15:245-255.

[23] Mark R. Withers, George W. Christopher, Steven J. Hatfill, and Jose J. Gutierrez-Nunez, Chapter 11, "Aeromedical Evacuation of Patients with Contagious Infections" In Aeromedical Evacuation; Management of Acute and Stabilized Patients. Eds. William Hurd, John Jernigan. Springer Press.

[24] Cieslak, Theodore J. and George W. Christopher (2007), "Medical Management of Potential Biological Casualties: A Stepwise Approach", In: Dembek, Zygmunt F. (2007), Medical Aspects of Biological Warfare, (Textbooks of Military Medicine), Washington, DC.

[25] https://en.wikipedia.org/wiki/Elizabeth_R._Griffin_Research_Foundation.

[26] Many Cases of Influenza, Health Authorities Differ. Danbury Evening News, Saturday, October 5,1918.

[27] Pandemic Influenza: Community Planning and Response Curriculum for District and Community Leaders. Humanitarian Pandemic Preparedness (H2P) initiative, July 2009. Available at http://www.coregroup.org/our-technical-work/initiatives/h2p (Accessed 18 September 2016).

SECTION

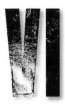

VI

DEVELOPING NEW SOLUTIONS
FOR PANDEMIC INFLUENZA PREPAREDNESS

21

INCREASING THE MEDICAL SURGE
CAPABILITY OF LOCAL AUTHORITIES

THE PANDEMIC APPLICATIONS OF BIOLOGICAL WARFARE DEFENSE

With respect to an individual city, a properly formatted biological war-fare attack represents a worst-case mass-casualty infectious disease sce-nario. This statement is not based on paper calculations.

On September 20, 1950, the United States Army conducted a sim-ulated Large-Area- Coverage Biological Warfare attack using live non-pathogenic bacteria (Bacillus globegii). This is the Niger variant of a common harmless soil bacteria called Bacillus subtilis. Under ideal me-teorological conditions, a converted naval minesweeper sailed a straight-line course approximately 2-miles off the coast of San Fran-cisco. As it sailed, the scientists onboard pressure-generated a small particle aerosol which disseminated 150-gallons of this liquid simulated biological warfare agent as a 2-mile aerosol line-source. An onshore breeze blew the invisible aerosol cloud over the city.

Several days before, the scientists had set up numerous all-glass impinger air samplers on government building roof tops and inside offices. Following the aerosol dissemination, these air samplers were retrieved and analyzed to see if any of the test bacteria had been captured. What they found was shocking. Nearly all of residents received a dose of at least 500 particle minutes per liter of air at a normal breathing rate of 10 liters per minute. This equated to a simulated Minimal Infectious Dose of 5,000 bacteria or more for virtually every individual in the 49-square mile city area.[1] The census for the San Francisco population at the time was 775,357 individuals. If a real bacterial biological warfare agent had been used and not a simulant, the economic impact of such an attack has been estimated to be $26.2 billion dollars for every 100,000 persons exposed (in 1997 dollars).[2]

The first wave of casualties to appear would be the high-dose exposures over the next 48-hours which would have involved all the individuals living close to the bay. Then even larger waves of casualties would appear over the next 7-days. A final wave would have occurred involving the inhabitants of Oakland who by being further away, would have received the lowest aerosol dose. Any case-fatalities that occurred past 7-days would be assumed to be due to a delay in treatment. It must be added that this simulated biological attack was conducted with late 1940's technology using a low-efficiency E-22 type of aerosol generator.

In the aftermath of a real Biological Warfare attack, there would be a reactive, rushed, response directed towards restoring the city infrastructure, managing the dead and dying, and attempting to triage and treat the casualties that received a minimal infecting dose of the biological agent. Hospitals inside the target area would rapidly become nonfunctional due to staff illness, failure to report for work, overwhelming casualties, a lack of drugs, and a slow or inadequate medical surge capacity.

The aftermath of such an attack would in many ways resemble the front lines of a large conventional battlefield. It would be a localized lethal epidemic, but with a highly compressed timeframe. Nevertheless, it is useful to examine the national response recommendations for an urban Biological Warfare attack. This could help assess where non-medically trained civilian volunteers could be used, and what type of training they would need to operate in an Influenza virus-contaminated environment such as a home with all the family members ill, or a deployed Federal Medical Station (FMS), an Alternate Care Site, or even within a hospital itself.

THE BIOLOGICAL WEAPONS IMPROVED RESPONSE PLAN (BWIRP)

From April 1998 to December 1998 the U.S. Army Soldier and Biological Chemical Command (SBCCOM) of the Department of Defense, formed a partnership with numerous multi-agency federal authorities and over 60 experienced emergency responders, managers, and technical experts, including Major General (retired) Donna Barbish who was an early visionary in recognizing the problem in local civilian authority domestic preparedness. This study was under the umbrella of the Nunn-Lugar-Domenici Domestic Preparedness Program and its goal was to develop a new Biological Weapons Improved Response Program (BWIRP).[3]

The team divided their response to a biological attack into phases with timelines for each response activity. Then they looked at how well the activities would work together to deal with the ever-changing conditions created by a Biological Warfare (BW) attack. The team then analyzed what personnel and resources would be needed to perform each part of the response. They recognized that an effective response to a major BW incident must be led by the local community. Local pre-planning before the event would be critical, and rapid implementation of the plan following an attack was the key to success. It acknowledged that the local community could best assess its own needs and develop a response.

This was more in line with the neighborhood-community-city-county-state "bottom-up" approach to pandemic Influenza planning that scientists had sought after for years. By using a "common response template" and existing resources, the cost for a city to plan and prepare for effective BW response was considered modest. The city or town's main effort would be to prepare and actually test their pandemic response plan using their existing emergency response infrastructure. The goal was to keep up with the onset of BW casualties in a coordinated non-chaotic manner.

The key of the BWIRP was to focus on enabling the local authorities to keep their main hospitals open and functional while dealing with the mass-casualties caused by a BW attack. The method used was to quickly establish local Neighborhood Emergency Help Centers and Alternate Treatment Centers (Acute Care Centers). This BWIRP document has great value when considering what personnel and skills would be required for an effective medical surge using what the BWIRP calls its Modular Emergency Medical System and its Community Outreach (CO) component.[4]

THE NEIGHBORHOOD EMERGENCY HELP CENTER (NEHC)

In the BWIRP protocols, the ability of local authorities can be enhanced by the rapid mobilization of two impromptu Emergency Medical facilities. The first is called a Neighborhood Emergency Help Center or NEHC. The second facility is called an Acute Care Center (ACC).

In a biological emergency, each City would act to establish a NEHC inside their various affected local communities. Predesignated NEHC personnel would be instructed to report at these sites at a specified time and location. Each NEHC would function to provide drug and vaccine prophylaxis if available, perform an initial medical assessment on symptomatic patients in its attached "Triage Clinic" to determine patient severity. The NEHC would act as a gateway for patients to directly enter the pandemic healthcare system by sending them to a second facility termed the Acute Care Center (ACC).[4]

It was envisioned that a NEHC could be established in an educational facility or appropriate community buildings such as a closed school. Each NEHC was designed to provide prophylactic medications and/or vaccines for up to 1000 to 2000 people per hour for dispensing medications and 600 people per hour for vaccination.[4] The local authority of a community would decide where its NEHC should be set up with Memorandums of Understanding with these facilities and pre-arrangements made with the local police to provide security if it is ever used.

Once set up, one entrance would be for "Not Sick" clients and the other for "Sick" clients. The NEHC would then function as high-volume triage center, where its staff would assess the patients and dispense prophylactic medications and vaccines (if any were available) and distribute self-help information to the walking "worried." A practical lecture room would teach home care and train family members how to don and doff personal protective equipment safely. This is vital if a family member that is brought to the NEHC is triaged to undergo care at home.

One important component of the NEHC is called "Community Outreach." This program would operate out of the NEHC and it would attend to people and families that could not come to the NEHC. When operated by local authorities the NEHC would also be the site where a multiphone Nurse Triage Line could be set up as discussed in an earlier chapter.

Several small Community Outreach teams would operate as directed by the Nurse Triage Line with each team composed of a local law enforcement officer, two members of a civilian volunteer organization, and a nurse. These teams would respond to locations identified by the Nurse Triage Lines to conduct specific house calls or to make door-to-door sector survey of the affected communities. This is similar to Philadelphia's Filbert 100 emergency call-line used in 1918. These small visiting health teams would act as a significant force multiplier for the doctors involved in a pandemic response.

Recognizing the BWIRP, the DHHS has issued planning guidance for local authorities that incorporates some of the BWIRP strategy and it is now promoting the use of the Neighborhood Emergency Health Centers.[5]

However, the local authorities are still dependent on a top-down State Public Health response controlled through a State Health Operations Center and a state NEHC Commander. All these will operate in compliance with the federal top-down National Incident Management System. The NEHC, will report up its state government's chain of command back to the DHHS. It is almost an axiom in that unless frequent exercises are conducted, the more federal and state agencies that are involved in a plan then the less likely it is to work correctly.

THE ACUTE CARE CENTERS/ALTERNATE CARE FACILITIES

The second component of a local BWIRP plan is the establishment of one or more Acute Care Centers (ACC) or "Alternate Treatment Facilities" at predetermined locations. Each ACC will need a local hospital to support it. However, a hospital may support multiple ACCs or in a community with several hospitals, each hospital may support their own ACC.

This could be part of a "surge discharge" strategy where non-Influenza patients that required in-patient hospital treatment but do not require intensive care with mechanical ventilation are relocated. Alternately, the ACC would just provide care for diagnosed influenza patients.

A third alternative is to treat Influenza patients that require critical care at the hospitals and use the ACC for the other influenza patients that need in-patient treatment but do not require mechanical ventilation. However, it is probably not a good idea to mix Influenza patients with non-infected patients inside the same facility. This is because of the risks for cross contamination when mixing sick people with well people, even when using full infection control methods.

The goal is to use the ACCs to temporarily enhance a community's capability to care for large numbers of casualties by converting non-hospital facilities into standardized mass-care centers (Figure 24). This response will hopefully ensure that the hospitals can continue to safely meet the needs of non-infected patients with other conditions.

The use of non-hospital sites for extra bed space may involve clinics, reconfigured outpatient facilities, home health care & hospice care facilities and designated Alternate Care Facilities set up in tents and in suitable buildings of opportunity. This will allow local hospitals to coordinate their medical operations at the community level while still keeping their emergency rooms open and functional (Figures 24 and 25).

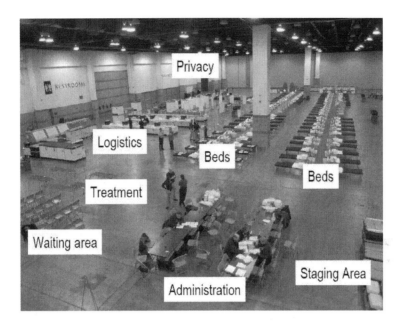

Figure 24. *Alternate Care Facility.* Source: Federal Medical Station Program.

As we have described, hospital capacity is only one factor in pandemic preparedness. With respect to the staffing of the Acute Care Centers, the BWIRP suggests that for every 50 patient beds, the following personnel would be required. These include; 1 Medical Doctor, Physician Assistant or Nurse Practitioner; 6 Registered Nurses or Licensed Practical Nurses; 6 Nursing Assistants; 2 Housekeepers; 2 Hospital Orderlies; 2 Clerks; and 1 Respiratory Therapist.

If a BWIRP-type medical response system is used by local authorities in their preparation for a 1918-type pandemic, the most critical health worker shortage will be the Registered Nurses, the Licensed Practical Nurses, and the Certified Nursing Assistants (CNA). In the US, the role of the traditional Hospital Orderlies has been gradually phased out of medical facilities and their functions are now replaced by the Certified Nursing Assistants.

So, for every doctor at an Acute Care Center, there would be a need for 6 Registered Nurses or Licensed Practical Nurses, and 8 Certified Nursing Assistants for every 50 non-critical patients.

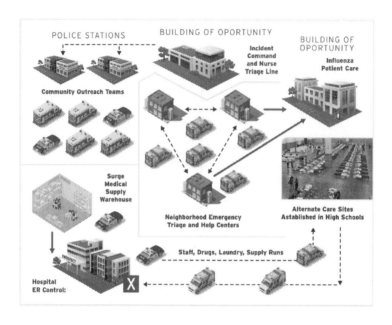

Figure 25. *Local Community Response Using Alternate Care Sites as Pandemic Influenza Treatment Centers.*

The BWIRP also calls for the rapid creation of a dedicated casualty transportation system to facilitate the movement of patients between various care centers (e.g., NEHCs, hospitals, and ACCs). The casualty transportation component is critical to the success of the entire system as it will expand the community's patient movement capacity, facilitate patient flow throughout the NEHC/ACC medical system, help support the small community outreach teams, optimize system-wide resource utilization, and ensure timely care.

The EMS personnel involved in this pandemic response would need to receive appropriate education, training, and equipment for upgraded personal protection. They should also receive prophylactic medications and/or vaccinations as available for the identified pandemic agent. They must also be able to safely perform a complete decontamination of their vehicle. The BWIRP staffing assessments suggest that pre-pandemic training of volunteers to serve as CNA's or Personal Care Assistants, might be able to provide a significant medical surge capability in a pandemic.

The concept of creating a 'just-in-time" emergency volunteer force to provide a specific surge capability is not new. In 1915, a volunteer Civil Defense force was created to counter the German zeppelin aerial bombings of the cities in the United Kingdom. By the Second World War this concept was expanded as local Civil Defense teams were formally organized and trained. In the United States, the Office of Civil Defense was formally established in May 1941 to coordinate a variety of civilian defense efforts with the Department of the Army and already established volunteer groups. One of these that still exists today is called the Civil Air Patrol. This originally had been created as a civilian auxiliary to the Army Air Corps that could be used for submarine hunting off America's coastal waters.

Following the development of thermonuclear weapons and the perceived threat of nuclear war, a large U.S. federal Civil Defense program began and ran from 1951 to 1994. This was authorized by Public Law 920 of the 81st Congress, but as the threat of a nuclear exchange with the Soviet Union appeared to ease, this law was repealed. However, small portions of the legislation were incorporated into the new *Stafford Disaster Relief and Emergency Assistance Act*, although the term "Emergency Preparedness" was now substituted for "Civil Defense."

The Stafford Act was a major change in U.S. civil defense policy, and it reflected a focus towards a more top-down "all-hazards" approach to disasters. The responsibility for local volunteer civil defense efforts now became shared between a variety of short-lived and ever-changing government departments, agencies, and federal-sponsored organizations. In a major change in 1979, the Federal Emergency Management Agency (FEMA) took over the duties of civil defense and FEMA was eventually absorbed into the new Department of Homeland Security in 2003.

During this process of constant bureaucratic shuffling, the original concept of local volunteers seemed to falter as enormous amounts of federal funding were appropriated for ever-increasing levels of top-down-directed emergency planning. Realizing that it needed to forge better links with the local authorities, FEMA eventually started its own "University" at the former closed St. Joseph's College in Emmitsburg, Maryland. Purchased in 1979, this 107-acre campus became the FEMA National Emergency Training Center (NETC), later renamed the Emergency Management Institute (EMI). One purpose of the EMI was to train local authorities in the structure and function of the federal response system, as well as to teach guidelines for local author- ities to be able to prepare and respond to multiple types of disasters. Yet despite this effort, when the levees in New Orleans collapsed in 2005, the careful federal and state paper planning fell apart when trig- gered by a failure of the city's local emergency plan.

There are lessons here for pandemic Influenza preparedness. Again, it must be stated; if the local authorities are not prepared to manage their own local area epidemics, the U.S. will not be able to manage a national pandemic.

LESSONS FROM THE MEDICAL RESERVE CORPS PROGRAM

As previously discussed, the goals of the Medical Reserve Corps (MRC) Demonstration Project was to determine if a dedicated medical surge response could be created by forming local MRC units composed of a range of medical and health professionals. It was also to demon- strate if the MRC as designed, could understand and function within the top-down FEMA federal disaster system. Finally, it was to assess if current and retired doctors and nurses would undertake additional training to understand working within an established FEMA/state/lo- cal Unified Incident Command System.

With respect to the use of the MRC in a severe pandemic, the con- cept was problematic from the start. While the MRC doctors and nurses might be released from their parent organizations for a temporary medical surge to another state, in a national pandemic they would be needed in their own area. Although stated as being able to bolster a local communities' medical response to a large-scale emergency, the Medical Reserve Corps was premised on the assumption that a major disaster would only affect one region of the United States at a time. As such, it was never suitable for use in a large-scale severe pandemic involving millions of ill individuals of all age groups throughout the United States.

The lessons of the MRC program suggested that somehow, an augmentation of medical surge capability had to be made using non-medical or minimally medical-trained personnel.

THE CONCEPT OF COMMUNITY EMERGENCY RESPONSE TEAMS (CERT)

Returning to the original idea of a trained volunteer Civil Defense force, in 1985 a local program was established by the Los Angeles City Fire Department to train civilians to help meet the city's future disaster needs. This was initially focused on earthquake preparedness and the Whittier Narrows earthquake in 1987 further underscored the need for such a local community Civil Defense program.

By 1993, this concept had garnered federal attention and FEMA began to supply both "Train-the-Trainer" as well as "Program Manager" courses for the fire, medical and emergency management organizations that these emergency volunteer teams would be attached to. The concept expanded nationally and an ever-increasing number of civilian "Community Emergency Response Teams" or CERT, have been formed. These volunteer CERT teams are now coordinated by the Department of Homeland Security.

Under the CERT concept, individual citizens are trained in basic disaster response skills and formed into neighborhood and community CERT teams sponsored by a local fire, police, or emergency management office. Each team's sponsoring agency liaises with, deploys, and may further train or supervise the training of its CERT members, and it receives Stafford Act grant funding for this process.

However, these teams are trained for conventional disasters and any type of pandemic training is non-existent. While the CDC offers an on-line Influenza volunteer training course that is focused on pandemic communications, there are no specific federal training programs for working in a lethal virus-contaminated healthcare environment.[6] It is important to remember that Influenza is only one of a number of lethal pathogens with pandemic potential and that potentially dangerous new viruses are now being discovered by scientists almost annually.

Outside of federal training, there is an outside pandemic training course that has been developed by the forward thinkers at the California Conference of Local Health Officers. They have developed a 2011 Community Emergency Response Team (CERT) Training Module for Pandemic Influenza.[7] This course provides a good introduction to understand some of the basic infection control procedures such as hand washing, masks and N-95 respirators, pandemic preparation, and basic home care; but it is not sufficient to enable a team member to function in a highly-contaminated biohazard environment. With added exercises and some expansion, this could be a model for a consistent, nationwide approach to basic pandemic volunteer training.

There are over 2,700 local CERT programs nationwide, with more than 600,000 individuals trained since the CERT concept was approved by FEMA. For pandemic planners to ignore this valuable volunteer resource would be foolish. Yet, when dealing with an infectious disease in a community the CERT volunteers would require additional training.

THE CONCEPT OF LOCAL VOLUNTEER PANDEMIC RESPONDERS

Unlike a natural disaster where minimally trained personnel can normally play a role; a severe infectious disease pandemic requires responders that have been trained to work in a biologically unsafe environment. There is also another factor to consider. It is the fact that all infectious disease epidemics instill a natural fear of becoming infected. Unlike a hurricane which is quickly over, a pandemic can continue for weeks. Recognizing this problem helps to determine how pandemic volunteers could be both recruited, trained, and retained, and the BWIRP helps to assess what standardized training such local volunteers would need, and what jobs they could be trained to perform to assist in a pandemic medical surge. Considering the continuing unpredictable problem of new emerging infectious diseases, these *Local Pandemic Volunteers* should be over-trained to enable them to operate during severe pandemics other than Influenza.

A severe pandemic would expose a volunteer worker to situations that might be well outside their previous experience. These include the following;

- Working in a highly stressful environment with reduced levels of sleep.
- Working in an environment that without precautions, will cause illness or death.
- Their safety at work is completely dependent on protective equipment and procedures.
- They will deal with difficult emotional situations with ill and critically ill patients in homes, Acute Care Centers, or hospitals.

As mentioned, previous studies have suggested that volunteers seem to be the least willing to report for work when dealing with technical disasters such as an infectious disease outbreak, an event involving ionizing radiation, or a toxic chemical event. This suggests that this fear may be based on an incomplete understanding of the technical threat and how an individual can be well protected by Personal Protective Equipment.

It is therefore reasonable to suggest that a pandemic education and training program along with constant realistic exercises, might instill enough confidence to significantly reduce this anxiety.[8] This is essentially how the U.S. military prepares its soldiers for the dangerous job of combat. The key is to understand the threat, (in this case pandemic Influenza), and then acquire a complete familiarization with equipment and procedures, and then perform enough drills and repetitions to ensure that an individual can perform accurately and confidently under stress. It also suggests that military veterans might make ideal, reliable, local volunteers for a pandemic response.

BASIC ROLES FOR A "LOCAL PANDEMIC RESPONDER"

The question now becomes, what contributions could volunteers play in a local severe infectious disease response? For this, it is necessary to return to the BWIRP and the DHHS derivative of this plan for a national pandemic. The basic idea would be to use community volunteers to perform many of the large number of tasks needed in a pandemic response. This would free up the more highly trained professionals for the more technical tasks.

We find that properly trained volunteers could be used throughout all aspects of a pandemic response. They could assist with the initial set-up of an NEHC in a suitable location and serve as escorts in the high-volume casualty reception center where medical staff would perform patient triage. They could assist in dispensing prophylactic medications and vaccines (if any are available) and distribute self-help information. They could assist with the radio communications with the dispatched community outreach teams, assist in the transport of clinical medical samples to laboratories, re-order supplies to maintain inventories, and serve as drivers and clerks. Select individuals could be valuable in leadership roles.[9,10]

Previously studied Influenza pandemics have caused national planners to believe that even in a severe Influenza outbreak, if families receive appropriate guidance they will be able to safely provide supportive care for most ill family members at home.[11,12,13,14] If an ill family member is brought to the NEHC and they are triaged to undergo Home Care, trained volunteers could assist in teaching the families the basics of providing this supportive care, as well as instructions for how to don and doff personal protective equipment in a safe manner.

As previously described, an important component of the NEHC is called "Community Outreach". This program would operate out of the

NEHC and could be attached to the Nurse Triage Line to serve that part of the community who are unable to access health care. A small Community Outreach team might consist of a local law enforcement officer, two civilian pandemic volunteers, and a nurse. These multiple, small, teams would respond to homes as directed by the Nurse Triage Lines to provide home care advice and other family assistance, including the collection of the dead.

During the severe 1918 Influenza pandemic in Philadelphia, many families were unable to feed themselves due to illness. In a modern pandemic, the problem may be a disruption of the food distribution infrastructure. In both cases, local pandemic volunteers would be essential to help create and operate classical "Soup Kitchens" in suitable locations. Pandemic volunteers could also assist social workers and public health personnel to operate a Mobile Training Facility designed to work closely with local community leaders and residents to improve their Influenza health-literacy. This is so they can effectively employ well-planned, evidence-based measures that minimize Influenza transmission in their community.

During a pandemic, as hospitals reach capacity and are no longer able to divert patients to other hospitals, they would request that the community activate their pre-planned Acute Care Centers at a predetermined location(s). Trained pandemic volunteers could serve in a variety of technical and non-technical roles at these sites. They could assist with the parent hospital's support of their ACCs by transporting supplies to the ACC and maintaining inventories. They could serve as admission clerks, perform housekeeping, help prepare and serve patient meals and assist with patient care.

For the "surge" Acute Care Centers the BWIRP recommends 8 Certified Nursing Assistants (CNA) for every 50 beds. The CNAs are professional healthcare workers that assist nurses by performing routine duties at hospitals and other care facilities. A significant medical surge expansion could be made in the form of pandemic volunteers trained to act as CNAs or "care assistants" who would work under the close supervision of a Registered Nurse.

LOCAL PANDEMIC RESPONDER TRAINING

It is likely that a tiered-system of training would be most effective in creating a local pandemic volunteer force, which could be tailored to each community's needs.[9] All pandemic responders should be trained to have a basic understanding of infectious diseases and their transmission to include historical pandemics, as well as a general understanding of bacterial and viral infections. The volunteers should be well-versed and practiced with respect to basic infection control procedures including the proper donning and doffing of Personal Protective Equipment, individual and team decontamination, vehicle disinfection, patient room disinfection, entering and leaving a biohazard area, and the management of biologically hazardous waste. They should also be trained in the use of body bags for the removal of the deceased from homes and care facilities. This would include practical training and exercises using a simulated contaminated room with fluorescent Glo-germ® and a black light box. Volunteers should also be trained in work/rest cycles and dehydration/heat illness avoidance while wearing Personal Protective Equipment.

Each member of the volunteer force should be trained to enable them to conduct a group educational program to teach families about personal biosafety, home care issues concerning hydration, fever, nutrition, the safe use of available medications, and when families should seek outside medical assistance. They should have a full understanding of Non-pharmaceutical interventions so they can effectively teach evidence-based measures that minimize Influenza transmission in the community.[15] This also sets the stage for individuals in the community to realize the importance of vaccination when a vaccine becomes available for their individual Tier group.

In addition, as many suitable pandemic volunteers as possible should be selected to undergo partial or full Certified Nursing Assistants training through potentially FEMA-funded Community College programs. These personnel would be capable of operating either in the Acute Care

Centers and well as in the community hospitals where they would help bathe and dress patients, check their vital signs and take other statistics like weight and height, and reposition patients who are unable to move themselves. They would also monitor patients and write chart changes in their health or behavior, escort patients, and obtain lab specimens.

Lower down on the healthcare provider scale are what are termed Personal Care Assistants who have no certification or licensure requirement and who usually receive on-the-job training. However, some states require passing a competency test prior to working. This is another opportunity for training volunteer pandemic workers. In summary, local pandemic volunteers would have a major role to play in helping a community develop a "medical surge" capability during a lethal pandemic. [16]

It is now a question of selecting which individuals in a community would be suitable as a reliable volunteer workforce in a pandemic environment. The personal qualities required of such individuals in such a workforce are courage, patriotism, the desire to help their community and country, self-discipline and a familiarization with working under a chain of command in a dangerous situation.

WHAT TYPE OF UMBRELLA ORGANIZATION WOULD BE SUITABLE FOR PANDEMIC VOLUNTEERS?

In another lesson from the Medical Reserve Corps, pandemic volunteers would require an organizational structure to manage and integrate them into existing emergency response systems. Without such a structure, pandemic volunteers may be turned away or assigned to duties that do not make the best use of their training and skills. In this respect, there are several options.

Local Pandemic Response volunteers could be attached to Local Public Health Departments or alternatively, they could be stood up as a separate unit within the existing "Citizen Corps" system. Another possibility is that they could be stood up as a "Public Health Corps Auxiliary" very similar to the Civil Air Patrol (CAP) which operates under 10 U.S.C. § 9442. This regulation clarifies that this CAP auxiliary status is only applicable when its members and resources are on a United States Air Force-assigned mission with an Air Force-assigned mission number. CAP members are covered by the Federal Employees Compensation Act (FECA) in the event of injury while participating in a mission. At all other times, such as when aiding civilian authorities, the CAP remains and acts as a private, non-profit corporation. Upon call up, the CAP becomes a civilian auxiliary of the United States Air Force.

This brings to light the possibility of the volunteer pandemic force being attached as an auxiliary to the National Public Health Service, but with the proviso that it is a local community resource designed to operate only in its own local community. This is to prevent the local volunteers being used for the larger metropolitan areas in a severe pandemic, leaving their own communities vulnerable. Like the National Guard, legislation could be enacted to ensure their civilian jobs were reserved in the event of a pandemic call-up.

There is an urgent need to create and properly train a dedicated volunteer Pandemic Response Force within the local communities and to have a well-rehearsed local community plan to activate these volunteers. With respect to the data on ocular Influenza virus transmission, there is an urgent need for an Integral Pandemic Respirator for both healthcare workers, pandemic volunteers, and homecare providers.

NOTES FOR CHAPTER 21

[1] Special Report No 142, "Biological Warfare Trials at San Francisco, California; 20-27 September 1950. U.S. Chemical Corps Biological Laboratories, January 22, 1951

[2] Kaufmann, A.F., Meltzer, M.I., Schmid, G.P., The Economic Impact of a Bioterrorist Attack: Are Prevention and Post-Attack Intervention Programs Justifiable? Emerging Infectious Diseases, Volume 3, Number 2-June 1997.

[3] Biological Warfare Improved Response Program, March 10, 1999, Summary Report on BW Response Template and Response Improvements, https://www.ecbc.army.mil/downloads/bwirp/ECBC_bwirp_executive_summary.pdf

[4] Biological weapons Improved Response Plan; A Mass Casualty Care Strategy for a Biological Terrorism Incident. https://www.ecbc.army.mil/downloads/reports/ECBC_comp_mass_casualty_care.pdf

[5] State of Delaware, Department of Health and Social Services, Division of Public Health; Neighborhood Emergency Help Center Plan: http://www.dhss.delaware.gov/dhss/dph/php/files/nehcplan.pdf

[6] CERC Pandemic Influenza Training https://emergency.cdc.gov/cerc/cerconline/pandemic/index.html

[7] http://lwrcert.org/resources/CERT-Pandemic-Influenza-Module-DECSRIPTION.pdf

[8] Koh D, Lim MK, et.al., Risk perception and impact of Severe Acute Respiratory Syndrome (SARS) on work and personal lives of healthcare workers in Singapore: what can we learn? Med Care. 2005 Jul; 43(7):676-82.

[9] Pandemic Influenza: Community Planning and Response Curriculum for Community Responders, Volunteers, and Staff. Humanitarian Pandemic Preparedness (H2P) initiative, July 2009 https://www.cdc.gov/nonpharmaceutical-interventions/toolsresources/publishedresearch.html).

[10] Centers for Disease Control and Prevention. Interim pre-pandemic planning guidance: community strategy for pandemic influenza mitigation in the United States—early, targeted, layered use of nonpharmaceutical interventions. Atlanta, GA: US Department of Health and Human Services, CDC; 2007. https://stacks.cdc.gov/view/cdc/11425.

[11] Hatchett, RJ., Mecher, C.E., and Lipsitch, M., Public health interventions and epidemic intensity during the 1918 influenza pandemic, PNAS, vol. 104 no. 18, 7582–7587, doi: 10.1073/pnas.0610941104http://www.pnas.org/content/104/18/7582.full.pdf

[12] Martin C. J. Ferguson, N.M., et.al. The effect of public health measures on the 1918 influenza pandemic in U.S cities, PNAS May 1, 2007, vol. 104, no. 1., 7588–7593.

[13] Home Care Guidance.https://www.cdc.gov/h1n1flu/homecare/caregivertips.htm

[14] Feb 15, 2017 Update Guideline for Isolation Precautions in Healthcare Settings https://www.cdc.gov/infectioncontrol/pdf/guidelines/isolation-guidelines.pdf

[15] Qualls N, Levitt A, Kanade N, et al. Community Mitigation Guidelines to Prevent Pandemic Influenza — United States, 2017. MMWR Recom Rep 2017;66 (No. RR-1):1– 34. doi: http://dx.doi.org/10.15585/mmwr.rr6601a1

[16] Fuh-Yuan Shih, MD, Kristi L. Koenig, Improving Surge Capacity for Biothreat Experience from Taiwan Academic Emergency Medicine 2006; 13:1114–1117

22

THE PROBLEM OF THE POOR, HIGH-DENSITY, LOW RESOURCE, URBAN AREAS

THERE IS ONE OTHER MAJOR FACTOR in pandemic preparedness that has been briefly mentioned but not fully discussed. This concerns the problems associated with the poor, high-density urban areas in the United States and the rest of the world. As previously mentioned, over the last century there has been a constant tendency for global human populations to move from rural areas to the cities for employment.

In 1918, for the first time there were more people living in cities in the United States, than in the rural areas.[1] Currently, over four-fifths of the U.S. population resides in urban areas, a percentage which is still increasing.[2]

One major risk of this urbanization is that any long-term industrial decline in a city can cause a cascade of increased area unemployment, lost tax revenue, slowly increasing poverty, and increasing crime. Faced with a depletion of its municipal resources, the city will raise taxes causing the more affluent residents to move out. Further retail and employment may also move outside the city making the problem worse.[3] This leads to a cascade of factors called Urban Decay in which a falling tax base leads to blighted neighborhoods, abandoned buildings, high unemployment, fragmented families with single parent mothers, criminals, street gangs, and drugs.[3,4] The eventual decrease in public school funding in these socially paralyzed areas creates catastrophic continuing consequences.

The city of Detroit is one good example and the same deficiencies are seen in other inner-city areas such as Philadelphia, Newark, Baltimore, and Chicago.[5,6,7] Most are in the Northeast or the Industrial Midwest which are the regions that have lost the most jobs with major demographic changes over the last 40 years.[8] There are currently 10 major cities with more than 20% of their inhabitants below the poverty level. These include Detroit with 32.5%, Buffalo (29.9%), Cincinnati (27.8%), El Paso (26.4%), and Milwaukee (26.2%), the East area of Cleveland (27.0%), Miami (26.9%), St. Louis (26.8%), Newark (24.2%), and Philadelphia (25.1%).

There are many other low-income areas in the US. However, most traditional urban ghettos have been largely demolished or abandoned due to gentrification and the increased use of Section 8 housing vouchers for 4.8 million low-income households. However, some cities can still be considered to have major urban slum areas including the Fifth Ward of Houston in Texas, Camden and Newark in New Jersey, most of Gary in Indiana, the South Suburbs of Robbins and Ford City in Chicago, Flint and Highland Park in Detroit, and major areas of St. Louis.

In other areas of the world, particularly in Europe, South America and in South Africa, the opposite may occur where the city center and inner-city areas remain clean and functional and the peripheral slums develop on the outskirts of the major metropolitan areas. While the U.S has disadvantaged areas, barrios, hoods, projects and run-down neighborhoods with few social services, these are nothing compared to the situation in other parts of the world as typified by the favelas of São Paulo, Brazil or the *basti* of Mumbai, India.

In addition to the described inner city and peripheral slum patterns, there is a third type of poor, high-density, low-resource community. In the United States, these are called *Colonias*. These are high-density, unregulated, ramshackle developments built on expanses of undeveloped land. Most of these communities have no water or sewage services and more than 2000 Colonias have been identified within the U.S., in Arizona, California and New Mexico. There are more than 1,800 designated Colonias in Texas, with 500,000 individuals living along the border in communities that lack clean drinking water, paved roads and electricity.[9] These make the southern U.S. border one of the poorest regions in the nation. Irrespective as to the cause and the pattern of high-density impoverishment, the high-density slums, ghettos and tenements, are a serious problem for public health and a vital consideration for pandemic Influenza planning.

Any city must be viewed as an ecosystem with its different populations interconnected with each other through normal daily activities. As previously mentioned, the 1918 Influenza pandemic killed more poor people than any other natural disaster that has ever occurred in the United States.[10] This same affinity for social inequity has been seen in other milder Influenza pandemics including the 2013 outbreak.

Each year, the Boston Public Health Commission issues an extremely well-researched report containing the latest demographics and health problems of the city. The 2013 Influenza outbreak was particularly noted in a report by the Boston Public Health Commission where the health officials reported that the low-income communities bore the brunt of the city's outbreak at that time.[11]

There are numerous reasons for this disparity in Influenza infection rates and mortality. Poorer areas tend to have high-density populations with more children. There are more person-to-person interactions among these households and their communities. Poor communities also tend to have a higher percentage of inhabitants with serious co-existing medical conditions such as heart failure, diabetes, and chronic obstructive lung disease. Poor communities traditionally have weak public health infrastructures and often a diminished lack of access to adequate medical care.

They also have less access to health information, including getting an Influenza vaccination. Even if the annual vaccine is effective that year, individuals that are living paycheck to paycheck may not have the money or insurance to pay for a vaccination(s) or they may not be able to miss work if they have to travel a distance to get a vaccination. They may also come into work when ill with an early Influenza infection.[12]

Staying home may not be economically feasible for persons in the lower wage occupations; these persons are less able to afford losing income from missed work or having the risk of job termination, or both. In addition to the spread of their infection with colleagues if they arrive at work coughing or sneezing, it must be remembered that individuals infected with Influenza are infectious roughly a day before they show any symptoms at all.

Given the great reliance of poor communities on public mass transit, the commute to work itself may cause active spreading of an Influenza infection across a broad age-group. Persons from low-income and minority households account for 63% of public transportation users.[13] The residents of poorer communities are much less able to stay away from work by telecommuting and may lack the necessary medical literacy to understand the importance of Non-Pharmaceutical Interventions (NPI). They may be less able to keep their children from interacting with other children (who may be infected) if the area schools suffer closure because of influenza.[12]

In the United States, low-income persons are more likely to obtain regular medical care at emergency departments and publicly funded clinics.[14] Because these locations typically do not segregate potentially infectious patients and are normally crowded, patients waiting for care in these settings are likely to have greater exposure to influenza viruses and other respiratory pathogens.[15]

Using data from the National Influenza Surveillance Network, an analysis of flu hospitalizations was made using data collected during the 2010-

2011 and 2011-2012 influenza seasons from 78 U.S. counties in 14 states (representing 9% of the U.S. population). This data showed that for both seasons combined, the incidence of influenza-related hospitalizations for high-poverty neighborhoods was nearly twice that seen in low poverty areas. In all sites and in all age and ethnic groups, there was an association of higher-level poverty with higher influenza-related hospitalization rates across all pediatric, adult ages, and ethnic groups.[16] Consequently, in all previous pandemics there has been an increased risk of influenza transmission, an increased rate of Influenza associated hospitalizations, and worse influenza outcomes in the poor, high-density areas of a city.

The high Influenza infection rates that typify the large poor, low-resource communities pose a health threat not only to the members of these communities, but also to society at large. More specifically, the health of the people who live in the surrounding metropolitan areas. The risk and significance of poor communities transmitting an influenza infection to other population groups has been explored using a sophisticated computer simulation model of the greater Washington, D.C., metropolitan region. This was developed in work with the Office of the Assistant Secretary for Preparedness and Response at the DHHS during the 2009 H1N1 pandemic. The scientists involved in this study explored the effects of a pandemic response based on different protective community vaccination rates using socioeconomic status as a factor.

Using a computer-generated baseline epidemic started by 100 randomly infected people in the simulated population of the greater Washington, D.C. region, the model contained 7,414,562 virtual individuals that encompassed the counties and demographics of Baltimore/Towson in Maryland; Washington/Arlington/Alexandria, District of Columbia-Virginia-Maryland-Virginia; Winchester, Virginia-West Virginia; Lexington Park, Maryland; and Culpeper, Virginia.[17] The simulated epidemic involved no vaccination or drug treatment, and it involved an Influenza strain with an R_0 number of 1.7, indicating the average infected person caused 1.7 other infections. The generated virtual outbreak covered a simulated period of 144 days with 106,429 new infections per day at the epidemic's peak (day 48), straining the capacities of public health and health care. The model showed 2,825,888 infections overall (38% of the total population of the region). Mortality and hospitalizations were not considered.

The computer runs were then repeated allocating the first protective vaccinations to the wealthiest counties first. The simulations in this case showed a reduction in total infections as expected, with 7,626 infections per day at the epidemic's peak. However, when the computer runs were repeated in a situation where the vaccines were quickly allocated to the poorest counties first, there was a significant drop in overall infections across all population groups. Also, there was a significant drop in the daily new infections at the epidemic's peak.

Further simulations revealed that any delay in vaccinating the poorest counties, served to increase the total number of infections over the entire region, as well as the number of new infections at the epidemic's peak. A 30-day delay in vaccinating the poorest counties increased the percentage of the regional population infected by 2.75% and only slightly diminished the number of new daily infections by a few hundred, even if the wealthier areas and counties received timely and abundant vaccine access.[18,19] Research in Europe confirms a similar argument for prioritizing vaccines to the low-income communities first, to minimize the infection rates in the higher-income communities.

If these studies are examined as a surrogate for a real-world, effective, all-aspect public health response, then there is a strong indication that in a severe Influenza pandemic, there should be an immediate strong, focused, early public health action directed at the major poor, high-density, low resource, metropolitan areas. This is not simply an issue of social justice, but a necessary requirement to reduce the infection rates over a wide region and reduce the number of new daily infections at the peak of the pandemic outbreak. Hopefully, resulting in enough case reductions that the outbreak can be managed by local authority medical surge efforts.

Following the doctrine established in the National Influenza

Pandemic Response Plan and the DHHS Guidelines, considerable financial resources have been devoted to pandemic influenza preparedness at the federal and state levels. However, as seen in the other chapters of this book, resources and planning at most local authority levels appears inadequate to implement a rapid and robust pandemic response.

Past experiences with natural disasters like hurricanes and the current socioeconomic disparities in healthcare in the United States, indicate that the poor, high-density, low-resource communities are a major target in a severe pandemic Influenza outbreak. These poor communities will proportionally suffer the most illness, hospitalizations, deaths, and post-pandemic sequalae. In addition, the population in these areas are expected to increase the Influenza infection rates throughout a wide region and significantly contribute to hospital overloading and the depletion of the limited medical resources in the area.[20]

It is therefore reasonable to suggest that these communities should have a higher focus in the national planning for a severe pandemic response. However, the National and DHHS Pandemic Influenza Plan and the government's Draft Guidance on Allocating and Targeting Pandemic Influenza Vaccine,[21] does not address social disparities in its exposure, vaccination, or treatment guidelines. While it is acknowledged that during an Influenza outbreak, certain population groups will be more vulnerable than others, it calls for faith-based and community-based organizations to develop plans "to care for dependent populations in need of medicine, or other essential needs."[22] This implies that attention to the needs of economically or socially vulnerable populations is more a matter for private charity. It is not.

The existing data strongly suggests that during a severe Influenza pandemic, it will be the poor, resource-limited areas that will be a major focus for the spread of the virus to other communities. This means that this is a strategic issue for local authorities who need to plan for the apparent fact that controlling an Influenza pandemic will require a rapid, massive, priority public health effort directed specifically at these poor communities.

However, there are problems with this concept. Many of the 61 largest U.S. cities are plagued with the same kinds of retirement legacy costs that sent Midwest cities such as Detroit into Chapter 9 bankruptcy. This includes several "too big to fail" cities like Chicago. There are a dozen major California cities that also have severe unfunded healthcare liabilities for their municipal workers. These struggling cities do not have the money or effective leadership to design and implement the public health pandemic preparations that are required, and they have set their own stage for a possible disaster like in Philadelphia in 1918.

Given the current limitations of the U.S. public health infrastructure and the disparities in health care, a severe pandemic influenza outbreak in the United States will disproportionately affect the poor, high-density, low resource, urban areas. The characteristics of these poor areas are as follows:

1. These communities are generally in the last tier for limited antiviral drugs and vaccine.
2. Least capable population group to prepare for a pandemic event.
3. Least capable population group to respond to the challenges of a pandemic.
4. Lack of sufficient health-literacy for widespread adherence to NPI strategies.
5. Historically will suffer the worst per capita illness rate.
6. Historically will suffer the worst per capita hospitalization rate.
7. Historically will suffer the worst per capita fatality rate.
8. These infections will contribute significantly to the overall urban disease spread.
9. These infections will contribute significantly to the overwhelming of medical resources.
10. The parent cities are generally unprepared for a pandemic. Some like Chicago are essentially bankrupt.

As discussed, the city of Philadelphia is considered to have been a worst-case scenario during the severe 1918 Influenza pandemic. For multiple reasons, such a scenario could be repeated in the poor, high-density, low resource areas in major U.S. cities during a modern pandemic. Such an event would be characterized by entire families requiring outside support, high numbers of the critically ill that will overwhelm the regional hospitals and intensive care units, insufficient mortuary services, disrupted lines of communication and transport, and a disorganized, overtaxed infrastructure. This is not taking into account the propensity for social unrest and infrastructure failures.

To minimize the overall number of peak infections, hospitalizations, and the deaths in the larger metropolitan areas, numerous studies indicate the poor, high-density communities should be singled out for early intervention efforts at the very start of a pandemic.

NOTES FOR CHAPTER 22

[1] United States Summary: 2010 (PDF). 2010 Census of Population and Housing, Population and Housing Unit Counts, CPH-2-5. U.S. Government Printing Office, Washington, DC: U.S. Census Bureau. 2012. pp. 20–26. Retrieved March 2013.

[2] Population Division Working Paper - Historical Census Statistics on Population Totals by Race, 1790 to 1990, and by Hispanic Origin, 1970 to 1990 - U.S. Census Bureau". Census.gov. Retrieved 2013-03-18

[3] Jackson, Kenneth T. (1985), Crabgrass Frontier: The Suburbanization of the United States, New York: Oxford University Press, ISBN 0-19-504983-7

[4] How East New York Became a Ghetto by Walter Thabit. ISBN 0-8147-8267-1.

[5] Edward Glaeser; Andrei Schleifer, "The Curley Effect: The Economics of Shaping the Electorate" (PDF), The Journal of Law, Economics, & Organization, 21 (1): 12–13

[6] Walter E. Williams, Detroit's Tragic Decline Is Largely Due to Its Own Race-Based Policies, 2012 http://www.investors.com/politics/perspective/detroit-collapse-was-due-to-racebased-politics/

[7] Lupton, R. and Power, A. (2004) The Growth and Decline of Cities and Regions. Case Brookings Census Brief No.1

[8] U.S. Census, Bureau, 2006 American Community Survey, August 2007

[9] Cisneros, Ariel. "Texas Colonias. Housing and Infrastructure Issues. Dallas Fed, June 2001. Web. 19 Mar. 2014.

[10] Sydenstricker E. The incidence of influenza among persons of different economic status during the epidemic of 1918. 1931. Public Health Rep. 2006;121(Suppl 1):191– 204.PubMed

[11] 2013-14 Influenza Season, Boston; http://www.bphc.org/healthdata/otherreports/Documents/InfluenzaReview_13-14.pdf#search=health%20of%20boston%202013%

[12] Williams DR, Jackson PB. Social sources of racial disparities in health. Health Aff (Millwood). 2005; 24(2):325–34. [PubMed: 15757915]

[13] Pucher J, Renne JL. Socioeconomics of urban travel: evidence from the 2001 NHTS. Transportation Quarterly. 2003; 57:49–77.

[14] Agency for Healthcare Research and Quality. National healthcare disparities report, 2004. Rockville (MD): US Department of Health and Human Services.

[15] Trzeciak S, Rivers EP. Emergency department overcrowding in the United States: an emerging threat to patient safety and public health. Emerg Med J. 2003; 20:402–5.

[16] Hadler JL, et. al. "Influenza-Related Hospitalizations and Poverty Levels -- United States, 2010-2012 MMWR 2016; 65(5): 101-105.

[17] Lee BY, Brown ST, et al. A computer simulation of employee vaccination to mitigate an influenza epidemic. Am J Prev Med. 2010;38(3):247–57.

[18] Lee TH., et.al. Rationing influenza vaccine. N Engl J Med. 2004; 351(23):2365–6.

[19] Bruce Y. Lee., Donald S. et.al. The Benefits to All by Ensuring Equal and Timely Access to Influenza Vaccines in Poor Communities, Health Affairs 2011 June; 30(6): 1141–1150. http://content.healthaffairs.org/content/30/6/1141.full

[20] Agency for Healthcare Research and Quality. National healthcare disparities report, 2004. Rockville (MD): US Department of Health and Human Services; 2004.

[21] http://www.pandemicflu.gov/vaccine/prioritization.pdf

[22] www.pandemicflu.gov/faq/pandemicinfluenza/pi-0001.html

23

MOVING TOWARDS AN IMPROVED NATIONAL PANDEMIC INFLUENZA RESPONSE PLAN

A S PREVIOUSLY DISCUSSED, THE BASIC STRATEGY outlined by the U.S. National Pandemic influenza Response Plan is to rapidly recognize that an Influenza pandemic is underway and quickly distribute anti-viral medications to the most vital fractions of the U.S. population. The second part of the strategy is to use behavioral-based Non-Pharmaceutical Interventions until an effective Influenza vaccine can be manufactured and nationally distributed.

We have already outlined the existing problems with this strategy, however new research indicates that a novel generation of effective anti-viral drugs and vaccines may be on the horizon. This brings new hope into salvaging the major premise of the basic National Pandemic Plan.

NEW VACCINE PRODUCTION TECHNOLOGIES

The 2017 National Pandemic Interim Update sets a broader DHHS / CDC vision of increasing Influenza vaccine production rates when a new pandemic Influenza strain emerges.[1] However, there is still much discussion over the actual effectiveness of the current seasonal Influenza vaccines, particularly for those aged 65 and older. These are precisely the age groups that are traditionally the ones most likely to die of Influenza or its complications.

There are currently two basic types of influenza vaccine that are available; inactivated influenza vaccines and live attenuated influenza vaccines. Traditionally, influenza vaccines have been produced to protect against 3 different seasonal influenza viruses (also called trivalent vaccines). However, recently vaccines which protect against 4 different viruses (quadrivalent vaccines), have now become available in some countries. The problem remains the length of time needed to produce a new vaccine.[2]

The traditional method for producing an Influenza vaccine involves growing the virus inside fertilized chicken eggs. This egg-based production method is well-established and cost-effective, but it requires millions of fertilized chicken eggs for vaccine production and it is not suitable for use in a fast-expanding pandemic. Another major problem of this system is that when RNA viruses are grown in eggs for vaccines, the viruses may adapt towards infection of the chicken embryo. When used as a vaccine for humans this cultured virus may then show less effectiveness to protect humans from infection by the original wild-type Influenza strain. Under the surveillance portion of the 2017 plan, HHS plans to better monitor the actual effectiveness of any approved new Influenza vaccines.

A second problem is that Influenza vaccine production and all vaccine production in general, is limited by the small number of factories that actually participate in this endeavor. Vaccine manufacture is largely done by private companies with a corporate culture that demands profit and a 15-20% annual net return on their sales. A one-time yearly Influenza vaccine injection is incapable of returning this type of profit compared to selling medications for chronic conditions like high-blood pressure or diabetes that are profitable for years.

With so few U.S. companies making vaccines, the majority are made overseas. This is a major strategic problem for the United States because in a pandemic emergency, the foreign country making the vaccine could nationalize its commercial production facilities to ensure it has enough vaccine for its own population. This has happened before.

In October of 2004, the United States lost half of its anticipated influenza vaccine supply when the United Kingdom suspended the manufacturing license of the California-based Chiron Corporation, a U.S. Company operating in England. At the time, Chiron had a contract to produce around 47 million doses Influenza vaccine for the United States and it was in production when the U.K. government halted the production because inspectors found bacterial contamination in some of the doses.[3] Apparently, the United States was given no advanced notice of the UK's coming suspension of Chiron's manufacturing license and apparently, the UK authorities acted to find another manufacturer to make the vaccine for their own population before they suspended Chiron's manufacturing license.

This development triggered a crisis for U.S. federal and state public health officials, who had to formulate trying to direct the remaining supply of influenza vaccine to the population groups most in need.[4] In addition, the vaccine problem associated with the 2009 "swine-flu" pandemic has already been discussed.

However, there is another method for influenza vaccine production that is based on using mammalian cells grown in large tissue cultures and then infected with a particular virus. The infected cells are then later harvested and broken apart to release the virus which is then concentrated, purified, and then inactivated and packaged into a delivery method for the vaccine.

Although the up-front costs for maintaining the operational readiness of these production plants is a significant consideration, these cell culture-based systems can be quickly scaled-up in an emergency. On August 31, 2016, FDA approved the use of a cell cultured Influenza vaccine for the production of *Flucelvax*, the first fully licensed cell-based flu vaccine in the United States.[5]

As mentioned in the 2017 HHS Pandemic Planning update, this production technology can produce vaccines that are much purer and they produce an immune response that is more directed against the wild-type virus isolates circulating in nature, than when the viruses for vaccines are grown and harvested from fertilized chicken eggs.

Modern molecular biology techniques can also now ensure that there is not a repeat of the SV-40 contaminated Polio cell-culture vaccine incident in the 1960's. This event was caused by the SV-40 virus (Simian Vacuolating Virus-40) that was discovered to cause cancer in laboratory monkeys. Between 1955 and 1963 around 90% of children and 60% of adults in the U.S. population were unintentionally inoculated with SV-40 contaminated Polio vaccines.[6] In addition, the Polio vaccines used in the former Soviet Union, China, Africa, and Japan could have been contaminated up to the year 1980, suggesting that millions of people were exposed to the virus. However, a later 35-year follow-up found no human excess of the cancers putatively associated with SV-40 in monkeys.[7]

NEW ANTIVIRAL DRUG DEVELOPMENT

Regarding antiviral drugs, DHHS has stated that a pandemic triggered by an anti-viral drug-resistant virus would pose an unprecedented challenge to the public health system, and the development of new safe, broad-spectrum antiviral drugs for seriously ill adults and children has been made a priority.

In this respect, the non-toxic drug *Favipiravir* has been stockpiled by the Japanese for the next severe Influenza pandemic. This antiviral agent selectively inhibits the Influenza RNA polymerase (Replicase) enzyme.[8] This drug should have gone into the U.S. stockpile as well, but DHHS shortsightedness selected Tamiflu before Favipiravir was fully developed. An additional antiviral drug called *Pimodivir* which acts on the Influenza virus in the same fashion has already been mentioned and is in fact under development.

Another drug (trade name Xofluza) is a medication developed by Shionogi Co., a Japanese pharmaceutical company, for the treatment of influenza A and influenza B. The medication is given as a single dose and may reduce the duration of flu symptoms by about a day. On October 24, 2018 the U.S. FDA approved Xofluza for the treatment of acute uncomplicated influenza in patients that are 12 years of age and older, and who have been symptomatic for no more than 48-hours. It is a new class of drug called a cap-*dependent endonuclease inhibitor* and it requires taking only one dose. Unlike neuraminidase inhibitors such as oseltamivir (Tamiflu) and Zanamivir (Relenza), Xofluza appears to prevent viral replication by inhibiting the endonuclease activity of the viral RNA polymerase (Replicase) enzyme. Other drugs are under development.[9]

It is the development of new and effective multi-modality anti-viral drug therapies that resurrect the premise of using antiviral drugs to cover the "vaccine gap", at least for a percentage of the population.

MOVING TOWARDS A UNIVERSAL INFLUENZA VACCINE

The Influenza Hemagglutinin protein is constructed like a small flower with a protruding "stalk" section topped by a small flower-like "cap" section. Traditionally vaccines are made against the top "Cap" section of the Hemagglutinin protein. The structure of this Cap is such that it can still function when the inevitable mutations in the genetic "blueprint" of an Influenza virus appear. This is a constant process because of the error-prone way the Influenza virus copies its genetic material.

These slight changes in the "Cap" section of the Hemagglutinin protein are enough so that each year the human immune system has difficulty recognizing it. Therefore, individuals must be re-immunized each year against the dominant circulating new viral strains that have new Hemagglutinin Cap mutations.

However, in contrast to the "Cap" section, the "Stalk" section of the Hemagglutinin protein is highly evolutionary-conserved and can tolerate only few mutations and still remain functional (Figure 26). As such, this "Stalk" section changes very little in the year to year strains that appear. This represents a new target for vaccination. Scientists are now researching to determine if a vaccine can be produced that will stimulate the human immune system to make an antibody that will attach to the "Stalk" section of Hemagglutinin. They have already demonstrated that isolated portions of the Hemagglutinin "Stalk" protein can stimulate the creation of antibodies that provide a broad protection against a variety of H1N1 and H3N2 strains in animals vaccinated with this preparation.[10]

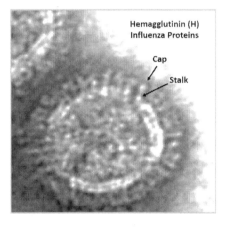

Figure 26. *Cap and Stalk Structure of the Outer Hemagglutinin Proteins of the Influenza Virus under an Electron Microscope.* U.S. Centers for Disease Control and Prevention.

Currently, there are several other innovative types of Influenza vaccines that are in preclinical or early clinical development. These may also be more potent, durable, and broadly protective than our currently licensed vaccine preparations.[11,12] In addition, there are U.S. domestic and international efforts to develop faster cell-culture based vaccine technologies that will be of enormous benefit in managing a future severe Influenza pandemic.

However, there are still major problems in pandemic preparedness that the U.S. has been slow to address. One of these is the ability to provide an early warning that a serious pandemic disease outbreak is underway. The major problems in this area are not technical, they are political and bureaucratic in nature.

A Background to Global Infectious Disease Surveillance and Outbreak Verification

The spread of infectious disease from one nation to another has been a historical global problem from the dawn of human civilization. However, in spite of devastating historical plagues every half century or so, it was not until the high-volume trade and movement of people in the 1800s and the devastating cholera epidemics of 1830 and 1847 in Europe, which made apparent the need for some type of global cooperation in public health. Consequently, the first international disease reporting system was formulated in Paris in 1851.

In 1920, following the catastrophe of the 1918 Influenza pandemic and the end of World War I, the newly formed League of Nations created the first global Health Organization and established International Sanitary Regulations to minimize the spread of serious infectious diseases. These laws made the presence of certain infectious diseases inside a country, notifiable to all the other signatory countries.

After World War II, the League of Nations transformed into the United Nations which absorbed all the other international health alerting systems in existence at the time. The United Nations formed the World Health Organization (WHO) in 1948.

In 1969, in an effort to improve its global disease surveillance, the WHO reformulated the basic international infectious disease notification protocols into *International Health Regulations* or IHRs. These international binding laws were designed to further facilitate the mandatory reporting of infectious disease outbreaks that were globally significant.

During the 1990s, scientists finally recognized the new threats posed by the increasing outbreaks of new, previously unrecognized infectious diseases and it became clear that a new approach to global public health surveillance was required. In 1995, the WHO agreed on the need to revise the IHR. To accompany these, the WHO established a formal mechanism for the investigation and follow-up of potential serious infectious outbreaks in early 1997. However, by the start of the 21st century, the WHO realized that it simply did not have the resources required to quickly recognize, respond, and contain the numerous potential pandemic situations that were occurring around the world.

Thus, a decision was made to form a *Global Outbreak and Response Network* (GOARN) among its signatory nations. This network was designed to amalgamate surveillance, technical, and response capabilities for combating new emerging infectious diseases. Primarily led by the WHO, the United States CDC is a notable partner which sends technical resources and staff to GOARN.

THE WHO GLOBAL INFLUENZA SURVEILLANCE SYSTEM

As previously discussed, Influenza viruses continuously circulate in nature, passing from birds to other susceptible animals, including other birds. These viruses are constantly making mistakes when they copy their genetic "blueprints" and they are mixing and exchanging these copied "blueprints" to create ever changing slightly new viruses. This is a survival strategy for the Influenza virus which has existed for millions of years.

In 1952, the WHO Global Influenza Surveillance Network was established to monitor which particular Influenza virus strains were changing, mixing, and widely circulating in nature at any given time. This surveillance system was necessary to help determine what the next seasonal flu strain was likely to be, and to detect any unusual strains that might indicate an increased risk for a global pandemic.

Today, this system is made up of four WHO "Collaborating Centers" and 112 National Influenza Centers (or NICs) that are located in 83 countries. The NICs constantly collect environmental samples of fresh feces from wild birds and domestic chickens. They also take nasal swabs from cows and pigs, and from humans that show signs of Influenza infection. In humans, nasal washings are preferred over throat swabs for samples. Then, the NIC laboratories try to isolate and identify any Influenza viruses in these samples. If an influenza virus is found, the NICs will ship this isolated strain to one of the four WHO Collaborating Centers for full protein and genetic analysis.

This constant process of sample collection and analysis allows scientists to determine which particular known or new strains of the Influenza virus are circulating in nature at any one time. This helps the WHO try and determine what viral strains should be included in the Seasonal Influenza vaccines that are prepared for the Northern and Southern Hemisphere each year.

Yet, this surveillance process is fallible as witnessed by the sudden 2009 emergence of the Influenza A/H1N1pan virus in Mexico rather than in Asia. Most alarmingly, this event was also accompanied by a severe vaccine production problem. It took 6-months to make a new vaccine for this H1N1 strain available and 8-months to produce it in large quantities. This was an unacceptable "vaccine gap" that could have had far reaching consequences had this Influenza strain had been more lethal than it turned out to be.

While many scientists are often critical of the WHO, particularly after the debacle involving its efforts during the West Africa and Congo Ebola outbreaks, the *Global Influenza Surveillance Network* (GISN) has been somewhat of a general success for over half a century. However, both the GOARN and the GISN still fall far short of developing a true integrated pandemic surveillance and management system. As a quick note, in May of 2011, the name of the WHO *Global Influenza Surveillance Network* was changed to the *Global Influenza Surveillance and Response System* (GISRS).

THE U.S. INFLUENZA SURVEILLANCE SYSTEM

The U.S. Influenza Surveillance System relies on international cooperation with the WHO Collaborating and National Influenza Centers as well as using an existing U.S. network of doctor's offices, hospitals, and health departments that volunteer to provide the CDC with information under the "ILINet" program.

The ILINet (Influenza-Like-Illness Network) is a voluntary program where selected physicians report their information on outpatient visits for influenza-like illness (ILI) throughout the United States. For surveillance purposes, an ILI is defined as a fever of 100°F or higher, accompanied by a cough, sore throat, or both. While these signs and symptoms are common to many diseases, a large, sudden increase in the number of ILI is often due to Influenza.

Currently the ILINet encompasses more than 2,700 voluntary healthcare providers in all 50 states, the District of Columbia and the U.S. Virgin Islands. These are referred to as "Sentinel Sites" and may entail healthcare clinicians from any specialty (e.g. family practice, pediatrics, internal medicine) and nearly any setting (e.g. private practice, emergency room, urgent care, school health center) who are likely to see patients with flu-like illness. This national network reports on more than 30 million doctor visits each year, and in New York State alone, the ILINet has 100 physicians in various specialties covering 34 state counties.

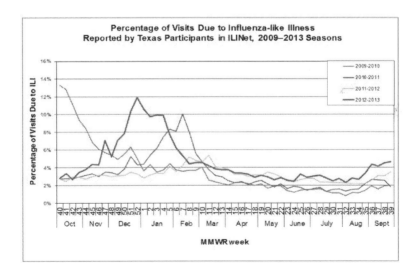

Figure 27. *ILINet Data Comparisons for Texas (October to September) (2009-2013).*
U.S. Centers for Disease Control and Prevention

Data collection and reporting is by a weekly count of patient visits due to influenza-like illness in five different age categories together with the total number of patient visits each week. This information is sent by the health provider by either the internet or facsimile, to the CDC on a weekly basis. Participating healthcare providers also send up to 11 clinical samples a year to a CDC-selected laboratory for virus isolation and sub-typing. This laboratory specimen collection is done by taking nasopharyngeal (nose) swabs or washings from a subset of ILI patients. The Department of Health in each state supplies the sample kits and pays for the sample shipping and testing.

Each sample provider is in turn issued a weekly feedback report summarizing their site's data, along with regional, state, and national Influenza data. This helps to create both a state and national picture of influenza activity each week (Figure 27). It cannot, however, be used to ascertain the actual total number of cases of Influenza in a particular state or the nation at any given time.

THE CURRENT PROBLEMS IN GLOBAL INFECTIOUS DISEASE SURVEILLANCE

The 2017 update to the U.S. National Pandemic Influenza Plan was designed to guide national preparedness activities over the coming decade.[1] The updates purport to reflect the lessons learned during the 2009 H1N1 pandemic and it gives a standard acknowledgement that there are still major problems in preparedness. It also incompletely outlines a new *"Pandemic Severity Assessment Framework"*. It states that DHHS has plans to double the number of sentinel sites that it uses to detect Influenza cases in the United States at any one time.

The 2017 DHHS plan focuses on the domains of Surveillance, Epidemiology, Laboratory Activities, Community Mitigation Measures, Medical Countermeasures, Healthcare System Preparedness, Communications, Scientific Preparedness, and Domestic/International Response Policy. It declares that these updated domains *"reflect an end-to-end systems approach to improving the way preparedness and response are integrated across sectors and disciplines, while remaining flexible"* and that this *"more nuanced and contemporary approach recognizes the interdependence of domain areas, which should lead to a better understanding of how the system will function as a whole."*

What this bureaucratic language is supposed to mean is open to question and the list of activities in the 2017 plan seem formidable for an organization whose past performance is reminiscent of the Red Queen's statement made to Alice in Lewis Carroll's *Through the Looking-Glass* that "it takes all the running you can do, just to keep in the same place."

The severe Influenza pandemics of 1957, 1968, and 2009, as well as the 2003 SARS pandemic, MERS, and the 2014 West Africa Ebola pandemic, have all been characterized by a failure to provide a timely pandemic warning to the general population, even though publicly-available information indicated that an infectious disease crisis was about to occur.[13]

One of the reasons for this failure involves the apparent inability of the WHO and the US Centers for Disease Control and Prevention to obtain verification of a new disease outbreak without formal laboratory diagnostics and a forensic-style epidemiological evaluation. To a large degree, this is understandable, and it is driven by concerns for false-positive alerts, the fear of causing socio-economic disruption, or less understandable, it is driven by political reasons. This seems to be compounded by the CDC's apparent negative bias and distrust with regards to the use of computer data mining of international media to trigger proactive pandemic investigations. This is in spite of the continuing proven value of these techniques on multiple prior occasions.

The CDC Influenza Division's surveillance response continues to be driven almost exclusively by laboratory-based surveillance data and its contacts through local and regional WHO offices. This is often time delayed. For example, the warning sequence of Suspicion / Verification and Public Notification for the 1957 Influenza pandemic took approximately two-months from local recognition to global awareness.[13] The Influenza pandemic of 1968 was associated with a one-month delay in global awareness. In the case of the 2009 influenza pandemic, verification through the IHR process took between one to two months, which suggests little notification improvement from 1968.[14,15] This and the problem of rapid ground-truth verification will be discussed further in the next chapter.

CONTINUOUS SCREENING OF COMMERCIAL AIR PASSENGERS FOR INFECTIOUS DISEASE SURVEILLANCE

While looking for possible methods to economically enhance the existing U.S. pandemic surveillance doctrine, we examined the fever (pyrexia) screening system set into place in Malaysia and Singapore during the 2002-2003 SARS pandemic. The WHO's delayed reporting of this outbreak by several weeks resulted in a significant number of cases occurring as far away as Canada and a small number of cases in the United States.

In healthy adult men and women, a fever is defined as a morning temperature of greater than 37.2°C (98.96°F), or an evening temperature of greater than 37.7°C (99.86°F). Fever is a common symptom of many medical conditions and it has been recognized as an important clinical sign since the time of the ancient Greek physician Hippocrates.

The most common cause for a fever is the inflammation caused by a bacterial or viral infection. In response to this, when activated, certain white blood cells in the human body began to release chemicals called pyrogens. These chemicals have a direct effect on the anterior hypothalamus in the deep brain. This causes the body temperature to elevate, much like raising the temperature setting on a thermostat. A continuous fever throughout the day is indicative of an acute infective process.

It is a basic principle in physics that all warm objects emit and radiate infrared radiation. The higher the temperature, the more infrared radiation is emitted. A thermographic camera (also called an infrared camera or thermal imaging camera) is a device that forms an image using the infrared radiation that is emitted from all objects based on their temperature, and digital infrared cameras can be used to take the temperature of the human body.[16] Individuals that are running a fever can easily be identified in a crowd and targeted for further individual Influenza screening including an interview, travel history, and confirmatory temperature measurement.

These thermal screening systems are already in routine use at some international ports of entry in various parts of the world. However, it is not used as a routine screening system for travelers arriving in the United States.[17] The question is why?

BREATH-SCREENING FOR INFLAMMATORY MOLECULES

Thermal cameras remain an accurate method for the non-contact screening of people with infections as elevated body temperatures, without disrupting crowd movement at airports, seaports, office buildings, high-volume pedestrian traffic areas, and other areas of mass gatherings.

However, as previously discussed, an individual in the early incubation phase of Influenza may be secreting infectious virus into the environment for 24-hours before they run a temperature or have any other symptom of the infection. Therefore, effective screening will require a second mechanism to screen high-risk groups or individuals traveling from infected areas. In this respect, there is some promising new technology.

During any respiratory virus infection, the viral-infected tissues in the upper airway send out chemical distress signals. This is much like when a ship at sea is in trouble and its captain sends out an SOS radio signal for help. In the human body, this SOS is in the form of special molecules that are released into the blood stream to signal the immune system that a virus is causing tissue damage. One of these molecules is a gaseous signaling molecule called nitric oxide (NO) which virally infected tissues start to manufacture within a few hours after infection.[18] Because NO is a type of gas, it can be found in the exhaled air of individuals suffering from airway inflammation.

In this respect, scientists and engineers have recently developed a prototype single-exhale sensing device like the breathalyzers used by the police to test automobile drivers for alcohol intoxication. An individual simply exhales into the device, which uses 3 small inexpensive semiconductor sensors to detect NO, isoprene, and ammonia biomarkers associated with Influenza infection.[18,19] The device can be used by personnel with minimal training and an individual selected for screening would simply exhale into the sensor system. Although still in the prototype stage, this suggests that the problem of screening still asymptomatic travelers is not an insolvable one.

> *The use of Thermal Scanners to trigger medical examinations and breath-testing stations would not prevent the spread of disease by air travel, but it might reduce the number of ill individuals that gain access to the high-density air transportation system. The goal in a pandemic is to delay the amplifying spread to allow more time for countermeasures to be implemented.*

NOTES FOR CHAPTER 23

[1] U.S. Department of health and Human Services. Pandemic Influenza Plan; 2017 Update https://www.cdc.gov/flu/pandemic-resources/pdf/pan-flu-report-2017v2.pdf

[2] New CDC guidelines on flu pandemic measures reflect 2009 lessons. Apr 24, 2017 http://www.cidrap.umn.edu/news-perspective/2017/04/new-cdc-guidelines-flupandemic-measures-reflect-2009-lessons.

[3] Sarah Lueck and Pui-Wing Tam, U.S. Uncovered Problems at Chiron Plant in 2003, Wall Street Journal, Oct. 11, 2004.

[4] U.S. Centers for Disease Control and Prevention, Fact Sheet: 2004-05 Flu Vaccine Shortage: Who Should Get Vaccinated, Oct. 7, 2004. www.cdc.gov/flu/protect/vaccineshortage.htm 206

[5] FDA-Approves Influenza Vaccine https://www.fda.gov/downloads/BiologicsBloodVaccines/Vaccines/ApprovedProducts/UCM522280.pdf

[6] Shah, K; Nathanson, N., (January 1976). "Human exposure to SV40: Review and comment". American Journal of Epidemiology. 103 (1): 1–12. PMID 174424.

[7] Carroll-Pankhurst, C; Engels, EA; Strickler, HD; Goedert, JJ; Wagner, J; Mortimer EA Jr. (Nov 2001). "Thirty-five-year mortality following receipt of SV40-contaminated polio vaccine during the neonatal period.". Br J Cancer. 85 (9): 1295–7. PMC 2375249 . PMID 11720463. doi:10.1054/bjoc.2001.2065.

[8] Y. Furuta, B.B. Gowen, D.F. Smee, and D.L. Barnard, Favipiravir (T-705), a novel viralRNA polymerase inhibitor. J. Antiviral Res. 2013 Nov;100(2):10.1016

[9] J. Arbuckle, et al. Inhibitors of the histone methyltransferases EZH2/1 induce a potent antiviral state and suppress infection by diverse viral pathogens. mBio. DOI: 10.1128/mBio.01141-17 (2017).

[10] Charles J Russell. Stalking Influenza Diversity with a Universal Antibody. N Engl J Med 365:16 October 20, 2011.

[11] Masar Kanekiyo, Chih-Jen Wei, Hadi M. Yassine, Patrick M. McTamney, et.al. Self-assembling influenza nanoparticle vaccines elicit broadly neutralizing H1N1 antibodies. Nature, 2013; DOI: 10.1038/nature12202.

[12] Qamar M. Sheikh, Derek Gatherer, Pedro A Reche, Darren R. Flower. Towards the knowledge-based design of universal influenza epitope ensemble vaccines. Bioinformatics, 2016; btw399 DOI: 10.1093/bioinformatics/btw399

[13] James M. Wilson V. Signal recognition during the emergence of pandemic influenza typeA/H1N1: a commercial disease intelligence unit's perspective. Intelligence and National Security, 2016 http://dx.doi.org/10.1080/02684527.2016.1253924

[14] Wilson, J. M., M. G. Polyak, J. W. Blake, and J. Collmann. "A Heuristic Indication and Warning Staging Model for Detection and Assessment of Biological Events." Journal of the American Medical Association 15, no. 2 (2008): 158–171. doi: 10.1197/jamia.M2558.

[15] Zhang, Y., H. Lopez-Gatell, C. M. Alpuche-Aranda, and M. A. Stoto. "Did Advances in Global Surveillance and Notifications Systems Make a Difference in the 2009 H1N1 Pandemic? A Respective Analysis." PLoS One 8, no. 4 (2013): e59893. doi: 10.1371/journal.pone.0059893.

[16] http:www.ferret.com.au/c/scitech/thermal-cameras-for-screening-people-with-elevated-body-temperatures-n2528870#X1Ff2Pu06oqulWuv.99

[17] CDC. Community Mitigation Guidelines to Prevent Pandemic Influenza—United States, 2017. MMWR 2017 Apr 21;66(1):1-34.

[18] F. S. Laroux, D. J. Kawachi, et.al. Role of Nitric Oxide in the Regulation of Acute and Chronic Inflammation. Antioxidants & Redox Signaling. July 2004, 2(3): 391-396. https://doi.org/10.1089/15230860050192161

[19] Pelagia-Irene Gouma, Milutin Stanacevic, et.al. Novel Isoprene Sensor for a Flu Virus Breath Monitor Sensors 2017, 17(1), 199; doi:10.3390/s17010199

24

MEDIA DATA MINING FOR IMPROVED EPIDEMIC SURVEILLANCE AND MONITORING

THE NEED FOR RAPID EPIDEMIC OUTBREAK DETECTION AND VALIDATION

Irrespective if the pathogen is a pandemic Influenza strain or the Ebolavirus, the basic management of any highly communicable lethal infectious disease involves the rapid detection of new cases, the isolation of these cases, the identification of any other people that the first cases may have been in close contact with, and the isolation of these contacts until it is confirmed that they are free of the disease. This is both a labor intensive and a time-consuming process that may easily become completely overwhelmed in a rapidly expanding epidemic/pandemic.

As seen in 2014 in West Africa, a rapidly spreading viral outbreak can become extremely difficult to control once a threshold number of infections have developed inside a high-density urban area. Most cities in the United States are within a 24-hour commercial flight from any other part of the world. This is less time than the incubation period for most known infectious diseases, even when a high-dose human exposure has occurred.

The problem is even more difficult when dealing with the outbreak of a previously unknown Emerging Infectious Disease. In this case, patient biomedical samples have to be taken to special laboratories to identify the type of infectious agent involved and how it is transmitted. This laboratory data must be combined with the clinical data derived from patients, to create a *Case Definition*. This then becomes the standard that is used to search for other cases of the disease.

At the same time, a search is made for effective drugs that can be used for prophylaxis and clinical patient management. As more is learned about the nature of the outbreak, public health authorities will assess the need for additional rapid mitigation efforts such as animal culling (common in avian Influenza outbreaks) or vector control (for insect transmitted diseases), together with the mobilization of "surge" medical resources if the epidemic continues to expand.

All of this requires time. Even a single week of delay in recognizing an epidemic outbreak, can have tremendous consequences depending on the infectious agent involved. Once a human-adapted pathogen has gained access to the international air traffic system, it can easily become pandemic. Therefore, it is essential that a lethal infectious disease outbreak be detected and confirmed as early as possible.

Note that vaccine administration has not been included as a factor here. This is because if the pathogen causing the disease is truly novel, the development of a new vaccine can take months or even years to create. Witness the years of development and testing that have gone into trying to develop an effective vaccine for Dengue and Malaria, still with little definitive results.

In recognition of these factors and the increasing threat of emerging infectious diseases associated with the travel and trade in the 21st century, a new WHO IHR revision entered into effect in 2005, along with internal hierarchical WHO protocols for outbreak verification.

THE PROCESS OF VERIFICATION

Upon the alert of a possible infectious disease outbreak, a designated WHO Outbreak Verification Team will communicate with the WHO Regional Offices, who in turn will seek further details from the Health Authorities in the affected country. This is usually done through the country's resident WHO representative. Additional information from organizations such as the International Red Cross or Médecins sans Frontières may also be sought.[1]

Upon receipt of this feedback, the Outbreak Verification Team confirms that the event meets the definition of an outbreak, its relevance to international public health is assessed, and if appropriate, further investigations are conducted. A final decision may require further consultations with the WHO regional office or the in-country health authorities. Once an outbreak is verified, this information is disseminated as an Alert to a network of partners (NGO's, and WHO Collaborating Centers) in the area and a weekly electronic bulletin is sent out to international public health officials to form a coordinated response.

This verification system follows the general principles of Surveillance: Data Collection, Data Collation, Data Analysis, and finally Data Dissemination to those who need the information for further action. This avoids the risk of false-positive alerts, but it is also associated with numerous potential delays in verification and may be subject to various political factors[2,3,4]

In fact, this is the system that completely failed in the 2014
West African Ebola Crisis.

THE PROBLEM WITH THE
WHO INTERNATIONAL HEALTH REGULATIONS (IHRs)

It is now recognized there is a delicate balance between the WHO's need to maintain trust with its signatory countries and its need for early outbreak reporting. Although common sense, it took a while to realize that compliant IHR reporting was not only dependent upon a nation's public health capability, but also upon a variety of political factors that could interfere with a nation providing WHO with an early alert of a serious infectious disease outbreak.[5] The most often cited case of this is the 2003 SARS outbreak in China.

To some scientists, this suggested that an alternate surveillance method was needed. One that was independent of any nation providing official voluntary information. They also recognized that a plethora of publicly available information was available that could alert to a sudden disease outbreak. The fact that numerous initial disease reports were originating in the electronic media and the Internet suggested this information could be garnered without having to rely on national government cooperation.[5]

THE DEVELOPMENT OF PROMED

In this respect, the *Program for Monitoring Emerging Diseases* (ProMED) is a large publicly available emerging diseases outbreak reporting system. Founded in 1994, ProMED pioneered the concept of internet-based disease reporting. The concept was to globally link a spectrum of infectious disease scientists, doctors and public health specialists together. Anyone with a computer and internet access could sign onto ProMED to report a possible disease outbreak or follow the progress of an epidemic. A first-line screening of reports was accomplished by using regional moderators scattered throughout the world. ProMED was able to demonstrate the importance of using unofficial sources of information for public health surveillance. This type of "event-based surveillance" or "epidemic intelligence" helps prevent the suppression of disease reporting by governments for bureaucratic or strategic reasons. With an average of 13 posts per day, ProMED continues to provide almost real-time information about infectious disease outbreaks on a global scale.[5]

THE DEVELOPMENT OF HEALTHMAP

Starting with the *WHO/UNICEF Joint Program on Health Mapping* in 1993, the HealthMap program evolved from the monitoring needs of the Dracunculiasis Eradication Program. Dracunculiasis is a parasitic infection and the cause of "River Blindness" in parts of Africa. The objective was to use a geographic information system (GIS) to assist in the eradication effort of the disease. This technology quickly expanded to the point where it could acquire data from a variety of electronic media sources and a formal collaboration with ProMED was established to obtain a global view of the state of infectious diseases. HealthMap represented the first freely accessible, electronic information system for monitoring, organizing, and visualizing reports of global disease outbreaks according to geography, time, and infectious disease agent. It currently monitors information sources in English, Chinese, Spanish, Russian, French, Portuguese, and Arabic. In March 2014, HealthMap was used to track early media reports of an outbreak of hemorrhagic fever in West Africa. This was eventually confirmed to be Ebola Virus Disease.

ADVANCED DATA MINING FOR INFECTIOUS DISEASE SURVEILLANCE

Despite the existence of the WHO IHR agreements, scientists discovered the initial intelligence concerning EID outbreaks were often observed first in the reports from the local, national, and international media.[6,7,8] As more and more global media began to appear on the world-wide web, the concept of automatic data mining for disease outbreak detection was developed. But first, scientists had to discover a method to filter out of the large amounts of "noise" across multiple languages to detect a true epidemic signal. The answer to the problem was to develop special computer algorithms to scan the "Big Data" on the internet for signs of an early disease outbreak.[9] "Big Data" is a term used to describe data sets that are so large and complex that traditional data processing methods are inadequate.

In this respect, the successful analysis of Big Data is defined by five "V" factors. These include Volume (the quantity of data that is collected), Velocity (the speed at which the data is collected and disseminated), Value, Variety (the multiplicity of sources that are used to compile the data) and Veracity (how much useless noise is in the data).

The tremendous amount of information in Big Data requires the use of special software algorithms for predictive analytics, behavior analytics, or other advanced methods that can extract both value and trends from many diverse data sets to reveal patterns or predictions of an event. This process is called "Data Mining" and in some applications, it requires the use of massively parallel software running on tens, hundreds, or even thousands of servers. This is seen in the SETI (Search for Extraterrestrial Intelligence) and Asteroid Mapping projects in which anyone with a computer can participate in through Internet links.

The Global Public Health Intelligence Network (GPHIN) is an existing automated electronic public health early-warning system. Designed for commercial applications it was developed by the scientists at Canada's Public Health Agency. It is now part of the *WHO Global Outbreak Alert and Response Network*.[10]

The GPHIN uses automated computers with automatic language translation and advanced data mining algorithms to continuously scan thousands of electronic sources of public information worldwide. This includes the news-feed aggregators such as *Al Bawaba* and *Factiva II*, and it constantly scans the Internet, websites, and digital copies of newspapers along with global news wires and other media sources, in twelve different languages. Custom algorithms identify potential signals of emerging public health events around the globe while filtering out obvious irrelevant data or "noise".

Potential indicators of outbreaks (termed "signals") are flagged and rapidly assessed by a multilingual, multidisciplinary human team. When a risk is identified, these analysts disseminate relevant information and alerts to senior officials and partners for further decision-making. The system has had remarkable success.

During the Asian SARS outbreak in 2002, GPHIN automatically discovered a financial report describing that a Chinese pharmaceutical company had a sudden increase in their sale of an antiviral drug in the Guangdong Province of that country. Consequently, the system alerted to the possible outbreak of a major new respiratory virus in that region. This report was coincident with the first outbreak of the deadly new SARS virus. Yet, it took the WHO an additional month to release its own first report of the SARS outbreak. By that time, the disease had spread to Hong Kong, Singapore, Canada, and the United States.[11]

In April 2012, the GPHIN identified eight cases of a severe, unknown respiratory disease with one death in the Mideast country of Jordan. Analysts determined the data to be reliable and the GPHIN issued an alert notifying its stakeholders and the WHO, about these cases. Following further investigation and the results of a retrospective laboratory analysis, an outbreak of the previously unknown *Middle East Respiratory Syndrome Coronavirus* (now known as MERS-CoV) was confirmed. An International Health Regulations (IHR) Notification by the WHO was eventually posted weeks later. Again, by that time, multinational disease spread had already occurred.

Use of the GPHIN has now been adopted by a number of nations as part of their obligations to meet the new IHR for early infectious disease detection and reporting.

BIG DATA USE FOR SITUATION MONITORING

There are indications that global media data mining can also play a role in the continuous monitoring of outbreaks as they unfold.[12,13] This would mean that the on-going evolution of an outbreak and the effectiveness of the response strategies implemented against it could be assessed in almost real-time.

As an example, during the 2014 response to the Ebola outbreak in

West Africa, the use of smartphones and Twitter data in Nigeria, helped to identify a new area Ebola outbreak almost three-days before it was recognized by the WHO.[13]

Other examples of relevant data that could be mined for situational awareness include the sudden cancellation of commercial air flights, the issuance of travel advisories or new health screening procedures that are suddenly implemented at a county's entry portals.

POTENTIAL ADDITIONAL SOURCES OF BIG DATA

Internet, smart phone capabilities and social media in general, have all expanded rapidly since the GPHIN was developed. Social media venues such as Linked-In, Twitter and Facebook have all witnessed a rapid growth over the last decade and they generate an enormous amount of user-generated content. New algorithms are already in development and specifically directed to access and analyze social media for early signals of a new infectious disease outbreak. It is possible that novel crowdsourcing applications could be applied to the internet and mobile phone networks to capture voluntarily submitted symptoms from the general public in near real-time.

However, there are problems in using social media as a data source for infectious disease surveillance on a global scale. This is because not everyone has access to a computer or smart phone. Consequently, the data derived from social media platforms only reflects the population that uses this modem of communication.

This is not only a possible source of bias in the collected data, but it is also a significant omission factor in the under-developed parts of the world where smart phones are rare. Unfortunately, as we have explained, many of these areas are also where new emerging disease outbreaks are likely to occur.

An examination of a database of 335 EID origins from 1940 to 2004, show a non-random pattern of emerging RNA viral disease associated with the "Biodiversity Hotspots" on the Earth.

A "Hotspot" is a region defined as containing 1,500 endemic species of vascular plants that have undergone at least a 70% loss of their primary vegetation. There are 34 areas around the world that qualify under this definition, with nine other possible candidates.[14]

Historical reviews show that a majority of the viral EID events have originated in wildlife. When these are plotted on a global map, the areas at greatest risk for a zoonotic viral emergence are the "Hotspots" associated with the equatorial tropics (Figure 28).

These ecological "Hotspots" are also home to 1.2 billion of the world's poorest people with a fast-growing population. The poverty and poor infrastructures in many of these tropical regions make it difficult to apply to any sort of data-driven outbreak surveillance system.[15, 16]

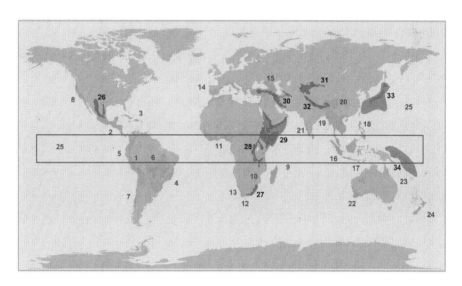

Figure 28. *Biodiversity Hotspots with Areas at the Greatest Risk for Outbreaks of Emerging Infectious Disease. Boxed Area.* Modified from Myers, N., et. al. (2000)[15]

It also compounds the problems associated with the rapid ground-truth verification of a data-driven outbreak alert.

Notes for Chapter 24

[1] CDC. Public Health 101 Series: Introduction to Public Health Surveillance. Accessed at https://www.cdc.gov/publichealth101/documents/introduction-tosurveillance.pdf

[2] World Health Organization. [Internet] Epidemic intelligence - Systematic event detection. Geneva: World Health Organization; 2015.

[3] Heymann DL, Rodier GR. Global surveillance of communicable diseases. Emerg Infect Dis.1998; 4:362–5.

[4] John S. Mackenzie (26 April 2000). "GOARN and One Health: lessons learnt" (PDF). WHO.

[5] Suthar AB, Allen LG, Cifuentes S, Dye C, Nagata JM. Lessons learnt from implementation of the International Health Regulations: a systematic review. Bull World Health Organ. 2018 Feb 1;96(2):110121E.

[6] Keller M, Blench M, Tolentino H, Freifeld CC, Mandl KD, Mawudeku, A., et al. Use of unstructured event-based reports for global infectious disease surveillance. Emerg Infect Dis. 2009 May;15(5):689-95.

[7] Brownstein, John S.; Freifeld, Clark C.; Madoff, Lawrence C. (21 May 2009). "Digital Disease Detection — Harnessing the Web for Public Health Surveillance". New England Journal of Medicine. 360 (21): 2153–2157. doi:10.1056/NEJMp0900702. PMC 2917042.

[8] Grein TW, Kamara KB, Rodier G, Plant AJ, Bovier P, Ryan MJ, Ohyama T, Heymann, D.L. Rumors of disease in the global village: outbreak verification. Emerg Infect Dis. 2000 Mar Apr;6(2):97-102.

[9] George G, Haas MR, Pentland A. Big Data and management. Acad Manag J. 2014;57(2):321

[10] Mykhalovskiy E, Weir L. The Global Public Health Intelligence Network and early warning outbreak detection: A Canadian contribution to global public health. Can J Public Health. 2006 Jan-Feb; 97(1):42-4.

[11] Heymann DL, Rodier G. Global surveillance, national surveillance and SARS. Emerg Infect Dis. 2004;10(2):173-5.

[12] Hay SI, George DB, Moyes CL, Brownstein JS. Big Data opportunities for global infectious disease surveillance. PLoS Med. 2013;10(4):e1001413.

[13] Gittelman S, Lange V, Gotway Crawford CA, Okoro CA, Lieb E, Dhingra SS, et al. A new source of data for public health surveillance: Facebook likes. J Med Internet Res. 2015 Apr 20;17(4):e98.

[14] Odlum M, Yoon S. What can we learn about the Ebola outbreak from tweets? Am J Infect Control. 2015;43(6):563-71.

[15] Myers, N., et. al. (2000) "Biodiversity hotspots for conservation priorities." Nature 403:853 858. doi:10.1038/35002501e

[16] Jones KE, Patel NG, Levy MA, Storeygard A, Balk D, Gittleman JL, Daszak P. Global trends in emerging infectious diseases. Nature. 2008; 451:990–993.

25

PROBLEMS IN RAPID GROUND-TRUTH VERIFICATION OF EMERGING DISEASE OUTBREAKS

HISTORICAL BACKGROUND

With World War II still fresh in the U.S. military's mind and with the Korean war underway a series of open-air Biological Warfare simulant tests were conducted on San Francisco in 1950. These were designed to assess the effect of a Large Area Coverage biological weapons (BW) attack on a high-density American city. The results of this test shocked the scientists involved and it gave rise to the creation of a special group at the U.S. Centers for Disease Control (CDC) called the Epidemic Intelligence Service or EIS.[1] The EIS was tasked to investigate any sudden outbreaks of infectious disease and to collect biomedical samples and quickly analyze these to determine if they were from the first high-dose exposure cases following a covert BW attack on America.

As this Cold War hysteria abated, the EIS medical intelligence unit found practical surveillance applications in public health with respect to environmental toxins, polio, food and water safety.[1] *However, the original goal pf the EIS was to rapidly provide ground truth verification that a metropolitan biological warfare attack had taken place.*

From the 1970's on, the Center for Disease Control slowly grew into a government bureaucracy eventually changing its name to the "Centers for Disease Control *and Prevention*". During this transition, an entire generation of infectious disease investigators and large blocks of institutional knowledge in the fields of bacteriology, parasitology, viral disease outbreaks, and entomology, simply disappeared from a lack of funding.

By the mid 1980's the leadership of the CDC realized that a variety of new infectious diseases were cropping up with an alarming frequency. The list of these "new" diseases was impressive; HIV in 1983, Hepatitis-E and Human Herpesvirus-6 in 1988, Hepatitis-C in 1989, Venezuelan Hemorrhagic Fever in 1991, a new more dangerous strain of Cholera in 1992, Brazilian Hemorrhagic Fever and Hantavirus in 1994, and Herpesvirus-8 in 1995. In addition, there were outbreaks of Cyclosporidia, Physteria, the Australian Hendra Virus, the Malaysia Nipah Virus, and a new Ebolavirus subtype out of Uganda. By the start of the 21st century, the rates of tuberculosis among some of the demographic groups in America's inner cities grew to record high levels.

Of the 183-million people who were dying every year on Earth, at least one-third were still succumbing to some type of an infectious disease. In a desperate response, the CDC's experts in chronic disease and occupational epidemiology, now had to orient themselves to investigate outbreaks of bacterial, viral, and parasitic disease. The Center eventually built new modern laboratories and in 1999 it established the Laboratory Response Network (LRN) to respond to emergencies. This network included state and local public health labs, with veterinary, military, and international labs all linked together for public health preparedness.

In an attempt to reestablish some type of an epidemic unit, the CDC created an emergency response branch within its new Division of Preparedness and Emerging Infections (DPEI). Called the National Center for Emerging and Zoonotic Infectious Diseases (NCEZID, this new unit was designed to provide a rapid epidemiological capability and laboratory support for new EID outbreaks. In addition, the CDC fostered closer cooperation with the WHO Global Outbreak Alert and Response Network.

During the 2014 Ebola crisis in West Africa it was hard to assess the effectiveness of the CDC because the U.S. Department of Homeland Security was inexplicably put in charge of the U.S. Ebola response. The CDC appeared to have been marginalized. After the U.S. Ebola fiasco, apparently the DHS has now been removed as the lead agency for any future pandemic response. Yet in 2019, it still seems to still have some say in the DRC Congo Ebola crisis, apparently with respect to screening illegal Congo immigrants crossing at the southern U.S. Border.

CURRENT PROBLEMS IN THE RAPID VERIFICATION OF INFECTIOUS DISEASE OUTBREAKS

The Global Outbreak and Response Network uses the new International Health Regulations (IHR) to require all of the 191 WHO member countries to have some capability for early infectious disease detection and reporting. Under contract, GPHIN continues the task of extracting disease outbreak information from the global electronic media. Yet unacceptable delays in alerting to potential pandemic outbreaks continue to occur.[2]

As discussed, the inadequate compliance to the IHRs by some nations has been a limiting factor in the current global surveillance system and not just with China's failure to timely report the new Severe Acute Respiratory Syndrome (SARS) outbreak in 2003. The slow response to the 2014 West Africa Ebola pandemic occurred not only because of the lack of a functional area public health infrastructure, but also because of a failure of the WHO to determine the ground-truth of the developing situation.

It must be noted that the West African Ebola outbreak occurred in a permissive foreign environment without on-going rebel activity to hinder viral containment efforts. The presence of low-intensity warfare in a future outbreak area will magnify the difficulties of outbreak containment. This is already being observed in the Congo where an Ebola outbreak continues to spread.

RAPID GROUND-TRUTH VERIFICATION IN REMOTE, CONTESTED AREAS

As outlined, there is a non-random global pattern of emerging disease outbreaks and a high percentage of Emerging Infectious Diseases are associated with "Biodiversity Hotspots".[3,4,5,6] These geographical regions are home to many of the world's poorest people with access to only a minimal medical and communications infrastructure. Of even more report, is the fact that some 90% of all the armed conflicts seen between the years of 1950 through to 2000, have also occurred within these "Hotspots".[7]

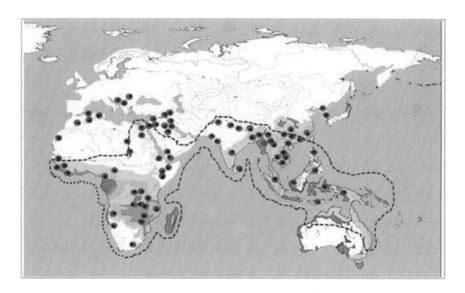

Figure 29. *Armed conflicts (colored dots), biodiversity hotspots (shaded) and the geographic range of bats associated with severe RNA virus disease including Hendravirus, Nipahvirus, and the Filoviruses (dotted line).* Adapted from[8,9,10]

The "Hotspots" may offer a tactical advantage to insurgent rebel groups via their remote and difficult terrain. Their infectious disease risk is derived from the fact that guerilla forces living in a remote insurgent camp have an increased probability of human–wild animal contact. In addition, dispersed civilian war refugees must also hunt for meat, gather firewood, and build camps, with additional pressure placed on the native wildlife in these regions.[7,11]

These activities place humans well inside the complex interplay of RNA viruses with their primary animal reservoirs and vectors in the area.[12] It also makes the verification of a new disease outbreak in these areas difficult. The lack of a communications infrastructure makes data mining efforts problematic and the presence of armed rebel groups make it dangerous to insert civilian teams for outbreak verification.

THE PROBLEM OF MEDICAL EVACUATION FROM CONFLICT AREAS

Many of these Biodiversity "Hotspots" are also a working environment for conservationists, missionaries, non-government aid workers, representatives of the U.S. Agency for International Development (USAID), and sometimes U.S. military special operations or Medical Civil Action Programs (MEDCAP). Consequently, these personnel also run a risk of contracting a known or previously unknown lethal emerging zoonotic viral infection.

The evacuation of an infected and critically ill U.S. citizen out of a "Hotspot" could easily require a mix of local liaisons, ground vehicle transport, rotary wing airlift, or even waterborne littoral transport before their final leg for aeromedical evacuation back to the United States. The potential for the secondary infection of any attending medical personnel is extremely high if protective equipment and isolation methods are not employed throughout the entire patient transport chain. Such multi-platform transport will also entail a dangerous delay in confirming a diagnosis and initiating any current or future antiviral therapies, possibly not until after the window for successful treatment has passed.

In addition, the final receiving medical facility may not have the necessary diagnostic reagents or recognize the true nature of the pa-tient's infection. In 1996, a nurse in Johannesburg, South Africa died from a secondary infection acquired from an unrecognized Ebolavirus Disease case that was air evacuated out of Gabon.[13]

The aeromedical transportation of an acutely ill patient with high viral shedding, from a third-world country to a high-level treatment facility, presents other special problems. These include the confined in-ternal space of a transport aircraft, the difficulties in ensuring complete interior decontamination, airframe vibration, the use of recirculated air for aircraft pressurization, and the risk of sudden cabin depressuriza-tion. All these combine to make this a special medical environment.

Following the first simultaneous 1976 outbreaks of Ebolavirus Dis-ease in Nzara, Sudan and Yambuku, Zaire, and a growing recognition of the threat of EID to overseas U.S. personnel, the Department of Defense created the *Aeromedical Isolation and Special Medical Augmen-tation Response Team* (AIT-SMART).[14,15]

Established in 1978, this was a rapid-response unit was composed of military veterinary technicians, two military critical care nurses, and 2 to 3 military physicians combined with a USAF worldwide airlift ca-pability and secure STU-3 communications. This team was designed to safely evacuate highly contagious U.S. patients out of outbreak areas under high-level biological containment. At the same time, it would provide critical care nursing for these isolated patients during their transport by a variety of global USAF rotary-wing and fixed-wing assets.

Back at Fort Detrick in Maryland, the AIT-SMART was associated with a specialized Medical Containment Suite (MCS) at the US Army Medical Research Institute for Infectious Diseases (USAMRIID). This was designed to provide ICU-level patient care under full Bi-osafety Level-Four (BSL-4) conditions (Figure 30).[16]

The MCS became operational in 1972 for use in the case of labora-tory pathogen accidents, and it became the destination for any highly contagious patient transported by the AIT-SMART. In this respect, the unit's Aircraft Transit Isolator could be attached directly to an access port situated on the external wall of the main USAMRIID building to provide continuously-contained movement of the patient into the MCS BSL-4 medical care suite. The evacuation team members wore protective Tyvek suits with HEPA-filtered Racal positive-pressure respirators and hoods sealed to provide a positive internal pressure inside a containment garment. For patient isolation, the team employed a Vickers Aircraft Transit Isolator with its interior maintained at a pressure negative to the external environment via a controlled air-flow through high-efficiency particulate air (HEPA) filters.

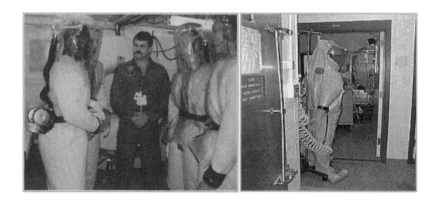

Figure 30. *(a) RACAL Powered Respirators. (b) BSL-4 Medical Containment Suite.*

Inside the 2-bed MCS suite, intensive care physicians and nurses from the Walter Reed National Military Medical Center practiced with simulated patients to provide clinical care under BSL-4 conditions.[16] This unique concept brilliantly combined BSL-4 level patient care with several suites of BSL-4 laboratories staffed by highly experienced researchers in exotic infectious diseases, along with BSL-4 clinical and pathology laboratories, a large experimental animal colony with strain mice, guinea pig, and non-human primate models, and scientists and physicians highly experienced in disease assessment, pathogenesis, and experimental vaccine development.

In 2010, the AIT-SMART was decommissioned, and this unified

capability was lost. As an alternative, the mission was handed over to one of the US Air Force's *Critical Care Air Transport Teams* (CCATT).[17] This USAF aeromedical unit is designated to use a Gentex® Patient Isolation Unit (PIU). The PIU is a temporary, single-use, portable structure designed to temporarily isolate a highly infectious patient. However, it provides only an enhanced patient isolation as the last step in the medical evacuation process (Figure 31). It does nothing to address the problems inherent in the evacuation of viral-infected patients from far-forward remote areas.

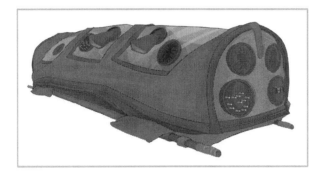

Figure 31. *Patient Isolation Container.*

There is one other important point to make. From its inception, the AIT-SMART was designed to only operate in permissive environments with readily accessible air evacuation routes. It was not suitable for insertions into remote rural geographical areas involved in asymmetrical warfare. As studies demonstrate, these are precisely the areas where new outbreaks of new highly lethal pathogens are most likely to occur.

In the next chapter we will discuss a possible solution to the problems of both ground-truth verification and the rapid aeromedical evacuation of infected U.S. personnel from conflict areas.

NOTES FOR CHAPTER 25

[1] Langmuir, A D; Andrews J M (March 1952). "Biological warfare defense. The Epidemic Intelligence Service of the Communicable Disease Center". American Journal of Public Health and the Nation's Health. 42 (3): 235–8. doi:10.2105/AJPH.42.3.235. PMC 1526024. PMID 14903237.

[2] Thomas W. Grein , Kande-Bure O. Kamara, Guénaël Rodier, Aileen J. Plant, Patrick Bovier, Michael J. Ryan, Takaaki Ohyama, and David L. Heymann Rumors of Disease in the Global Village: Outbreak Verification EID Journal Volume 6Number 2—April 2000

[3] Daniel J Salkeld, Kerry A Padgett, and James Holland Jones, A meta-analysis suggesting that the relationship between biodiversity and risk of zoonotic pathogen transmission is idiosyncratic. 2013, Ecology Letters. Volume 16, Issue 5, pages 679–686.

[4] Hanson, T., Brooks, T.M., Gustavo, A. et.al. Warfare in Biodiversity Hotspots. Conservation Biology, 2009. Volume 23, No. 3, 578–587. \

[5] Draulens ,D. & van Krunkelsven, E. The impact of war on forest areas in the Democratic Republic of Congo. 2002. Cambridge Journals, Tervuren, Belgium.

[6] Hart,T., Mwinyihali R., Armed Conflict and Biodiversity in Sub-Saharan Africa: The Case of the Democratic Republic of Congo. 2001. Biodiversity Support Program / WWF, Washington, D.C.

[7] Morse, S.S. Factors in the emergence of infectious disease. Emerg Infect Dis. 1995; 1:7-15. [PMC free article] [PubMed]

[8] Interim Version 1.1; Ebola and Marburg virus disease epidemics: preparedness, alert, control, and evaluation WHO/HSE/PED/CED/2014.05

[9] Sulkin, S. & Allen, R. 1974. Virus infections in bats. Monographs in Virology, 8: 1-103.

[10] Mackenzie, J., Field, H. & Guyatt, K. 2003. Managing emerging diseases borne by fruit bats (flying foxes) regarding henipaviruses and Australian bat lyssavirus. Journ Applied Microbiology, 94.

[11] Taylor, L.H., Latham, S.M., Woolhouse, M.E.J. 2001. Risk factors for human disease emergence. Royal Society Philosophical Transactions Biological Sciences, 356(1411): 983-989.

[12] Smith, KF, Goldberg, M. et.al., Global Rise in Infectious Disease Outbreaks. 2014; J.R. Soc. Interface 11: 21140950. http://dx.doi.org/10.1098/rsif.2014.0950.

[13] Sidley P. Fears over Ebola spread as nurse dies. BMJ. 1996 Nov 30;313:1351.

[14] Mark R. Withers, George W. Christopher, Steven J. Hatfill, and Jose J. Gutierrez-Nunez, Chapter 11, *"Aeromedical Evacuation of Patients with Contagious Infections"*

In; Aeromedical Evacuation; Management of Acute and Stabilized Patients. Eds. William Hurd, John Jernigan. Springer Press.

[15] Christopher, G. W. and E. M. Eitzen, Jr, "Air evacuation under high-level biosafety containment: the aeromedical isolation team"; Emerg Infect Dis, 1999: Mar-Apr; 5(2): 241–246.

[16] Marklund, LeRoy A., "Patient care in a biological safety level-4 (BSL-4) environment"; Crit Care Nurs Clin N Am: 15 (2003), 245– 255.

[17] Beninati W, Meyer MT, Carter TE., The critical care air transport program. Crit Care Med. 2008 Jul; 36 (7 Supp.): S370-6.

26

EMERGING INFECTIOUS DISEASE THREATS AND U.S. NATIONAL SECURITY

SEVERAL SUMMARY HISTORICAL REVIEWS demonstrate an alarming and continuing increase in the number of emerging infectious diseases that are jumping from wild animals to humans worldwide.[1]

There is also a disturbing number of previously unknown viral sequences found in biomedical samples taken from wild animals during general surveys.[2] As we have mentioned, there is an average of one or two novel EID outbreaks every year and it is estimated that 10 to 40 new viruses are expected to emerge into human populations over the next 20-years. The pathogenic severity of these viruses and their epidemic/pandemic potential are currently unknown. Multiple unrecognized lethal species-crossing viruses still exist in nature and the zoonotic transfer of RNA viruses from wildlife represents a continuing and increasing threat to global human health.[3,4,5]

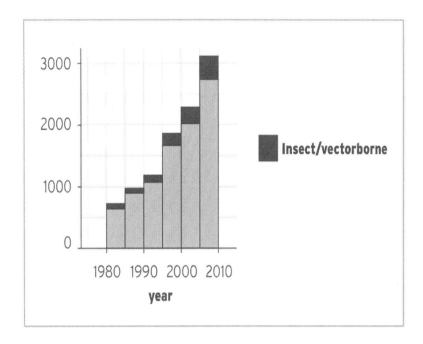

Figure 32. *Global number of human infectious disease outbreaks 1980-2010.* Total global outbreaks left axis. Diseases transmitted by insect vectors (dark color). [6]

In 2000, the United States National Intelligence Council published a National Intelligence Estimate titled, '*The Global Infectious Disease Threat and Its Implications for the United States*". This was the first time the U.S. Intelligence Community had publicly confirmed that infectious disease threats were now a national security issue. Unfortunately, a number of the assessments made in this Intelligence Estimate have now been validated.[6]

THE NEED FOR AN INDEPENDENT
U.S. DISEASE INTELLIGENCE COLLECTION ENTITY

There is a general public assumption that the WHO, the CDC, and other international public health organizations are capable of effectively monitoring the world for developing health security issues and that timely warnings will be issued along with appropriate countermeasures. This is an incorrect assumption on all accounts.

The failure of the WHO and the CDC to provide early pandemic alerting is a constantly recurring theme for the last two decades. It was witnessed by the West Nile virus outbreak in New York City, the significant delay in realizing the emergence of the SARS virus in southern China, the MERS virus in the Mideast, the Ebola crisis in West Africa, the Chikungunya virus in Puerto Rico, and the Zika virus in Florida.

The US capability for global disease surveillance and a rapid response appears to be dramatically faltering.[7] There is little proactive effort in improving response times and a new, untreatable, extremely lethal, and highly contagious Emerging Infectious Disease can appear and begin to spread in the United States at any time. It is clear that the United States must develop new, more direct methods to derive rapid actionable intelligence pertaining to global disease outbreaks.

This has prompted scientists to continue to explore open-source data mining efforts for the rapid detection of new emerging disease outbreaks.[8] In 2008, a new state-of-the-art web harvesting platform was designed by former senior Microsoft engineers. Subsequent venture capital was used to create the *Veratect Corporation*. Like GPHIN before it, this company was focused on producing early warning disease intelligence for commercial clients. Operating out of two separate data mining operations centers, it employed language-fluent analysts to continuously monitor global media traffic in fifty-languages. Its senior analysts were experienced in monitoring global media for disease activity and their leader was well versed in the framework of the WHO IHRs.

Veratect focused on reducing the extraneous 'noise' in the outbreak-related information on the World Wide Web, including the data derived from electronic discussion groups. Its media data mining effort was focused on acute, rapidly evolving, and unusual disease events with the potential for a threat to U.S. national security.[7] Detected events were reviewed in daily meetings. Occasionally, a disease event would be referred to outside parties for their opinion and to gather further information such as:

- Is a serious infectious disease outbreak actually underway?
- What is the microorganism involved?
- Is it a known pathogen or is it one that is potentially new to science?

This process is called *ground-truth verification* and it is a major rate-limiting factor for the rapid early warning of emerging outbreaks with potentially serious pandemic potential.

Under normal daily operations, Veratect's scientists reviewed up to 80 computer alerts coming from as many as 40 different countries, involving up to 35 potentially serious infectious disease outbreaks *every single day*. The company was essentially a 21st century electronic sheepdog, constantly watching over its human flock by searching for the early signs of the next possibly catastrophic global pandemic.

It did not have long to wait.

On 23 February of 2009, Veratect's data mining system intercepted a news media report describing the outbreak of an undiagnosed disease that had killed fourteen individuals in Santorales in Mexicali, Mexico. Children were among the victims and hundreds of women had gathered to protest this event on a highway into the city. There was no 'persistent signal' (further media reports) so the assumption was that the event was due to a brief outbreak of a bacterial or rickettsial infectious disease. That same day, the Veratect computers triggered to a non-specific report of an abrupt increase in respiratory disease among children in Ciudad Juárez, Chihuahua State. This was located roughly 500 miles east of Mexicali. Again, there was no 'persistent signal' over the next few days.

Then on 6 April, Veratect's data mining system alerted to multiple local and national media reports from Mexico that described an unusual outbreak of an undiagnosed respiratory disease in La Gloria in Veracruz State.[9] This was roughly 160 miles southeast of Ciudad Juárez where the outbreak had occurred 12-days before. This new outbreak in La Gloria also involved pediatric deaths and there was a reference of a possible connection to pigs, but no further reporting was noted.

La Gloria is a tiny Mexican town with a population of 1092 men and 1151 women and during the weekdays, over half the population transiently live and work in the high-density capital of Mexico City located some 120 miles to the west. The town of La Gloria is also situated only 5-miles from the *Granjas Carroll de Mexico* farming operation, which raises nearly 1,000,000 pigs annually. Many of the town's residents had already protested this pig farming operation because of the odor emanating from the facility.

In an ideal world, this should have been the time when a small official U.S. medical verification team could have been dispatched to work with the Mexican health authorities to clarify the reports that triggered the Veratect computers. However, Veratect did not have such a team and it was forced to use interpersonal contacts to try and gain some degree of ground truth verification of what was happening.

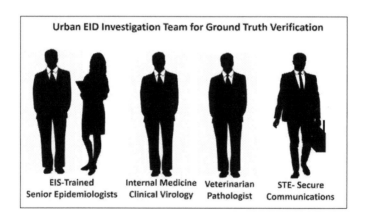

Figure 33. *Small Ground-Truth Verification Team.*

Had it existed, such a multi-disciplinary team might have included a veterinarian specializing in animal infectious diseases, two epidemiologists to collect and analyze data, and an internal medicine physician with experience in tropical diseases and clinical virology. A fifth member of the team would have a variable specialty depending on the situation. The team would carry a STE encrypted communications package for secure "landline" and satellite communications (Figure 33). It would be dependent on the host country's cooperation and the country's own diagnostic laboratory capability. However, the team would also be capable of collecting biomedical samples and safely transporting them back to U.S. laboratories if necessary.

Ten-days later on April 16, Veratect's computers triggered to reports from the Oaxaca State in Mexico that referred to an outbreak of 'atypical pneumonia' and an attempt by the Mexican health authorities to rule out SARS. The U.S. President was in Mexico City on that day and a member of the U.S. delegation was infected with the now spreading A/H1N1 Influenza virus. The delegate later transmitted this infection to his own family.[10]

On April 20, Veratect was informed that scientists from the Canadian Public Health Service had been urgently requested to fly to Mexico to evaluate a cluster of unusual respiratory disease fatalities in Mexicali and Veracruz.[9] Two-hours later, Veratect informed multiple groups within the CDC of the situation. Incredibly, the CDC had no awareness of the events in Mexico but related that several unusual H1N1 influenza cases had appeared in California and Texas. The discovery of these cases in California was made incidentally by a US Navy research laboratory.[9]

With the realization that there was a complete lack of integrated situational awareness at the CDC Director's Emergency Operations Center, Veratect again advised the CDC of the situation in Mexico, emphasizing that the situation required immediate attention.[9]

On 22 April, the CDC issued a public announcement for its two confirmed H1N1 cases in California. It made no mention of Mexico. Veratect then began to pressure the CDC for the laboratory results from Mexico. Canadian scientists had this laboratory data with them when they returned to the Canadian National Microbiology

Laboratory and on 22 of April the following day, Canada issued a Public Health Alert for the presence in Mexico of a novel Influenza A/H1N1 strain with pandemic potential.

The WHO would not declare the presence of this novel A/H1N1 Influenza strain in Mexico a *Public Health Emergency of International Concern* until 25 April. The CDC did not issue its own public warning until after the WHO announcement.

The independent disease surveillance system operated by Veratect played a key role in the early reporting of unusual media patterns describing an 'atypical pneumonia' in Mexico that was later referred to as the "swine flu". This ultimately became the 2009 A/H1N1 Influenza pandemic.

The company Veratect remained operational until after the 2009 H1N1 Influenza outbreak when it became a commercial casualty of the global recession. But this was not before it proved the necessity and advantages of a public/private-independent partnership for global disease surveillance and the necessity for improved rapid verification of data mining alerts.

KEY LESSONS LEARNED FOR FUTURE PANDEMIC SURVEILLANCE

During the evolving 2009 Influenza pandemic, the CDC Director's Emergency Operations Center (EOC) had a complete lack of situational awareness about the events that originated and were currently taking place in Mexico. This is alarming because the CDC-EOC was designed to act as a fusion center for all incoming data pertaining to a developing infectious disease event. This indicates that the CDC's current system for global disease surveillance is not optimally functional in its current form.

The CDC Influenza Division insists on using the WHO *Global Outbreak Alert and Response Network* and its IHR partnerships, or the laboratory-based surveillance data it obtains through its own actions. As seen in the 2009 episode in Mexico, the acquisition of this data is most often accompanied by a significant time-delay.[11]

In spite of the requirements of the WHO IHR's, every nation is quite capable of delaying or under-reporting an infectious disease out-break within their borders. This may be due to concerns over diagnostic uncertainty, political reasons, or a fear of potential socioeconomic dis-ruption. Consequently, under the current global surveillance system, the alert of an evolving infectious disease event can be delayed for days to weeks, depending on the WHO and the CDC's ability to obtain la-boratory and epidemiological evaluations for ground-truth verification.

Veratect demonstrated that a system for independent media data mining outside of the WHO/CDC system can be a key source of early pandemic outbreak information. However, to issue a national U.S. public alert, the company had to have a ground-truth verification from Mexico in the form of credible laboratory and epidemiological data.[9] This is in conflict with the need for an early warning for any rapidly evolving public health emergency.

Canada's independent decision to alert their nation before a formal WHO pandemic warning was most probably a learned response fol-lowing their own alarming experience with the WHO-caused delays during the SARS pandemic in 2003.

Once the Mexican Authorities realized they had a definite infectious disease outbreak, there was little IHR coordination between Canada, Mexico, the WHO, and the U.S. Centers for Disease Control. The current international system essentially failed for the United States. Cases were already inside America's border by the time the WHO and CDC issued their own alert. This emphasizes that there needs to be a better consolidation of disease surveillance and verification operations.

The 2009 H1N1 influenza pandemic demonstrated that independ-ent continuous intelligence-driven data mining is a valuable bio-sur-veillance tool. It is not dependent on other countries effort in partici-pating in the WHO system and it demonstrated an enhanced early de-tection capability sufficient to address public health crises posing a risk to U.S. national security.

On the other hand, the traditional risk-averse, forensically driven surveillance culture favored by the CDC was actually able to pick up the first cases of A/H1N1 in the Continental US through its participating laboratory network.

The 2009 Influenza pandemic was a watershed moment because it showed that both surveillance approaches were complimentary and that both approaches are probably necessary. It also emphasized the need to match both methods with a dedicated asset that is tasked to provide rapid ground-truth verification a possible early outbreak when alerted to by either system.

It is now time to directly and decisively address this threat. The first step is to improve early pandemic detection by establishing an independent disease surveillance effort based on continuous media data mining. The second step is to create a well-funded, highly mobile team of specialists for rapid on-site ground-truth verification of suspected disease outbreaks that could represent a threat to U.S. national security.

One of these teams should be a U.S. military unit capable of conducting conflict inserts into contested areas to garner epidemiological data, collect biomedical samples, and evacuate any ill U.S. personnel under appropriate biological containment.

NOTES FOR CHAPTER 26

[1] Jones KE, Patel NG, Levy MA, Storeygard A, Balk D, Gittleman JL, Daszak P. Global trends in emerging infectious diseases. Nature. 2008; 451:990–993. [PubMed].

[2] Turmelle, A.S. & Olival, K.J. 2009, Viral richness in bats, Ecohealth, 6(4):522-539.

[3] Lederberg J. Infectious disease/an evolutionary paradigm. Emerg Infect Dis 1997; 3:417-23.

[4] Woolhouse M, Scott F, Hudson Z, Howey R, Chase-Topping M (2012) Human viruses: discovery and emergence. Royal Society Philosophical Transactions Biological Sciences, 367: 2864–2871.

[5] National Intelligence Estimate (NIE 99-17D). The Global Infectious Disease Threat and Its Implications for the United States. McLean, VA: National Intelligence Council, 2000.

[6] Smith, KF, Goldberg, M. et.al., Global Rise in Infectious Disease Outbreaks. 2014; J.R. Soc. Interface 11: 21140950. http://dx.doi.org/10.1098/rsif.2014.0950.

[7] Grein, T. W., K. B. Kamara, G. Rodier, A. J. Plant, P. Bovier, M. J. Ryan, T. Ohyama, and D. L. Heymann. "Rumors of Disease in the Global Village: Outbreak Verification." Journal of Emerging Infectious Disease 6, no. 2 (2000): 97–102. doi: 10.3201/eid0602.000201.

[8] Wilson, J.M., Polyak, M, Blake, J., et.al. A Heuristic Indication and Warning Staging Model for Detection / Assessment of Biological Events. JAMA 15, no. 2 (2008): 158–171.

[9] James M. Wilson, Signal recognition during the emergence of pandemic influenza type A/H1N1: a commercial disease intelligence unit's perspective. Intelligence and National Security, 2016. http://dx.doi.org/10.1080/02684527.2016.1253924

[10] Politico Staff. "W.H. Memo on Swine Flu." Accessed October 4, 2016. http://www.politico.com/story/2009/04/wh-memoon-swine-flu-021941.

[11] Zhang, Y., H. Lopez-Gatell, C. M. Alpuche-Aranda, and M. A. Stoto. "Did Advances in Global Surveillance and Notifications Systems Make a Difference in the 2009 H1N1 Pandemic? A Respective Analysis." PLoS One 8, no. 4 (2013): e59893. doi: 10.1371/journal.pone.0059893.

27

THE NEED FOR AN INDEPENDENT NORTHCOM PANDEMIC FUSION CENTER WITH CENTRALIZED COMMAND / CONTROL

THE ADMISSION THAT PANDEMICS can have critical national security implications brings the U.S. Armed Forces and NORTHCOM into the area of disease surveillance and pandemic outbreak response.[1]

For over a decade and a half, the federal government has put out numerous *Requests For Proposals* for various types of bio-surveillance strategies in support of other Federal Agencies such as the DoD, DHS, USDA and USAID. Civilian biosurveillance efforts by HealthMap, ProMed and EcoHealth Alliance, have added privately to the early detection of infectious disease outbreaks. However, all of these systems are stove piped in one way or another. They vie for resources and the amount of costly, duplicative effort is massive with incomplete cross communication. After numerous repeated surveillance failures, it seems clear that this continuing fragmentation of responsibility and authority must be resolved, and the system reorganized back into a single integrated organizational framework.

In the last chapter it was suggested that an independent media data mining intelligence system should be created and operated in conjunction with the current existing WHO and CDC pandemic warning effort. Because ground-truth verification has constantly been a rate-limiting factor in the outbreak warning process, any new independent media data mining system should have the capability to rapidly deploy its own highly trained, on-site, outbreak verification teams.

DEVELOPING A DEDICATED
MILITARY PANDEMIC WARNING, COMMAND, AND CONTROL SYSTEM

Traditional infectious disease surveillance has shown significant problems for the last 100 years. Despite multiple iterations of WHO and CDC cooperation and a plethora of new U.S. government departments and reorganization attempts, the problems remain. Clearly, the present system is not meeting the dynamic changes occurring with respect to Emerging Infectious Diseases. We propose that the U.S. Military should now become involved in global disease surveillance. Why propose such a thing when the United States already has the Centers for Disease Control and Prevention?

> The answer to this question is simple. Why do we have a civil
> Federal Aviation Administration (FAA) to control American
> airspace; yet we also have the military's NORAD (North
> American Aerospace Defense Command) to provide aerospace
> warning and protection?

It is because many National Security issues need to be addressed rapidly and decisively by the military and not by plodding, civilian agencies that may have lost sight of their primary function or have become inhibited by internal or extrinsic political considerations.

There is a large degree of consensus that the basic architecture of a warning system will help determine its overall effectiveness and that the most effective structure is a warning system that is closely integrated with a pre-established response.[2]

In this respect, the U.S. military has an exceptional half-century history in the design and operation of an integrated national strategic surveillance system. Outside of England during the WW II Battle of Britain, this was quite possibly the very first real defensive "fusion" center ever created. The US system collated the vast amounts of data from ground-based early warning radars scattered across the Arctic Circle. It monitored satellite thermal detection systems and radiation-warning VELA satellites. It received tracking data from a worldwide multibillion-dollar network of 29 dedicated optical and radar sensor stations as well as a large space-based orbiting optical telescope. Gigantic pyramid-shaped phased-array radars in North Dakota and Florida constantly scanned the heavens while more conventional large radars on a Pacific atoll and in Turkey, further refined the data.

This world-wide system still exists, and it continues to make 420,000 daily observations as it monitors over twenty-thousand objects presently in Earth orbit. During the early Cold War, the system was used by the U.S. Air Force for defense against Soviet bombers. Later it was upgraded to defend against incoming foreign nuclear Intercontinental Ballistic Missiles (ICBMs). This integrated system has two qualities that have made it continuously successful.

The first was that its designers were careful to fully integrate the strategic warning part of the system into two other subsystems. One of these was a *Management* subsystem that used multiple modalities to rapidly verify any warning of a possible incoming bomber or missile attack. This subsystem became even more necessary with the advent of Soviet ballistic missile-launching submarines that reduced the effective U.S. response time down to a 15-minute window from the time of an alert. In addition to verification of an attack, a portion of the Management subsystem could predict target locations and tally projected casualties from any incoming nuclear strikes.

A second integrated subsystem then was used to deal with the *Response*. Primarily, this was in the form a verified Alert sent from the *Warning and Management* subsystems to the *Response* subsystems of the National Command Authority. This response subsystem involved the US President and it was used to authorize a retaliatory nuclear counterattack by U.S. land, sea, and air platforms.

The major factor involved in the system's success, was that the relationships forged between these three integrated subsystems (*Warning*, *Management* and *Response*), were painstakingly maintained, the subsystems drilled, and the system routinely exercised to maintain a constant high degree of reliability and readiness. Numerous checks and balances were built-in to avoid false-positive determinations or actions.

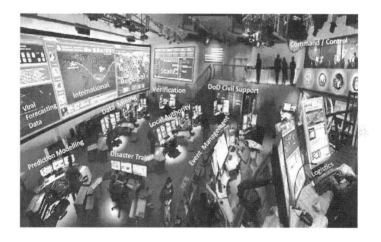

Figure 34. *A full-scale, multi-faceted Fusion and Command Center mockup. Demonstrating advanced tools and techniques for distributed collaboration, data fusion, visualization, and adaptive planning.* Credit: U.S. Air Force Research Lab. Adapted to outline a Pandemic Fusion Center.

These same basic principles should guide the formation of a new Pandemic *Early Warning* System as it is integrated into its own *Management* and *Response* subsystems that we will shortly describe.[3]

For the Warning subsystem, this new independent Fusion Center would use advanced Media Data mining techniques as previously described. Although independent, it would still communicate with the existing CDC and WHO surveillance systems during its daily operations.

Throughout the warning process, the military would play a supportive role to existing civilian efforts at pandemic preparedness. Only in the case of a catastrophic failure of civilian local authority planning, would the military assume a more prominent role. An analogous event of this type would be the 2005 Hurricane Katrina debacle in New Orleans.

The Pandemic "Fusion" Center is envisioned to be operated by the U.S. military Northern Command (NORTHCOM) as its own system. It would be composed of four integrated subsystems involving:

- Rapid Event Detection by a media data mining *Warning Subsystem*
- Rapid Verification, disease assessment and modelling by a *Management Subsystem.*
- Civilian Response monitored and assisted by a *Response Subsystem*
- Catastrophic Management Assets deployed by the *Response Subsystem* if required.

MANAGEMENT SUBSYSTEM FOR DATA MINING VERIFICATION AND OTHER EPIDEMIC INTELLIGENCE

We have already discussed the Media Data Mining Warning Subsystem. However, any outbreak alert by this system, must be verified as an actual infectious disease event of national security significance. This is one of the jobs of the integrated Management subsystem.

Upon receiving a *validated* media data mining alert, one of several, small mobile, Ground-Truth Verification Teams under the command of the Fusion Center would attempt a rapid verification. Initially this would take the form of traditional communications via the CDC and

WHO with the health authorities of a foreign nation. However, the Fusion Center would also seek information from the Defense Intelligence Agency, and it would stand ready to deploy the small "ground-truth" verification team to the actual event site if necessary. In this respect, there would be three categories of rapid verification team deployment.

The first would involve the verification of an outbreak in a friendly, foreign country. This is not a difficult undertaking. We have already outlined the composition of such a verification team in Chapter 26 during the discussion of the 2009 pandemic Influenza outbreak in Mexico. This team would be dependent on the host country's cooperation and the country's diagnostic laboratory capability. However, the team would stand ready to take biomedical samples and transport these back to designated United States laboratories for analysis if required.

LABORATORY SUPPORT FOR GROUND-TRUTH VERIFICATION

The second type of verification deployment would involve confirming an outbreak in a rural or urban area in a friendly Third-World country with a *limited* health infrastructure. In this case, the verification team could use a U.S. military transport aircraft and ideally, biomedical samples would be brought back to the U.S. mainland to the high-containment laboratories at Fort Detrick and the CDC for disease assessment, full pathogen characterization, and a search for effective drug treatments.

However, in some circumstances, the verification team might be accompanied by an advanced containerized laboratory with a small team of scientists and technicians. This has been done for years in the support of military Tier-One assets participating in Weapons of Mass Destruction (WMD) missions. This containerized laboratory was operated with the technical support provided by an accompanying Walter Reed Medical Research Unit.

In this respect, a new modernized and advanced airmobile Disease Assessment and Support Laboratory could be constructed. If based on the Patient Transport Container already designed and built for FEMA, it would feature a high-level of biocontainment with a Magnahelical-controlled negative pressure interior (Figure 35). This laboratory would remain on-board the aircraft.

For rapid pathogen isolation and disease assessment, this laboratory should be capable of insect and mammalian cell-line tissue culture, transmission electron microscopy, basic bacteriology, ELISA serology and an RT-PCR Nucleic Acid Microarray system to allow for pathogen strain identification to the strain and sequence level.[4,5] As an example, the Affymetrix Axiom® DNA Microarray system provides unprecedented ability to conduct microbial surveys in remote areas and nucleic acid microarrays can be constructed to allow identification down to the viral Family level.

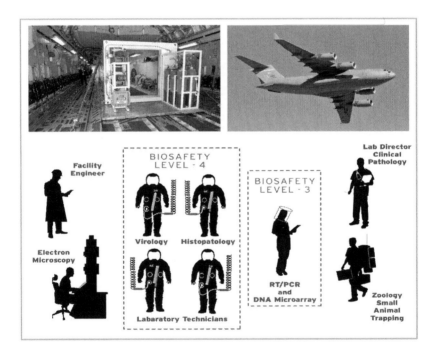

Figure 35. *Airmobile Laboratory and Proposed Verification Team.*[6]

Collected biomedical samples could include animal or human blood, skin swabs, stool, saliva, crushed insect samples, soil, water and vegetation, and hundreds of different pathogens can be scanned for simultaneously with 23-hours from sample to results. This technology promises to revolutionize field epidemiological studies. For novel emerging disease agents, the laboratory should also be capable of random multiplex (RT)-PCR using 3'-locked random primers followed by rapid Ion Torrent genetic sequencing.[7]

For disease assessment studies, a separate section of the laboratory would feature a small clinical area with a patient exam bed, monitors and a point of care clinical laboratory for blood chemistry determinations together with a hematology section. The patient exam bed would double as an autopsy table with nearby tissue processors, a microtome, and staining. The lab would feature light and fluorescent microscopy, TEM specimen preparation and an electron microscope mounted on an anti-vibrational platform.

Powered by a long-duration aircraft APU or one of three small standby emergency diesel generators, the laboratory could be accompanied by a small support-module with food, communications and hygiene facilities to allow the lab staff to live and work on-board the aircraft while it is parked at an airfield.

The main mission of the verification team in a permissive Third World country, would be to land in the capital city, insert into an outbreak area, and confirm that an EID outbreak was underway. The team would collect clinical samples for analysis back in the mobile laboratory and in U.S. laboratories. They may work with the locals to construct an isolation treatment center and teach basic case-contact tracing and isolation to help disrupt the epidemic cycle while the pathogen is being identified. Infected US casualties would be subjected to early treatment (if one is available) and flown back to the United States under biocontainment and medical support.

OUTBREAK VERIFICATION INSIDE
NON-PERMISSIVE, CONTESTED, LOW-INTENSITY CONFLICT REGIONS

This is the most difficult scenario. As previously discussed, there is a high association of lethal emerging RNA viral diseases with

"Biodiversity Hotspots" that have limited medical and communication infrastructures.[8,9,10,11,12]

Some 90% of all low-intensity conflicts over the last half-century, have occurred inside these "Hotspots."[13,14,15,16] Such regions may also be the working environment for a small number of U.S. civilians and U.S. military. Consequently, these groups run a low but definite risk of being in the middle of an EID outbreak and could conceivably require medical evacuation.[17]

The presence of armed rebel groups may make it difficult to insert a civilian verification and medical evacuation team and it would likely require the participation of U.S. military Special Operations forces who are trained to insert and work in such areas.

RECONSTITUTING A MILITARY AEROMEDICAL ISOLATION TEAM FOR OUTBREAK VERIFICATION

Emerging outbreaks of new pathogenic viruses must be recognized, characterized, and contained as rapidly as possible. The reasons for this are multifold.

1. Following an EID outbreak, there is a narrow window for containment using contact tracing, quarantine, rapid lab diagnosis, and positive case isolation. If this window is missed, a local EID outbreak may expand faster than local resources can manage.

2. If antiviral drug therapy is available, there is a very narrow treatment window for patients suffering from a severe infection.[18,19,20]

3. The aeromedical evacuation of an EID patient may involve a variety of transportation platforms and this should be performed under high-level biological containment throughout the entire Tac Evac process.[21]

4. Finally, as repeatedly discussed, the response to any potential pandemic virus requires a sufficient lead time to mobilize the necessary "surge" public health and medical resources in the event that cases appear in the United States.

It is therefore reasonable to suggest that a dedicated military *Aero-medical Isolation and Special Medical Augmentation Response Team* (AIT-SMART) be reconstituted with an upgraded capability particular to the EID environment and Pandemic "Fusion Center" requirements.[22,23] It is reasonable that this team be composed of Special Operations medical personnel with the ability to conduct conflict inserts into a contested area using a variety of ground and air platforms to investigate a suspected outbreak. It is envisioned that this AIT-SMART be under the direction and funding of the NORTHCOM Fusion Center and the command of JSOC "North" co-located with NORTHCOM. Such a team could be trained to be capable of:

- Employing on-site rapid point of care diagnostics to attempt rapid on-site pathogen identification.
- Collect and transport biomedical and possible environmental samples.
- Initiate time-sensitive antiviral drug therapy to designated individuals.
- Provide initial high-level supportive medical care during the patient evacuation process.
- Perform a biological-secure TacEvac for up to 4 casualties from an operational area.
- Initiate and teach initial local epidemic control measures.

Such an idea is not without precedent. In late 1965, the U.S. Army Special Forces obtained funding from the Walter Reed Army Institute of Medical Research to establish a *Field Epidemiological Survey Team* (FEST).[24]

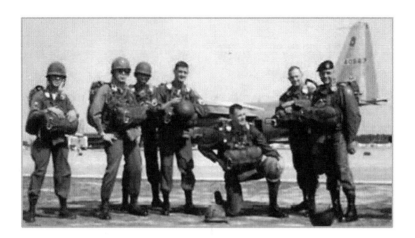

Figure 36. *U.S. Army Special Forces-Walter Reed Army Institute of Research Field Epidemiologic Survey Team (Airborne).* Photo Credit LTC Louis Dorogi, Journal Special Operations Medicine. Volume 9, Edition2/Spring 2009 pp54-71.

All team members were Airborne and Special Forces-qualified medical personnel with an attached entomologist, a veterinarian and several laboratory technicians. This unit underwent an additional fifteen-week pre-deployment training program and new equipment items were developed for remote area operations.[23,25] In 1966, the unit was deployed to Vietnam with the 5th Special Forces Group (Airborne). There it conducted a number of diverse important epidemiological studies and collected biomedical samples for later study, often under combat conditions.

The FEST was deactivated in October 1968 as a result of increased aeromedical evacuation capability, but not before it had proved conclusively that practical epidemiology could be performed in remote, hostile areas by a team that combined medical research skills with Special Operations military qualifications.

For the reasons we have described, it is reasonable to suggest that an AIT-SMART / FEST team be created with the ability to insert into contested areas to verify suspected EID outbreaks, obtain and securely transport biomedical samples, train indigenous personnel in basic epidemic management, initiate initial antiviral therapy and conduct a safe biocontained tactical evacuation of the affected U.S. personnel. (Figure 37).

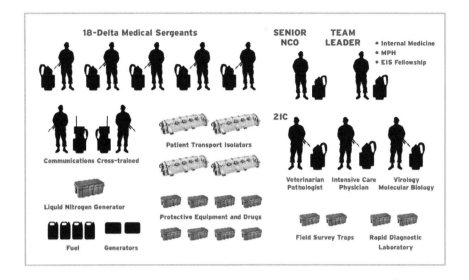

Figure 37. *Proposed Special Operations Aeromedical Isolation-Special Augmentation Response/Field Epidemiological Survey Team and equipment.*

The four medical officers of the team should be selected from the Special Operations community. The eight enlisted team members should be Special Operations 18D30 medics with additional clinical training rotations in internal medicine and critical care. Two of the enlisted 18D personnel should be cross trained as Special Force 18E Communications Specialists.

In addition to their MOS, all personnel would undergo a highly specialized three-phase 15-week core training program covering virology, medical microbiology, tropical medicine, epidemiology, contact tracing, patient *Case Definition* construction, rapid field point-of-care viral diagnostics, current antiviral pharmacology, biomedical sample collection, biologically-contained patient transport, small mammal trapping, and other training in the techniques and procedures necessary to study a wide variety of infectious disease agents, animal reservoirs, and vectors. On operations, the team would carry provisions for 14-days without resupply to remove them from the local money and food chain during their deployment to an outbreak area.

Along with this effort, direct funding should be provided for the further development of accurate, ruggedized, rapid Point-of-Care diagnostics for known emerging disease agents. For outbreaks of new infectious agents currently unknown to science, biomedical field samples could be collected by the team and securely transported for later laboratory rapid genetic sequencing.[6] The team may or may not be accompanied by the airmobile Diagnostic Laboratory and technicians which would remain in a secure location such as the main foreign capital airfield.

The normal mission for this team would be to insert into a contested rural or urban area to confirm the ground-truth of an EID outbreak and collect clinical samples for transport back for infectious agent isolation and disease characterization. Depending on the findings, part of the team might work with the locals to construct an isolation treatment center and teach the local inhabitants the process of contact tracing and isolation to disrupt the human epidemic cycle. This would include establishing proper burial practices in the area and the establishment of a drop zone for the aerial delivery of additional supplies and equipment for expanded containment efforts.

Another primary mission of the self-contained AIT team would be to rapidly insert into a remote conflict area to provide supportive medical care to infected U.S. personnel, initiate suitable anti-viral therapy (if any exists), and conduct a biologically-secure transport of up to 4 U.S. casualties back to a dedicated infectious disease care unit for continued management.

Finally, as part of their continuous training, such a team could act as the "tip of the spear" for established worldwide Navy BURMED / Naval Medical Research Units and assist in any research / field survey efforts by USAMRIID, the CDC, or NATO partners. These would be excellent practical training missions which could also collect select epidemiologic intelligence for other users, such as assessing a select region for drug-resistant Malaria. These constant training deployments would reinforce any perishable skills. Additional tasks could involve the team's attachment to other major agencies to assist in conducting approved clinical field trials of appropriate vaccines and drugs for diseases of military significance.

This team with its unique capabilities would also be of major assistance to the *DoD Global Emerging Infections System (DoDGEIS)* while improving U.S. national biological security and enhancing the fulfillment of *Presidential Decision Directive* NSTC-7.

When assessing the costs of training, maintaining, and deploying this 12 to 14-man *Aeromedical Isolation Transport and Field Epidemiological Survey Team*, it is useful to compare the total projected 5-year cost of this effort, directly with the $750 million cost that was incurred by having to deploy the 101ˢᵗ Airborne Division (Air Assault) to execute *Operation United Assistance.* This was during the West Africa Ebola crisis and in direct support to the USAID (United States Agency for International Development).[26]

This is in addition to the USAID's own expenditure of more than 2.3 billion dollars against this infectious disease outbreak.[27] This does not include the cost of screening for cases of Ebolavirus disease at US airports and the panicked incident management of the 11 cases of Ebolavirus disease that eventually appeared in the United States.

The early deployment of an upgraded AIT-SMART/FEST at the very beginning of the 2014 West Africa Ebola outbreak, would have provided significant ongoing medical intelligence to USAID. It could have made a significant impact on this event before it required an expensive deployment of over 3,000 U.S. military personnel to build, train, and staff a large number of Ebola treatment Centers in Liberia.

MANAGEMENT SUBSYSTEM FUNCTIONS

In addition to the main Rapid Warning/Verification Surveillance Subsystem the predictive epidemiological section of the Management Subsystem of the Pandemic Fusion Center will estimate disease spread and identify any geographical areas projected to potentially have the most trouble.

As the disease agent is better understood by the assessment information coming out of the CDC and USAMRIID laboratories, this data (transmissibility, R_0 number, virus environmental stability and concentration in various body fluids), will be incorporated by the Management subsystem into advanced epidemiologic computer models to simulate the new infectious disease agent's potential spread. (Figure 38). These predictive computer models would entail population density, population movements, age-based contacts, transmission parameters, various estimated viral reproduction numbers (R_0), the outbreak start date and location, predictive epidemic spread and the effect of various mitigation measures if initiated at specific times.

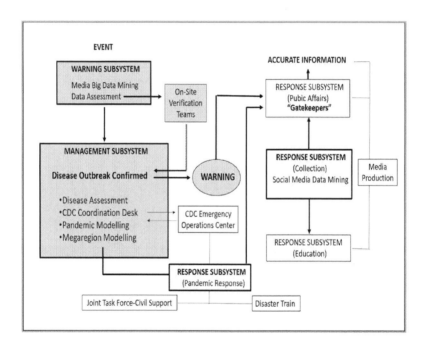

Figure 38. Warning and Management Subsystems of the Pandemic Fusion Center.

Ideally, the pandemic plan and status of any individual Local Authority in the U.S. could be called up from CDC / State-shared data in near real-time. The Management subsystem will use this data to monitor the on-going civilian Public Health response and compare this to its computer projections. The goal is to provide an early warning to the

States concerning their worst affected local communities. This would be done in cooperation with the CDC (Figure 38).

A final *Response* subsystem would be the last piece of the Pandemic Fusion Center. One function of this subsystem would be to providing guidance and a strategy for the timing and direction of Public Affairs. Again, Big Data Media-Mining can play a vital role in this area.

NOTES FOR CHAPTER 28

[1] National Intelligence Estimate (NIE 99-17D). The Global Infectious Disease Threat and Its Implications for the United States. McLean, VA: National Intelligence Council, 2000.

[2] Mileti, D. S., and J. H. Sorenson. Communication of Emergency Public Warnings: A Social Science Assessment. Oak Ridge National Laboratory Report (ORNL-6609). 1990.

[3] James M. Wilson, Signal recognition during the emergence of pandemic influenza type A/H1N1: a commercial disease intelligence unit's perspective. Intelligence and National Security, 2016. http://dx.doi.org/10.1080/02684527.2016.1253924

[4] Eunice C. Chen, Steve A. Miller, Joseph L. DeRisi, Charles Y. Chiu, Using a Pan-Viral Microarray Assay (Virochip) to Screen Clinical Samples for Viral Pathogens J Vis Exp. 2011; (50): 2536. Published online 2011 Apr 27. doi: 10.3791/2536 PMCID: PMC3169278 PMID: 21559002https://www.ncbi.nlm.nih.gov/pmc/articles/PMC3169278/

[5] Renois F, Talmud D, Huguenin A, Moutte L, Strady C, et.al. Rapid detection of respiratory tract viral infections and coinfections in patients with influenza-like illnesses by use of reverse transcription-PCR DNA microarray systems. J Clin Microbiol. 2010 Nov;48(11):3836-42.

[6] https://www.af.mil/News/Photos.aspx?igphoto=2000534023

[7] Clem, A.L., Sims, J., Telang, S., Eaton, JW., Chesney, J., Virus detection and identification using random multiplex (RT)-PCR with 3'-locked random primers, Virol Journal, 2007, 4:6

[8] Russell A., Norman Myers and Cristina Goettsch Mittermeier, Hotspots: Earth's Biologically Richest and Most Endangered Terrestrial Ecoregions, Conservation International, 2000 ISBN 978-968-6397-58-1.

[9] Mittermeier, R. A., Myers, N., Thomsen, J. B., et.al. Biodiversity hotspots and major tropical wilderness areas: approaches to setting conservation priorities. Cons. Biol. 12, 516– 520 (1998).

[10] Daniel J Salkeld, Kerry A Padgett, and James Holland Jones, A meta-analysis suggesting that the relationship between biodiversity and risk of zoonotic pathogen transmission is idiosyncratic. 2013, Ecology Letters. Volume 16, Issue 5, pages 679–686.

[11] R.S. Ostfeld, Biodiversity loss and the rise of zoonotic pathogens. 2009. Clinical Microbiology and Infection Volume 15, Issue Supplement s1, pages 40–43.

[12] Parrish, C.R., Edward C. Holmes, E.C., David M. Morens, D.M., Park, E.C., Burke, S., et.al. Cross-Species Virus Transmission and the Emergence of New Epidemic Diseases, Micro and Mol Bio. Rev.2008.

[13] Hanson, T., Brooks, T.M., Gustavo, A. et.al. Warfare in Biodiversity Hotspots. Conservation Biology, 2009. Volume 23, No. 3, 578–587.

[14] Draulens, D. & van Krunkelsven, E. The impact of war on forest areas in the Democratic Republic of Congo. 2002. Cambridge Journals, Tervuren, Belgium.

[15] Hart, T., Mwinyihali R., Armed Conflict and Biodiversity in Sub-Saharan Africa: The Case of the Democratic Republic of Congo. 2001. Biodiversity Support Program / WWF, Washington, D.C.

[16] Woolhouse M, Scott F, Hudson Z, Howey R, Chase-Topping M (2012) Human viruses: discovery and emergence. Royal Society Philosophical Transactions Biological Sciences, 367: 2864–2871.

[17] Myers, Russell A. Mittermeier, Jennifer Kent, et.al.*Biodiversity hotspots for conservation priorities,* (2000) Nature 403, 853-858 (24 February)

[18] Warren TK, Wells J, Panchal RG, Stuthman, KS, et.al. *Protection against filovirus diseases by a novel broad-spectrum nucleoside analogue BCX4430.* Nature. 2014 Apr 17; 508(7496):402-5.

[19] Qiu X, Kobinger GP. *Antibody therapy for Ebola: Is the tide turning around?* Hum Vaccin Immunother. 2014 Feb 6;10(4).

[20] Qiu X, Audet J, Wong G, Fernando L, Bello A, Pillet S, Alimonti JB, Kobinger GP. *Sustained protection against Ebola virus infection following treatment of infected nonhuman primates with ZMAb.* Sci Rep. 2013 Nov 28; 3:3365.

[21] Clayton, A.J., "Containment aircraft transit isolator"; *Aviat Space Environ Med,* 1979: Oct;50 (10):1067-72.

[22] Mark R. Withers, George W. Christopher, Steven J. Hatfill, and Jose J. Gutierrez-Nunez, Chapter 11, *"Aeromedical Evacuation of Patients with Contagious Infections"* In; Aeromedical Evacuation; Management of Acute and Stabilized Patients. Eds. William Hurd, John Jernigan. Springer Press.

[23] Christopher, G. W. and E. M. Eitzen, Jr, "Air evacuation under high-level biosafety containment: the aeromedical isolation team"; Emerg Infect Dis, 1999: Mar-Apr; 5(2): 241–246.

[24] Dorogi, L.T., The United States Army Special Forces-Walter Reed Army Institute of Research Field Epidemiologic Survey Team (Airborne) Journal of Spec Ops Medicine. 2009, Volume 09, Issue 2, 54-71.

[25] Disposition Form – The Office of the Surgeon, U.S. Army Center for Special Warfare, Ft. Bragg, NC to G-3, U.S. Army Center for Special Warfare, POI, *Pre-deployment Training U.S. Army Special Forces-WRAIR Field Epidemiologic Survey Unit (Airborne),* 10 December 1965.

26 Operation UNITED ASSISTANCE: The DOD Response to Ebola in West Africa. 6 Jan. 2016. Joint and Coalition Operational Analysis (JCOA), Joint Staff J-7. http://www.dtic.mil/doctrine/ebola/OUA_report_jan2016.pdf

27 US Agency for International Development (USAID), "West Africa Ebola Outbreak FactSheet #3, 2016", 6 November 2015, http://www.usaid.gov/sites/default/files/documents/1866/west_africa_fs03_11-062015.pdf.

28

DEVELOPING A CONTINUOUS FEEDBACK LOOP FOR PANDEMIC PUBLIC AFFAIRS MANAGEMENT

S. Zadrick; *Media Corp of America*
S.A. Rodriguez, R. Rodriguez; *Natcom Global*
S. Aukstakalnis; *AlertsUSA, Inc.*
N. Andrade; *Koeppel Direct*

INTRODUCTION TO THE PROBLEM

The *Response* subsystem represents the final integrated portion of the proposed NORTHCOM Pandemic Fusion Center. This *Response* subsystem is envisioned to have two components. The first component would operate in close conjunction with the CDC and it would deal with assisting in the coordination of a national pandemic response.

This includes a catastrophic response component that will be discussed in detail in the next chapter.

The second part of the *Response* subsystem is a proactive Public Affairs component that would deal with the fact that during a severe pandemic event, individuals, families, and entire communities will be desperate to understand what is happening. Herein lies a number of significant challenges that must be addressed early on.

In this respect, the national/international mass media has undergone a fundamental and radical change over the last 40-years. The older, more traditional methods for educating the public by radio, broadcast television and cable news, have largely been supplanted by new mediums of communications. In addition, America as a society is changing, and the traditional news audience is growing older and giving way to a new generation that is habituated to 24/7 news access outside the traditional 3-day cycle of news content.

This information revolution has been accompanied by a severe fragmentation in news content and the appearance of overt bias with respect to various news channels, newspapers and internet platforms that support various causes and government parties. An ever-increasing fraction of the population now mass around the use of social and on-line media with feuding blogs, forums, Instagram, Facebook, Twitter and more.

The recipients of the news can now also become newscasters themselves, even with only a rudimentary knowledge of what they are posting and discussing. The "noise" of this uninformed, biased, or false information can be deafening and sometimes inhibitory to real news content. In addition, media news is no longer just local, regional and national. It can be disseminated on an international scale with either genuine or misleading information. Either may garner a large enough following to begin to influence public opinion.

When managing a severe public health crisis, the senior authorities must maintain their credibility at all times. Unfortunately, politicians have a history of misleading the public in matters that concern public health. This was a prime factor in the deaths and cancers caused by the wildly toxic aerosol cloud generated during the 9/11 World Trade Center event. The EPA was pressured to lie about air quality safety and the National Media backed this ridiculous assumption.

Based on every major national poll conducted since July 2007, the majority of the US population does not trust the Federal government. Public confidence has fallen from a high of 73% in 1958 to the present, when fewer than three-in-ten Americans express trust in their elected officials.

This distrust must be overcome in order to successfully manage an outbreak of a severe, lethal pandemic disease. It is essential that a trusted information feedback-loop be established between the pandemic authorities and the public. In this respect, recent surveys by Pew Research Center reveal that public confidence in the scientific community as a whole has remained stable for decades at around 44%. Currently the one segment of society with the most trust is the Department of Defense with eight-in-ten Americans expressing confidence in the U.S. military.

Therefore, based on these demographics, it is reasonable to propose that the most trusted spokespeople during a severe lethal pandemic will be senior military scientists led by someone with the same nature, stature, respect and trustworthiness as exhibited by Charles Everett Koop, the former 13th Surgeon General of the United States.

REAL-TIME MONITORING OF PUBLIC PERCEPTIONS DURING A SEVERE PANDEMIC

While the use of Social Media as a method for early outbreak detection is problematic, the use of these platforms to understand a population's current attitudes and beliefs during a pandemic is quite practical. This is a possible tool that requires further exploration for the proactive management of infectious disease outbreaks.

The Big-Data "mining" of Social Media can help authorities understand the major changing public perceptions and attitudes that are prevalent at any stage of a developing severe pandemic. This information can be used to refine further official public communications. It can identify any major circulating rumors early, and counter these through the Internet and Social Media channels at any time during an outbreak.

The overriding pre-requisite for using this type of a "public-government-public" feedback loop, is that the pandemic authorities must maintain their credibility at all times. The authorities *must* strictly adhere to the truth without any "spin" or distortion. In a severe pandemic, sources such as Wikileaks or non-authorized leaks from federal agency employees will illuminate any falsehoods or half-truths that are present in any official government statements or communications. Any delayed or misleading information or over-promises of the availability of a limited vaccine or anti-viral drug by a given date, will only tend to create distrust, outrage, and possible social unrest that will only further compound the existing problems.

THE PROBLEM OF "VIRAL" INTERNET COMMUNICATIONS

Much like the Influenza virus which can spread within seconds of contact, information can quickly spread through the electronic Social Media. If popular or controversial, this information can go *"viral"* almost instantaneously. To avoid confusion, the word *"Viral"* when used in the context of media, refers to information that is circulated rapidly on the Internet. In this book we will use the term *"Internet Media Dissemination"* (IMD) to describe this process.

In the 21st century, IMD can circumnavigate the globe without the requirement and limitations of person to person contact. Only the touch of a button on a computer or smartphone is needed. In addition, inaccurate IMD is much harder to contain than the more traditional forms of communication and there are no real geographic boundaries. The only limiting factors are the socioeconomic variables that can impact access to information, since computers, notepads, and smart phones are not as prevalent in the underdeveloped countries.

The International Telecommunications Union estimates that as of April 2019, over half of the world's population, (56.1%), has internet access although this over-indexes to 81% with the access that is derived from the developed world. In the 21st century, the print and broadcast media channels are not enough—nor are they trusted, read, or viewed by all members of the public. According to a 2018 Pew Research Center survey, Social Media is now the primary source for online news with over 2.4 billion users.[1] The majority of these users gravitate to just a handful of platforms which include Facebook, Twitter, Instagram, YouTube and Snapchat.

This alternative news delivery by Social Media now occurs at the expense of the more traditional media. This is because people want to access news and information in microbursts at their convenience—when they feel inclined to scroll or click through breaking news notifications on their phones or computers. Therefore, to be maximally effective, a Public Affairs strategy for a severe pandemic must be able to harness this almost instantaneous global spread of information via the Internet and Social Media channels.

As discussed, Social Media outlets can be used to spread truth and educate, or they can be used almost as a weapon to create fear and deliver misinformation. For example, #FakeNews became a trending hashtag and a talking point surrounding the 2016 U.S. presidential elections. Before that, it was the media frenzy during the 2014 Ebola outbreak which quickly spread fear across the globe, although geographically, the virus was largely contained in West Africa.

In a pandemic, how can rapid Internet Media Dissemination be leveraged to ensure that accurate and vital information is given to the populations groups that need it the most? What preemptive actions are available to the national authorities to inform, educate, and empower individual citizens, groups and communities during a pandemic response? What is the best way to disseminate essential information such as basic practices for controlling the spread of infectious disease between individuals and within a community? Is there a way to control the Internet dialogue to ensure the strict spread of truth about a pandemic situation?

The basic answer is that IMD *cannot* be controlled, it can only be countered as different falsehoods and rumors appear and change. This will require the use of Big Data Mining to constantly take the "pulse" of the US population via the current opinions circulating over the pandemic event. This approach could identify the most common misconceptions, rumors and falsehoods, and then just as quickly allow the pandemic authorities to respond back to the public with expert factual information sent through the Social Media venues.

There are already several "Reputation Management" companies that have attempted to do this as part of privacy and reputation protection solutions for both businesses and individuals. However, these have had mixed results. Governments could most certainly do this to a very high degree using advanced capabilities including tasking the National Security Agency to delete entries in select IMD sites or use robotic messaging to completely overwhelm any negative postings on social media. However, any inadvertent disclosure of these acts could violate the trust that the national authorities must establish with their population subgroups. It is not worth the risk.

However, there is a solution. Many experienced disaster managers realize that in a crisis, the use of a single knowledgeable spokesperson to disseminate official information, has many advantages. In this context, one practical mechanism would be for the NORTHCOM Pandemic Fusion Center, to create a system of "truth" *Gatekeepers*.

This would be in the form of a unified collection of military and civilian public health and infectious disease specialists working in tandem with various humanitarian agencies across the globe. The job of these *Gatekeepers* would be to proactively release factual information concerning the pandemic. They would be the only individuals authorized to communicate information about the pandemic. To curb speculation and fear, they would try to get ahead of the news, drive the news and become a trusted source of real news, while combatting sensationalism and the creation of hysteria.

This would entail having a preformed shortlist of established, trained, and drilled *Gatekeepers* ready to act as the trusted experts in a pandemic response. These military and civilian subject matter experts would receive training in public speaking and be well briefed with respect to the latest facts of a pandemic situation. Based on the poll results of "trust demographics", the two Chief *"Gatekeepers"* should be a senior military subject matter expert together with a senior civilian scientist or Public Health expert. Because of the historically variable effectiveness of the position of Surgeon General of the United States, the prominence given to this position would be decided at the time or addressed by a trained *"Surgeon General in Waiting"*.

All *Gatekeepers* would use common language and understandable terms in their explanations and messaging to the public. Select members of the team that show a talent, would provide Panel Press Conferences. This *Gatekeeper Panel* would be current on the facts with pre-planned messages rehearsed before each interview. Panel members would be trained to avoid being led by the interviewers and every opportunity would be used to introduce these truthful pre-planned messages.

The *Gatekeepers* would demonstrate concern and empathy for the impact of the pandemic and their focus would be to accurately relate the situation at the time and avoid a communications vacuum. There will always be some questions that will not be answerable at a given time. However, speculation would be avoided, and the message kept focused on the facts. The *Gatekeepers* would clearly outline the steps being taken to proactively manage the situation, as well as demonstrate the government is not just reacting to events.

In a severe 1918-type pandemic, the *Gatekeepers* would operate inside the Fusion Center, although with modern teleconferencing they will not all have to be physically present. It is envisioned the *Gatekeepers* would be supported by an expert multimedia production team working in a multimedia rapid-production facility.

Several times a day, the national *Gatekeepers* would disseminate "real" news through the dominant IMD channels. The Internet streaming of multiple video content and images of pandemic supplies being moved and community assistance teams going into the poor resource areas, would reinforce the fact that there is an on-going public health response. Video footage of Alternate Care Sites being set up or actually in operation could be supplied by DoD television media staff deployed to different localities. This would be very much like what the National Media already do when reporting on hurricanes.

The high-quality and constant rapid production of new video material and video updates would serve to complement the IMD commentary by the *Gatekeeper* subject-matter experts. This would tend to override the traditional 3-day news cycle approach taken by the National Media and it could be a critical part of a pandemic communications strategy for the twenty-first century.

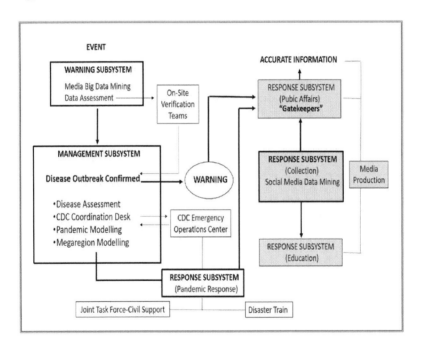

Figure 39. *Public Affairs Response Subsystems of the Pandemic Fusion Center.*

In today's media climate where there is room for manipulation and news reinterpretation, it's imperative to lead with real news in a direct-to-consumer approach. Social Media is a venue that uniquely allows this, and it is an IMD strategy that could potentially save lives. A real-time social media feedback system between the *Gatekeepers* and the public would address the ever-changing perceptions and complaints of the various population segments in the United States. Inaccurate rumors could be quickly quashed, and accurate pandemic data disseminated along with constant reminders of the specific actions that the individual public must take to avoid infection.[2] This would be a vital component of the *Response* subsystem of the Pandemic Fusion Center. (Figure 39).

One question that arises is how could such an approach be applied to the pandemic response in the underdeveloped countries in the world? During the 2014-15 West Africa Ebola outbreak, rioting occurred in some areas because the population was frightened and completely uninformed. Health workers were killed, and rudimentary hospitals looted based on public rumors and superstitions.

In this respect, FM/AM terrestrial radio is a form of mass media that is still operative in even the most underdeveloped of countries where authoritarian governments use it for propaganda and rudimentary entertainment. Representatives from select international agencies such as the WHO, the USAID, the Red Cross / Red Crescent, and Médecins Sans Frontières, could deploy small Public Affairs teams on the ground to work with foreign national and local authorities to target these underdeveloped regions of the world.

In this fashion, useful information could be shared beyond the reaches of the internet. This represents more than just humanitarianism. With modern global air travel, it is essential to contain minimize or contain a remote pandemic as quickly as possible before it can spread to the high-density Megaregions of the world.

A ROLE FOR "INTERNET INFLUENCERS"

We have mentioned that the *Gatekeepers* would be supported by an expert full media production team. Consequently, the Pandemic Fusion Center should have its own staffed on-site media production facility which it can use to quickly create both National Media and multimodal IMD advertisements and public service announcements to counter false or egregious misinformation.

To reinforce public perception of the on-going public health response the *Gatekeepers* would work with their liaisons in the CDC to disseminate "factual" pandemic news, multiple times a day with streaming video content and images of pandemic response activities. In addition, the media production facility could create multimedia pandemic content consisting of national radio and television advertising, public messaging presentations with adaptable pandemic information directed to specific demographic groups (elderly, 20-60 age group) and minorities, all with frequent message repeating.[3]

Short Feature Informational "Filler" Videos

In the early days of television in the United States, most of the output was live. When an equipment breakdown occurred during a live broadcast, a standard recording filled in for the normal content. Similar short films were also used as interludes or" interstitial programs" shown between televised movies to fill gaps in TV schedules. The word "interstitial" is derived from the word interstices, meaning a small interval between things. This short programming became known as a "filler". If a normal live program finished earlier than expected, a short extra interstitial program was inserted to fill the time until the next scheduled program was due to start.[4]

With the recognition that Emerging Infectious Diseases now represent a significant issue for National Defense, it may be time to start educating the general U.S. population about this threat.[5] In this respect, the Media Production Facility of the Pandemic Fusion Center could begin to create short interstitial video programming that would demonstrate what the current worldwide-deployed *Naval Medical Research Teams* are doing to fight Emerging Infectious Disease (EID) around the world. In addition, not everyone wants to join the U.S. military and fight in a low-intensity conflict. This interstitial programming could easily be adapted for wider military recruiting applications that reach a broader audience. This could be oriented to include recruiting efforts aimed at technical-trained recruits and possibly post-Master or PhD level scientists.

Other interstitial programming might deal with what the *US Agency for International Development* (USAID) is doing to fight EID in developing countries. This could be alternated with programming that actually outlines actually why infectious diseases previously unknown to science are now a national security threat.

This idea is not without precedent. During the Cold War and the early days of the "space age" the Department of Defense, the National Aeronautics and Space Agency (NASA), and Civil Defense, all created multiple short interstitial programs that ranged in length from 5 to 20-minutes or more, which covered various topics such as the space program, nuclear fallout protection, nuclear casualties, and military preparedness.[6] These "fillers" were too short to be shows and too long to be commercials. They were designed to educate the public on important strategic topics.

The Rapid Media Production Facility could easily begin to construct a library of various length multimedia interstitial programs designed to educate the public on the threat of EID and explain some of the ongoing work involved in countering this threat. Cross-over budget utilization could be used for this process which would obviously entail joint discussions with the major television broadcasters and cable channels. Of course, with mobile devices projected to surpass TV in consumption time in 2019, digital media will have to be a major component of this as well.[7]

THE USE OF PUBLIC MESSAGING

Another role for the Media Production Facility of the Pandemic Fusion Center, is to quickly create reactive Public Service Announcements (PSA) for use by commercial radio stations and Public Information Films (PIFs) for use in broadcast and cable entertainment television. These would be created in response to any major pandemic misconceptions revealed through Media Data Mining. A PSA or PIF refers to a message or video in the public interest that will be disseminated by the national media without charge.[4] We discussed this within the context of "Fillers", but in the specific context of Public Messaging, it is to raise public awareness and change public attitudes or behavior on an important social issue.

Government created PSAs are traditionally supplied to broadcasters free of charge and they represent a cost-free means to fill the gaps in fixed-duration commercial breaks that are left unsold. Although much rarer in the 21st century, they are still sometimes produced.

During a severe Influenza pandemic, public messaging could be used to inform local communities of the phone numbers for the Nurse Triage/Assistance Lines as described in Chapter 15. These telephone numbers would be a local community central contact point for Influenza information and help. By dialing this number, the caller could learn the location of their closest Alternate Care Site. The Duty nurses operating these lines could offer antiviral medication prescriptions to the callers per a standard protocol with their orders approved by a State-licensed physician. An additional Nurse Triage Line would be provided for the un-insured or for individuals whose health plans were not participating in the Triage Line concept. The Duty Nurses and attending physician could answer questions on the home care of Influenza patients, dispatch home visit teams to incapacitated families, or arrange ambulance transport to Alternate Care Sites. The key would be for the local government authorities to pre-contract their own local area radio and television stations for airtime to take the place of paid media that has expired.

LEVERAGING THE NATIONAL WIRELESS INFRASTRUCTURE

The national wireless infrastructure and SMS messaging is a tremendously powerful communications medium available to pandemic public affairs managers. According to the Cellular Telecomm Industry Association (CTIA), as of 2017 there are there are at least 273 million smartphones in use within the United States alone. This astounding level of penetration of technology into the general populace provides an enhanced ability to exert additional influence over public perceptions during a pandemic emergency.

In 2012, the FCC, a collaborative effort among the FCC, the Department of Homeland Security Science and Technology Directorate (DHS S&T), the Alliance for Telecommunications Industry Solutions and the Telecommunications Industry Association, all partnered to create the *Wireless Emergency Alerts system* to distribute vital information regarding hazardous weather conditions, missing children and other life-threatening conditions to the public via their mobile devices.

Today, through the use of the *Wireless Emergency Alert* (WEA) network, government agencies and approved State or Local Authorities, can disseminate and coordinate rapid emergency information, including updates, warnings, vital information regarding hazardous weather conditions, missing children and other life-threatening conditions to the public via their mobile devices. This can be programmed to cell phones and pagers within a defined geographic area, or nationwide. However, there is one word of caution.

In 2019, researchers from the University of Colorado at Boulder, demonstrated that it was possible to easily spoof wireless emergency alerts within a confined area, using open source software and commercially-available software-defined radios. They recommended that steps be taken to ensure that all alerts are verified as coming from a trusted network, or using Public-key cryptography upon reception.[8]

Private companies have stepped up to contribute their resources to supporting public health and safety. Google Public Alerts (launched in 2012) partners with a select group of government agencies like the US National Weather Service.[9] Similarly, Twitter Alerts (launched in 2013), posts emergency information from public agencies in the form of tweets or text messages to platform users.

However, early warnings are just one component of an effective EID notification system. Unlike the threat of a hurricane or other weather-related events of an immediate nature, an infectious disease outbreak will require more than just forewarning. Such an event will require ongoing education to aid in disease prevention and provide information to help people identify early symptoms to ensure they receive the proper diagnosis and avoid further spread of the disease.

Like the multimedia interstitial programs that would be developed for linear television stations, variations of this same content could be created for placement on digital media platforms. A consumer searching for symptoms related to an infectious disease could be greeted with a sponsored ad on Google.com informing them of potential outbreak

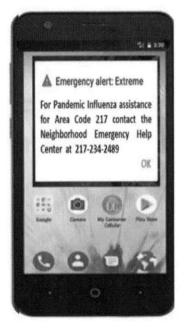

in their vicinity along with an ad that when clicked on, would take the searcher to a website with more information.

Similarly, a user browsing their Facebook feed could be greeted with sponsored post in the form of an informational video related to the potential outbreak. That said, an even more interesting application of digital media platforms and the data they possess, would be to aid the national authorities in their pandemic modelling. This idea has precedent.

In 2008, Google.org launched Google Flu Trends (GFT), a project that hoped to accurately predict flu activity based on Google.com search queries. Although the project was ultimately unsuccessful after showing initial promise (missing estimates of flu activity in 2013 by 140 percent), it did serve to highlight the potential benefits of a collaboration between the public and private sector in amassing and interpreting enormous data sets for the purpose of identifying health trends.[10] Although GFT was sunset in 2015, it served to spawn projects such as the *HealthMap Flucast*, a website from Boston Children's Hospital that combines data from the CDC with data from *Flu Near You* (a crowd-sourced system that aggregates user-generated health data).

Just as meteorologists fly specially instrumented aircraft into hurricanes to gather real-time data to improve hurricane tracking-predictions, the Pandemic Fusion Center would be able to use this user-generated social data to refine it's near real-time epidemiology computer models of pandemic disease spread. In a lethal pandemic, this could allow a preemptive direction of resources to the predicted worse-infected areas first. Such an almost real-time system would be critical for rapidly allocating scarce resources to where they are needed most and then rapidly re-directing them to the next developing critical area. More specifically this is in reference to the "Pandemic Disaster Trains" that will be described in Chapter 29.

INTERNET-BASED "HOW-TO" PANDEMIC INFORMATION

Another task of the Rapid Media Production Facility would be to create a series of multi-media instructional videos to teach the population of the United States the Non-Pharmaceutical Interventions (NPI) that must be taken by individuals and businesses to slow the transmission of a lethal viral pandemic for which there is no treatment or immediate available vaccine.

Instructional videos have a strong visual appeal, and video-based learning has proven to be an effective method for corporate training. As attested by the popularity of *YouTube*, it also has value for teaching individuals to do home repairs or hone new skills. For learners unfamiliar with electronic distance-learning, their fear of technology can be overcome by educational videos where all the learner needs to do is press a 'start' icon to receive instruction. There are several different types of Distance-Learning Videos and their effectiveness can be tailor-made for varying needs and different learner demographics.

Demonstration Videos are actual recorded demonstrations or animations that show learners how to perform a specific task. Some of the topics that could be covered in this type of a Pandemic Preparedness video would include:

- The different types of personal protective equipment.
- How to don personal protective equipment and decontaminate this before doffing.

- How to prepare an oral rehydration solution.
- How to prepare a home-made hand sanitizer lotion.
- How to daily sanitize paper and coin money.

Contextual Videos are used to visually represent real world situations in which the different techniques learned in previous video instruction are brought together for practical applications. This type of video is useful when learning actual pandemic-mediation activities.

- Individual precautions to take when in public areas or at work.
- Grocery shopping during an Influenza pandemic.
- Individual precautions to take when using Mass Transit.

Illustrative Videos using drawings, outlines, and other graphics can be used to effectively group different topic or points together under a common heading. A recognized example is a narrated PowerPoint® slide lecture.

Combined Illustrative / Contextual Videos use a combination of graphics and narration mixed with short video segments demonstrating multiple activities. These are a highly effective training tool for multi-factorial scenarios such as:

- Introduction to Influenza and its transmission and treatment
- What steps should a Local Government take during a lethal pandemic outbreak?
- How to recognize an Influenza infection.
- How to practically nurse a family member with Influenza at home.
- How to avoid Influenza infection while nursing an ill family member at home.
- The early recognition of Influenza complications.
- Businesses actions to take to reduce the Influenza risk to employees.

The use of Internet Media Dissemination would have widespread use for training the population in basic Non-Pharmaceutical Interventions through individual computers, mobile and connected devices as well as in formal classroom or auditorium settings.

DIRECTED NATIONAL MEDIA ADVERTISING

Stated once again, in a severe lethal pandemic, the authorities must maintain credibility and public trust. Corporate entities do this every day with media advertising, and the pandemic authorities should be prepared to do this as well. During a severe pandemic, the Federal Government needs to advertise what it is responsible for and outline what it is doing. In addition, and most importantly, the Federal Government must outline what the State and Local Authorities *should* be doing.

There is a good reason for this because response planning and pandemic preparedness begins at the local authority level, A particular local authority that has failed in its disaster planning and has consequently suffered an out of control situation, will tend to blame the higher levels of government. This happened in 2005 when the Local Authorities in New Orleans failed in their portion of the response to Hurricane Katrina. The local government immediately and very vocally used the national media to blame the state and federal authorities for their own mistakes. Early advertising by the national authorities can counter this type of event and prompt the local authorities for increased preparedness efforts.

In addition, frequent advertisements can also be used to educate the public on the need to use individual methods to prevent self-infection and constantly emphasize what small and large businesses should do to decrease their employee's Influenza risks.

For the federal government, specialized companies exist that can negotiate pre-purchased media using buying methodology to purchase airtime at a fraction of what would normally be paid (*cents on the dollar*) for commercial advertising. The resulting pandemic media messages would be analyzed for indications of their effectiveness as the advertising campaign progresses.

There are several mechanisms to do this. For example, Digital Ad Ratings can analyze an ad's audience across computer, mobile and connected devices in a way that is comparable to the Nielsen TV Ratings. It can provide audience reach, frequency, gross rating points, and on-target percentage across digital platforms. Metrics are reported by demographic (age/gender), by device and by publisher and country. Alternately, the advertisement's viewability can be measured by duration in-view by demographic, mobile viewable demographics, sophisticated invalid traffic filtration, and multiple audience qualifiers. When combined with Nielsen Ad Ratings, this can give a cross-platform measurement of the audience for an advertising campaign.

THE ANTI-VACCINATION DEBATE

During a pandemic the population will search multiple radio and television channels for the latest updates. Cable news networks and Internet news sites are sure to spread unverified rumors which when repeated, have the risk of being wrongly turned into fact. Many members of the public will log onto Social Media and Discussion Forums and read about conspiracy theories. Even accurate news reports may become overly sensationalized by the press.

In the confusion, people may be given contradictory guidance. Most particularly with respect to vaccination. This leads to the concept of a *Twitter Troll*.

A *Twitter Troll* is a relatively new slang term. It refers to an individual which for aberrant psychological reasons, is compelled to frequently cast false accusations, lies, or conspiracy theories through the Twitter fraction of Social Media. Taking this a step further, they may use specialized computer software to control a Twitter account via the Twitter Application Programming Interface (API). Known as a *Twitter bot*, this software may autonomously perform actions such as tweeting, re-tweeting, liking, following, unfollowing, or direct messaging other accounts.

A recent study by scientists at the George Washington University, outlined that in 2018, *Russian Twitter Trolls* attempted to fuel the U.S.

anti-vaccination debate.[11] Russian operatives employed sophisticated Twitter bots in a campaign to sew confusion and misinformation surrounding vaccinations. In 2019, significant chickenpox and measles outbreaks plagued the U.S. and at least three states saw simultaneous outbreaks of the measles virus. The CDC has blamed this occurrence on misinformation caused by the rise of anti-vaccination movement, which many officials said directly led to these measles outbreaks.

The George Washington University study concluded that this Russian trolling experiment mimicked other trolling efforts used in the past to intensify widely debated issues in the United States by inflating different viewpoints. Considering that a severe EID pandemic can represent a strategic threat to the United States, this Russian experiment in manipulating U.S. public opinion on vaccination cannot be considered trivial.

Situations like this can only be minimized if trusted, accurate information is given to the public by both the U.S. government and the U.S. press. There is no room for media entities to spread unverified rumors in their rush to be the first to announce so-called *"Breaking News"*. This is particularly important for the inhabitants of the poor, low-resource communities so that their leaders, supported by the organizations working with them, can take the appropriate pandemic actions without conflicting guidance.

Informing the public truthfully about a pandemic situation will serve as a precaution advocacy to emphasize the vital need for individuals to implement and strictly adhere to Non-Pharmaceutical Interventions until a drug treatment or vaccine becomes available.

NOTES FOR CHAPTER 28

[1] Perrin, A., M. Anderson, M. Share of U.S. adults using social media. Pew Research Center. April 10, 2019. https://www.pewresearch.org/topics/social-media

[2] Mileti, D. S., and J. H. Sorenson. Communication of Emergency Public Warnings: A Social Science Assessment. Oak Ridge National Laboratory Report (ORNL-6609). 1990.

[3] Perry, Ronald W.; Michael K. Lindell; and Marjorie R. Greene. 1982a. "Crisis Communications: Ethnic Differentials in Interpreting and Acting on Disaster Warnings" Social Behavior and Personality 10(1):97-104.

[4] "Public Service Advertising". www.psaresearch.com.

[5] National Intelligence Estimate (NIE 99-17D). The Global Infectious Disease Threat and It's Implications for the United States. McLean, VA: National Intelligence Council, 2000.

[6] The Charlie Dean Archives
https://www.bing.com/videos/search?q=charlie+dean+archives&view=detail&mid=8CC8AE09B655476189F8CC8AE909B655476189F&FORM=VIRE

[7] https//www.emarker.com/content/mobile-time-spent-2018 Accessed 9 July 2019

[8] Bode, Karl; Koebler, Jason (2019-06-26). "How the U.S. Emergency Alert System Can Be Hijacked and Weaponized". *Vice*. Retrieved 2019-07-07
https://www.vice.com/en_us/article/evy75j/researchers-demonstrate-how-us-emergency-alert-system-can-be-hijacked-and-weaponized

[9] https://www.google.org/publicalerts Accessed 9 July 2019

[10] htpps://www.wired.com/2015/10/can-learn-epic-failure-google-flu-trends/

[11] Russian Trolls Fueled Anti-Vaccination Debate. The Washington Time. May 31, 2019 https://thewashingtontime.com/russian-trolls-fueled-anti-vaccination-debate-study-finds-2

29

ADDITIONAL FUNCTIONS OF THE *RESPONSE* SUBSYSTEM OF THE PANDEMIC FUSION CENTER

THE FINAL FUNCTION OF THE integrated *Response* subsystem would be to ensure that the Federal portion of the pandemic response was working at a maximum operational effectiveness. Much like a severe weather-watch by a radar system, the constantly updated and refined results of the on-going computer modelling by the Management subsystem would be fed into the *Response* subsystem (Figure 40). There, skilled personnel would use this information to provide early impending local area warnings to the CDC and individual States to help ensure that the local authorities have their pandemic volunteers, surge personnel and Alternate Treatment Centers ready and functional.

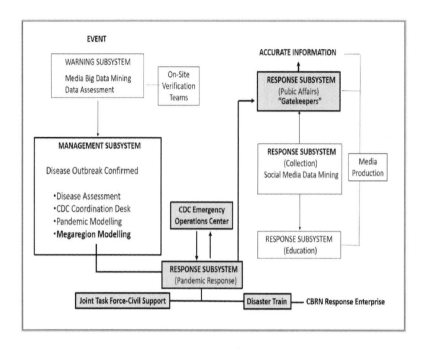

Figure 40. *Active Pandemic Response Component of the Pandemic Fusion Center.*

The Federal government has repeatedly stated that its domestic role in a national pandemic is essentially drug and medical item stockpiling, facilitating new vaccine and drug production and delivering all these items to the States. The logistics of the Strategic National Stockpile system is already well thought out and practiced. It could easily be co-ordinated by the *Response* subsystem and directed to the highest priority regions as identified by the Fusion Center's pandemic modelling. Working in conjunction with the CDC, the Fusion Center would release 6-hourly reports along with any other pertinent epidemic/pandemic information.

A final function of the Response subsystem is to deploy a waiting backup in case of a catastrophic preparedness failure with national security implications. As will be described, this capability would also give the CBRN Response Enterprise its own "All-Hazards" tool for a powerful response to a catastrophic but localized CBRN or explosive event, or if authorized, even a natural disaster such as a Cat 4 to 5 hurricane.

In a pandemic, it is the responsibility of a State's own local city authorities to manage their local disease outbreak themselves. This includes the problems of medical surge and patient care. However, if the local authorities fail in their pandemic planning, there will be little backup. Like with Hurricane Katrina in 2005, it will be the poor, high-density, low resource communities that will suffer the most in such a failure. The local Authorities cannot really manage these areas now, even under even normal circumstances. They will most certainly not have the resources to manage these areas during a pandemic crisis.

Speed is everything when responding to this type of situation and any delays in implementing countermeasures can have serious consequences. As the residents of an impoverished, low-resource community suffer a preparedness failure and they watch their neighbors, coworkers and family members become ill and some die around them, and all there will be is Federal and State advice to stay away from others, to frequently wash their hands, and if sick, stay home from work.

As we have outlined, these low-economic areas will have the worst per capita illness, hospitalization and fatality rates and will significantly contribute to a widespread dissemination of Influenza or other pandemic RNA viruses throughout the rest of a larger metropolitan area via daily personal interactions and the use of mass transit.[1]

Such a large-scale event might represent a threat to national security which would invite some degree of participation by NORTHCOM, the CBRN Response Enterprise and the Joint Task Force for Civil Support. Therefore, the *Response* subsection of the Pandemic Fusion Center needs a backup resource that is ready to be staffed and deployed within hours.

The front line of a military battlefield has some analogies to a large civilian mass casualty event, and it is useful to examine how the military has traditionally managed mass-casualties during wartime. More specifically during the human carnage generated by the two World Wars of the 20th Century.

It was not until the 1850's during the Crimean War, that a large scale, systematic method was developed to rapidly redistribute war casualties from an area of high concentration on the battlefield to a low concentration in the rear areas. The method used was the train, and an 8-mile military railway was constructed between Balaklava and Sevastopol to carry wounded soldiers from the front camp hospitals to definitive treatment hospitals in the rear.

Other armies adopted these British innovations in military medical treatment, and an organized system for railway ambulance transport was in extensive use by the time of the Italian-Austrian War of 1859, the Schleswig-Holstein war of 1864, the Austro-Prussian-Italian Conflict of 1866, and the Zulu War of 1879. Initially, these used a primitive "paillasse" system of thick straw-covered mattresses, to cushion wounded soldiers from the horizontal and lateral g-forces associated with rail transportation. By the late 1800's, the bamboo framed Collis-Dandy System had been developed for this purpose. The metal frame Bre'chot De'spres-Amelines or BDA stretcher-cushioning system later succeeded this.

By the close of the 19th Century, the British Empire found itself involved in an almost continuous series of small wars around the globe. By the time of the Boer War (1899-1902), advanced ambulance trains had been developed and placed at strategic intervals all along the South African railway system. There, they would gather the sick and wounded from the various military posts along the line.

By the outbreak of WWI, the first state-of the-art hospital trains had become operational. These were called "Trains Sanitaires", the early concept of the ambulance train had now effectively become a "hospital on wheels."

Each ambulance train was more like a small holding hospital made up of 5 ward coaches with 24 beds each, a kitchen coach, orderly room, and a first-class saloon coach for 2 doctors and 2 nurses.

The staff and kitchen coaches were fitted with 1800-gallon water tanks and the ambulance/hospital assembly could be hitched to a passing train locomotive and the patients offloaded down-rail at higher-level medical treatment facilities.[2] Each train could carry 800 patients and definitive medical treatment was provided on-board as the injured were transported to hospital locations on the west coast of France (Figure 41).

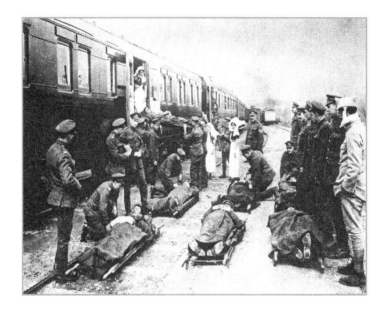

Figure 41. *Unloading a Hospital Train at a Definitive Care Site on the French Coast.*

By the first Battle of Ypres, over 1500 casualties a day were being evacuated by hospital trains passing through Villeneuve. This included patients with frostbite, infectious diseases, stretcher trauma cases, walking cases, and as well as patients requiring critical care. As the war progressed, hundreds of thousands of injured soldiers were transported by train from the battles of Neuve Chapelle, Loos, and the second battle of Ypres.[2]

However, it was during the Battle of the Somme that the hospital trains were used to their fullest advantage. During the 4-days encompassed by 1-4 July 1916, a total of 133,392 casualties were treated while moving from the battlefield to hospitals on the coast. These trains were made up of rail cars standardized to perform specific functions: surgery, surgical dressings, and a kitchen car which could serve 700 meals, stores, an office, a dispensary car, mess room, and accommodation for orderlies, nurses and doctors.

After WWI, hospital trains were put into service throughout the world. Greece adopted an adaptable system of covered hospital trailers which could be driven on and off railroad flatcars. In Romania, a special epidemic hospital train was used for service with the Serbian Divisions in South Russia. There some 1800 troops a day were bathed, and their clothing disinfected to stop a typhus epidemic.

Hospital trains were deployed in East Africa, Canada, India, and Sweden. They were used in 1922 by the British Red Cross in Turkey to alleviate refugee suffering where they provided a comprehensive service of tent, clothing and food drop offs, with health care delivery performed from the train. In May 1935, the Quetta earthquake killed over 23,000 people and two hospital trains were used to evacuate the seriously injured to Karachi. These early ambulance trains proved so successful that the concept was further refined. Consequently, Hospital trains found widespread use throughout the entire Second World War.

Four specially constructed trains were sent to France with the first British Expeditionary Force. Situated on special sidings, the trains were made up of different specialized railcars. Each train included 14 ward coaches for bedridden and sitting patients, kitchen cars, pharmacy cars, medical stores, general stores, office, and living quarters for doctors, nurses and orderlies. During the 10-day route and evacuation of British Forces from France. From 30 May to 10 June in 1940, these four hospital trains carried and managed an incredible 31,000 casualties.[2]

It was during WWII that developments in military aviation lead to the situation where mass casualties could be generated on home soil. Consequently, the British Ministry of Transport used 30 special casualty evacuation trains to quickly move civilian hospital patients from the cities subjected to heavy aerial bombardment.

The Casualty Evacuation trains designed for this purpose, were a standardized collection of 10 ward cars capable of carrying a total of 300 patients with a staff and kitchen car, a security car, and 2 break cars containing 300-gallon water tanks and medical item storage. Each train was staffed by a Medical Officer in Charge, a hospital staff officer, a hospital train officer, and 3 nurses, 10 auxiliary nurses, and 8 orderlies from the ambulance brigade. These trains were kept on 5 different sidings in the greater London area with their crews billeted in nearby accommodation. Subsequently, over 7,000 hospital patients were moved to the west of England.

By the end of World War II, from D-day to the end of the conflict in Europe, a total of approximately 250,000 civilian sick, infirmed, homeless, and post-fighting casualties had been transported by rail within the confines of the country.[2]

From 1952 onwards, the British Army of the Rhine maintained 3 hospital trains in Europe. Each train consisted of 11 special rail cars comprising an operating theater and ward, 1 kitchen car, 1 pharmacy coach, 5 general ward coaches, 1 compartment ward coach, and accommodation for medical officers and other ranks. The 51-foot long x 9-foot wide ward coaches were fitted with 36 bed frames modified to take stretcher cases and each train and could handle 200 lying and 50 sitting patients. These hospital trains remained in active service until 1964, when aeromedical evacuation techniques superseded rail transport for seriously injured soldiers.

With respect to modern times, a catastrophic infectious disease outbreak whether the result of a natural event or a biological warfare attack, is a problem of both rapid resource availability and medical command and control. The response requirements will vary depending on whether the infectious biological agent is highly person-to-person transmissible or not, and if a specific drug treatment, vaccine, or both are available. Therefore, any system that is employed must be flexible, largely self-contained, and operate directly under a streamlined, efficient, chain of command for deployment, relocation, and resupply.

A study of the use of Hospital Trains during the First and Second World Wars reveals several commonalities with other types of large-scale mass casualty events. This suggests that specialized "Disaster Trains" can provide a more simplified, cost-effective approach to dealing with not only severe pandemics, but also other natural large casualty-generating events as well.

Such a centralized "All Hazards" approach would make the "Disaster Train" a versatile, rapidly deployable, centralized, mass casualty response system affordable by even small states and nations.

The concept of a prepackaged "Disaster Train" is designed to provide a rapid response to an ongoing civilian mass casualty event before the local area medical services become overwhelmed.[3] This assistance is provided by rapidly bringing in the appropriate personnel, vehicles, emergency supplies, drugs, vaccines, and mortuary functions as a single mobile package.

The basic function of the Train is to rapidly provide a large coordinated medical "surge" capability if the hospitals in the disaster area are still functional, and to provide a "surge discharge" capability by transporting and relocating all existing stable hospital patients to care facilities outside the affected region (Figure 42). Conversely, the train can also be used as a stand-alone hospital facility while providing other capabilities such as augmenting the local area mortuary services.

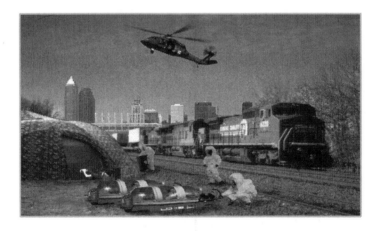

Figure 42. *The "Disaster" Train Rapidly Configured for a Response to a Large-Scale Chemical Incident.* Figure Credit; S. Hatfill, R. Coullahan

To accomplish its "surge discharge" function, the Disaster Train brings with it a series of specialized medical cars capable of quickly and safely transporting existing hospital patients en masse, including bed-ridden and critical cases without any interruption to their care. In this respect, the train carries its own supply of ambulances, along with fuel and support mechanics, to transport patients from full-capacity hospitals in the affected region back to the train for medically secure transport to alternate care facilities well outside the affected region.

Should the disaster area lack functioning hospitals, the Disaster Train can use its own commercially available *Expeditionary Force Provider Kit* to provide immediate housing for 150 patients or staff. This commercially available facility can be set up in as little as four-hours after the Train's arrival and it can support 150 people for a month without significant resupply. Its use is to temporarily house patients for re-triage before they are loaded onto the Train for re-location out of the affected area, or to house extra surge personnel that may later be brought into the disaster area.

Although rarely used, every "Disaster Train" that is created, will be a national strategic asset. As such, its caretakers should be composed of assigned military personnel operating within a rigid system of accountability and chain of command. Outside of its deployment for intermittent field exercises, the train would be kept at a guarded secure siding/warehouse location ready to respond at any time to a sudden national disaster.

The "Disaster Train" could be activated for a variety of federal requirements or rotated through parts of full-scale exercises for public health or CBRNE (Chemical, Biological, Radiological, Nuclear and Explosive) response programs.

Such a system not only provides an "All-Disaster" capability, but it can be specifically modified to provide a self-contained, comprehensive, on-site pandemic response to poor high-density low-resource inner areas during a severe Influenza pandemic.

This would be accompanied by a significant positive Public Affairs perception during a time of crisis.

THE COMPONENTS OF A SELF-CONTAINED "DISASTER TRAIN"

As seen in Figure 43, the design of a basic "Disaster Train" is centered around a *Core Component* capable of entering a metropolitan area with

240 highly trained *"surge"* response professionals on board. These would most likely come from the military's CBRN Response Enterprise.

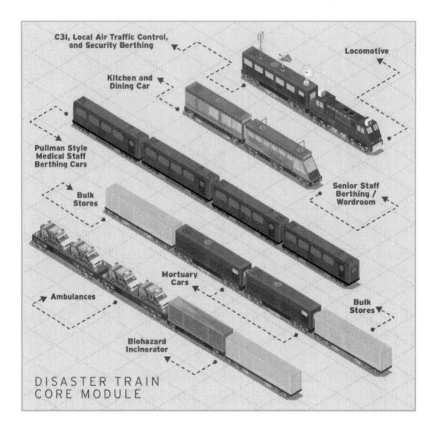

Figure 43. *Major Components of the Disaster Train.*

The front *of* the *"Disaster Train"* is composed of a Locomotive Control Car (Driving Trailer in Europe and the UK) that allows the train to be run in reverse with the locomotive at the back. This is common on commuter trains in the US and Europe and is important for serving areas without extensive switching facilities or having a turn-around.

The Locomotive Control Car is followed by a Command Car with state-of-the-art communications linked to the National Authorities and several consequence management databases for patient tracking and patient flow prediction. Communications with a national military-based logistical system is provided for a rapid and efficient resupply co-ordinated by the National Authorities. A small but well-armed National Guard security force is also carried on-board.

Once on site, the fully assembled Disaster Train could manage and relocate 280 ambulatory patients at a time, along with 512 general and surgical ward hospital patients and 40 critical care patients on life support. At the same time, the operating theaters of the Train are designed to support 12 simultaneous emergency surgical procedures. The Basic "Disaster Train" also transports two Mortuary cars with all the supplies and equipment necessary to process and embalm a total of 2700 fatalities at the disaster site; 20 at a time without resupply.

Depending on the nature of the event, the train can support emergency surgery while transporting casualties, or it can leave this surgical capability behind at its deployed *Expeditionary Force Provider* camp.

First Responder Berthing Cars

These "Pullman Sleeper-style" articulated passenger cars share passageways and are more-or-less attached to make movement between the cars safe and easy. These single-level cars have a minimum design-life of 40 years with an HVAC system that maintains each car interior between 68-72° F within the continental United States and Europe. Power can be supplied by either the train or an external source. The Berthing Cars transport and provide accommodations, hygiene, and feeding for the junior and senior operational, medical, and administrative staff of the on-board response. These personnel will provide a "surge" capability during a disaster. Some Pullman cars can be left at the disaster site for temporary on-site housing for the medical teams if necessary.

Hospital Bed Cars

Attached to these Critical Care cars are standardized Hospital Ward cars capable of safely transporting stable but bed-ridden patients, including orthopedic cases.

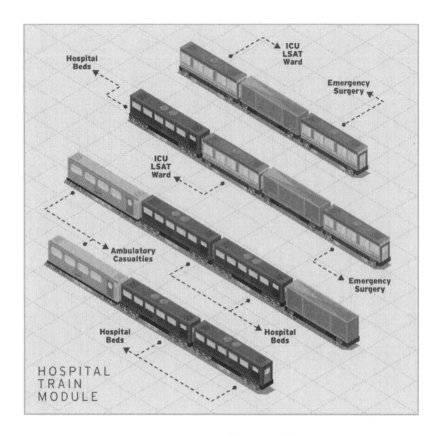

Figure 44. *Hospital Train Module.*

Mortuary Facility Cars

The core module of the Disaster Train can also transport multiple civilian or military *Mortuary Response Teams* (MRT) tasked to provide victim identification, body preparation and rapid embalming for the later dignified disposition of remains.

The core train transports two MRT cars with all the supplies and equipment necessary to process and embalm a total of 2700 fatalities without resupply (Figure 43).

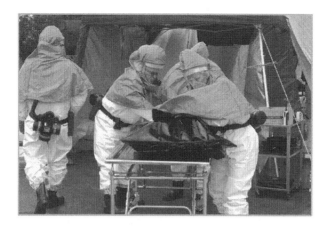

Figure 45. *DMORT Morticians and Pathologists wearing RACAL-Type Positive-Pressure Air Purifying Respirators while loading cadaver bags.* Photo Credit: Linda Wisniewski phe.gov

All MRT personnel would be trained to operate in a BSL-3 environment using BSL-4 procedures with strict whole-body decontamination (Figure 45). Bodies are identified, embalmed and placed into body bags for later dignified burial. Supplies include a pallets of low-cost flat-pack disaster coffins that can be quickly assembled.

Critical Care/ Surgery/ Hospital Bed Module Cars

The core portion of the Disaster Train will also contain 4 specialized modules, each with 3 operating rooms to perform stabilizing trauma surgery, and a high-level *Critical Care Car* (ICU) which can effectively manage 10 patients on modified Life *Support for Trauma and Transport* (LSTAT) stretchers.

The Life Support for Trauma and Transport (LSTAT™) (Figure 46) is a self-contained, stretcher-based miniature intensive care unit designed by Northrop Grumman for the US military to provide care for critically injured patients during transport and in remote settings where resources are limited.[4]

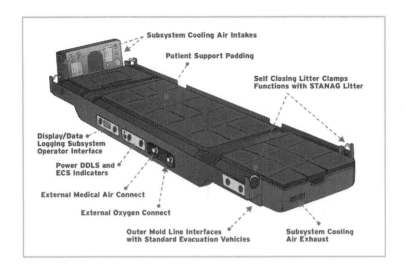

Figure 46. *The LSTAT (Life Support for Trauma and Transport) Stretcher. Northrop Grumman.*

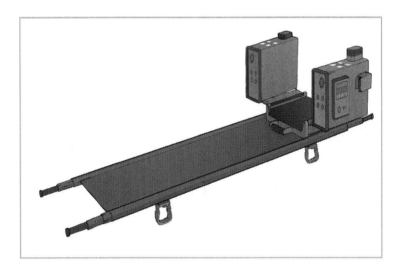

Figure 47. *A lower-cost abbreviated version for mass-casualty intensive care*

The LSTAT contains conventional medical equipment that is integrated into one platform and reduced in size to fit within the dimensional envelope of a North Atlantic Treaty Organization (NATO) stretcher. The system consists of a stretcher frame with a power module, mechanical ventilator, defibrillator, fluid drug infusion pump, oxygen, and non-invasive sensors for patient monitoring with data recording.

The LSTAT system is the basis for managing the redistribution of critical care patients on life support. For hospital relocation transport, critical care patients are brought to the on-site location of the Disaster Train already on the LSTAT stretchers carried by the ambulances the Train has brought with it. These patients on their LSTAT units are brought into the Critical Care Car and their stretcher is attached to a shock-absorber holding frame spanning the length of the unit. A 3-foot wide connecting thruway allows patient access on each side of stretcher holding frame.

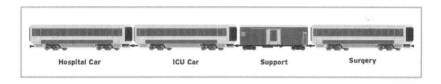

Figure 48. *Integrated Surgery, Recovery / ICU and Hospital Bed Unit.*

A total of 10 intensive care patients can be loaded on each Critical Intensive Care Car (ICU). Inside is a small workstation shared by 2 doctors, 12 nurses and 3 orderlies, and the patients are monitored from the displays on their individual LSTAT stretchers *crash cart* can be pulled out of this workstation and slid along a central floor track to an individual patient in distress.

The Critical Care Car is connected as a unit to a central pharmacy/storage/sluice room built into a connecting car. This Support Module also accesses the Surgical Car with its 3 small operating rooms through a central corridor (Figure 48). The Critical Care Car can also serve as a patient recovery area for post-surgical patients.

The Surgical Care Cars
Patterned after the *Lifeline Express Hospital Train* developed in India

for remote rural health care, each Disaster Train Surgical Care Car features 3 surgical operating theaters designed to U.S. Healthcare Code compliancy that can be state licensed and Joint Commission accredited. Each Operating Room (OR) on the train would meet a U.S. Class "C" standard for performing major and minor surgical procedures, Each OR is integrated with a Medical Gas System (O₂, Medical Air, and Vacuum) and a HEPA filtration system with 20+ air exchanges/hour.

The layout maximizes the internal space and the smaller previously described attached Support Car provides a lavatory (Optional), a Soiled Utility Room, a Clean Utility Room, medical storage and a Janitor's Closet.

Ambulatory Patient Cars

Up to 280 ambulatory patients can be transported in the core train's four PRIIA 305-003/Amtrak 964 Single-Level coach passenger rail cars. These cars have ground-level access at track-bed height for facilitated passenger movement.

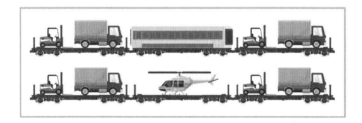

Figure 49. *National Stockpile Push Packs and Delivery System.*

Self-Contained National Pharmaceutical Stockpile

The "Disaster Train" carries a portion of the Strategic National Stockpile (SNS) sufficient for the train's area of responsibility, including a bulk store of standardized pharmaceuticals sufficient to supply a 200-bed hospital. An on-board pill packaging capability is combined with 4 delivery trucks and a helicopter for rapid pharmaceutical distribution to any still functioning local medical facilities (Figure 49). This stockpile can be resupplied by helicopter, ground, or by pallets air-dropped from military cargo planes. To avoid waste, all stored pharmaceuticals are drawn from the Strategic National Stockpile, stored on the train, and returned to the VA hospital system for use a year from their expiration date.

The Expeditionary Force Provider Kit

This portion of the Disaster Train can provide almost immediate housing for 150 surge support personnel or alternatively for its use as an Alternate Treatment Site. This is in the form of a military *Expeditionary Force Provider Kit*. Upon arrival at a selected site, this facility can be set up in the field and ready for occupation within *4 hours*.

The prepackaged containerized kit includes seven HVAC conditioned Air-Beam supported tents, satellite TVs, a dining facility tent, a hygiene tent with four washers/dryers, four seated latrines with showers, a kitchen and dining facility, and two power generators with a 30-day fuel supply.

Designed by the U.S. Army's Natick Laboratory, each $5 million kit is designed for weather ranging from 15 below zero to +120°F.

All system components are prepacked for efficiency in 25 TRICON containers with 3 units secured together to yield the same footprint and mobility as a 20-foot ISO intermodal container.

The *Expeditionary Force Provider Kit* is commercially available, and all subsystems have thirty-days of repair parts for initial operation.

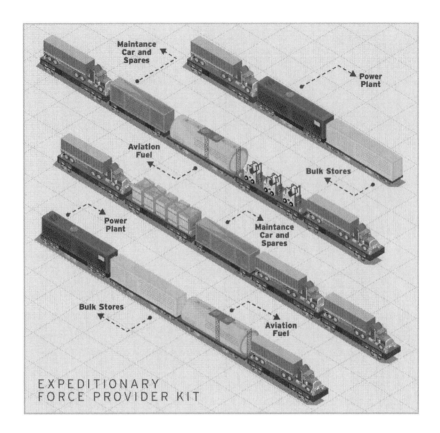

Figure 50. *Expeditionary Force Provider Kit*

The On-Site Logistics Module

This provides the Core Hospital Train with fuel, power, water, hazardous waste incinerators, and sewage facilities once it arrives on site. Depending on the scenario and incident severity, this basic provision can be supplemented before the train departs for the disaster area. For example, a rapid earthquake response would include extra rail cars carrying water, food, and tentage for survivors. These would be rapidly loaded from the associated warehouse at the train's permanent siding.

For self-sufficiency, this module also carries a variable number of low-bed trailers for drive-on-drive-off ambulances and other vehicular transport. These can be refueled from the on-board gasoline and diesel stores of the Logistics Module.

This gives the Disaster Train a self-contained capability to remain at a site for an extended period for direct medical support.

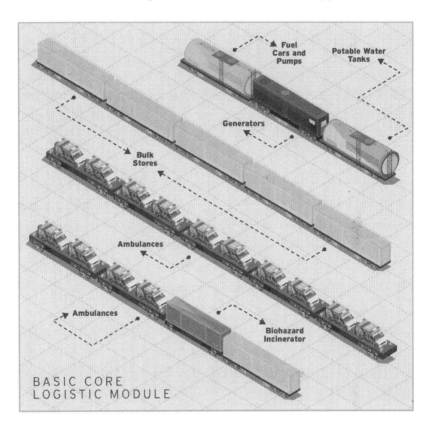

Figure 51. *Basic Core Logistic Module.*

OPERATION OF THE "DISASTER TRAIN" AS A COMPREHENSIVE MOBILE PANDEMIC RESPONSE UNIT

In this configuration, the train is designed to provide comprehensive on-site support to poor, high-density, low-resource communities during a severe 1918-type pandemic. Consequently, while it maintains a basic "Disaster Train" capability, its on-board personnel and capabilities are modified to accommodate this type of mission. As seen in Figure 52, during the very early stages of a pandemic, the prepackaged train will use a normal rail network to locate itself inside a poor community or as close to it as possible. Pre-selected streets are blocked off and a perimeter is set up. Within 4-hours of the Train's arrival, floodlights are set out, armed security is put in place, and the *Expeditionary Force Provider Kit* has been unloaded from the train, erected inside the perimeter, and is fully staffed from the train based on guidelines provided in the *Biological Warfare Improved Response Plan* (BWIRP).

The NEHC will also disperse small teams for door-to-door service for house calls on patients undergoing home care or patients too ill or to immobile to come to the Triage Clinic.

Again, these community outreach teams work closely with local community volunteers. This service would also supply meals prepared in the train's own kitchens to distribute to families where the household members are too ill to look after each other. Critically ill patients can be taken to the Intensive Care Cars of the train for ventilator support provided by the LSTAT stretcher beds. A separate train car is used for palliative care for severely ill patients that are expected to die. Upon death, the bodies are embalmed on-site using the train's Disaster Mortuary Facility.

The local NEHC is also where suspected Influenza cases arrive by either personal transport or by being picked up by the train's ambulances. These cases are registered and triaged at an on-site "Triage Clinic".

A "*Medi-Tag*" is attached for individual patient identification and history. This data is entered in a Medical Care Repository Database and transmitted to the National Authority. Personal effects are collected, inventoried and bagged. Patients that have been segregated with suspected influenza cases are assessed in one air-beam tent. The "worried well" and individuals with other medical conditions are assessed in a separate tent. Thus, the NEHC with its attached Triage Clinic serves as the gate point for patient entry into the nearby Acute Care Center (*Alternate Treatment Center*) where patients requiring definitive medical or palliative care are sent to be nursed. The Expeditionary Force Provider Kit is used for this purpose.

With periodic resupply, the train can function for weeks in a severe Influenza pandemic to provide a coordinated medical surge response to impoverished areas including the essential community outreach service.

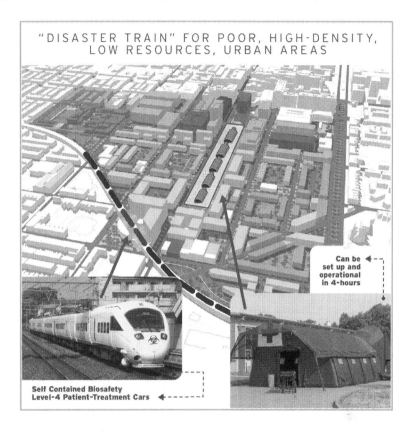

Figure 52. *Deployment of a Pandemic Disaster Train and Its Expeditionary Force Provider Kit to Set up an Alternate Treatment Center in a Poor, Disadvantaged Urban Area.*

There are other concerns that may be associated in a severe pandemic, and in some areas, food availability may be a major problem. The city of Chicago already has what are known as "Food Deserts" where there are no supermarkets or corner grocery stores within a reasonable distance of a poor high-density areas.[5] While there may be fast-food outlets in the area, these are dependent upon just-in-time deliveries which are highly vulnerable in pandemics.

To address this problem, the train would carry two dedicated Kitchen

Cars and one freezer car, together with delivery vehicles and multiple small portable propane-powered mini-kitchen sets that can be used to set up classical "Soup Kitchens" in buildings of opportunity. This is another example of the inherent flexibility of the disaster train concept and its ability to tailor-make a disaster response package that is specific and responsive to a particular catastrophic event.

When configured for a pandemic response, the train provides much more than just an Acute Care Center. The train's extensive communications systems in the Command Car and the emergency managers that it carries on-board, allows it to serve as the center of a Unified Incident Command System for the entire affected area.

Even more importantly, the train also carries on-board social workers and public health personnel that will work closely with local community leaders and residents to improve their Influenza health-literacy. This would greatly assist the rapid introduction of well-planned, evidence-based community measures needed to minimize Influenza transmission until a definitive drug treatment or a vaccine can be disseminated.[6,7,8,9]

The Problem of Casualties with Biosafety Level-4 (BSL-4) Emerging Infectious Diseases

Biosafety Level-4 (BSL-4) represents the highest level of precautions designed to protect scientists and health workers from contracting severe or fatal infectious for which there are no vaccines or treatments.[10,11] At the time of the 2014-16 West African crisis, the United States Army's small BSL-4 patient treatment facility was not available. Consequently, the risk of managing BSL-4 patients at a lower biosafety level quickly became apparent. Out of the 11 cases of Ebolavirus disease inside the United States, 2 were caused by the secondary infection of health care workers operating under lower biosafety conditions.

To deal with this problem, a "Disaster Train" could easily deploy with manufactured mobile BSL-4 containment facilities, each capable of transporting and managing 6 patients at a time. These have already been designed and built for FEMA, each as a self-contained

Magnahelical-controlled negative pressure container designed to operate at a minimum -0.10 Inch WC (-25 Pa) below the surrounding ambient air pressure (Figure 53).[12]

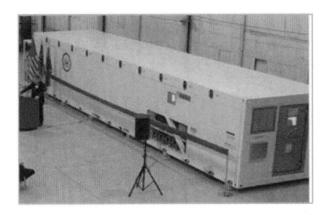

Figure 53. *FEMA Mobile Biological Patient Isolator (fema.gov).*

Although of limited use in their present configuration, with some modifications these FEMA isolators could be used for BSL-4 level care and transport. The medical personnel inside each isolator would wear an air-supplied full-body airtight protective suit kept under positive pressure, and they enter and leave the containment chamber through a decontaminating airlock via electrically interlocking doors. As previously mentioned in Chapter 27, they could also be adapted for use as a biologically secure laboratory.

Each of these modified isolators feature secure waste management, "dunk tanks," and pass-through autoclaves. Airflow is managed with HEPA (High Efficiency Particulate Air) filters with bubble tight isolation dampers. Duplicate stand-by power and air-handling systems are present for each container.

When combined with the deployment of a *second* Expeditionary Force Provider Kit, the "Disaster Train" could rapidly be configured into a mobile BSL-4 Isolation and Treatment unit capable of quickly deploying a self-contained 300 Bed Alternate Treatment Facility for patients with a suspected or confirmed BSL-4 level infection.

Alternatively, special Pullman cars could be constructed and connected to serve as fully mobile small BSL-4 Facility that could be brought into an outbreak area and left behind when the train departs. This would include a BSL-4 Level Diagnostic and Clinical Laboratory and a backup BSL-4 physical plant to include an incinerator unit for biohazardous waste and sewage.

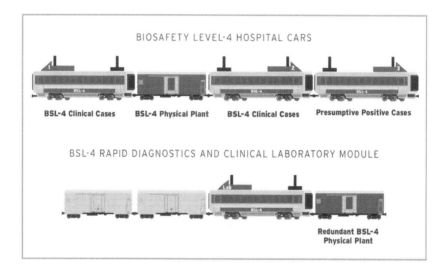

Figure 54. *BioSafety Level-4 Hospital Cars.*

While designed primarily for large-scale biological warfare attack on a major metropolitan area, the "Disaster Train" concept could provide an *All-Hazards* response with a rapid reconfiguration into a chemical, conventional explosive, hurricane, or radiological response with a large-scale burn management capability.

With its origin in biological warfare defense, the "Disaster" Train concept is easily adaptable to provide a comprehensive pandemic response to a large, poor-resourced disadvantaged metropolitan area. Such a system would have the following advantages over existing pandemic response planning efforts:

1. The Train would provide a secure central location to maintain and keep a constant inventory of a portion of the Strategic National Stockpile of medical supplies and equipment. This process includes a strict bi-annual Military Inspector General Audit with a recycling of drugs and other shelf-date supplies back into the Veterans Affairs Hospitals and Tri-Med health care systems before their expiration date.

2. The Train would provide a quick, secure method to transport a large supply of antibiotics, vaccines, protective equipment, medical equipment, and other supplies, into an affected urban area within a few hours of notification. For other rare types of catastrophic urban scenarios, the train could also transport refugee supplies of food, water, tentage, and other mass care items and supplies. This self-contained capability is envisioned to operate under a rigid and coordinated area Command and Control System under NORTHCOM and the National Guard Bureau and staffed via the CBRN Response Enterprise.

3. The Train would be able to transport large numbers of surge personnel into or close-to a disaster area in a physically secure manner, along with their self-contained long-term accommodations and ambulances for independent ground transportation.

4. The Train gives the ability to provide a rapid medical / surgical "surge discharge" capability to a local hospital by moving large numbers of sitting, stretcher, and critical care patients on life support, from congested poorly functioning urban hospitals to health care facilities well outside the affected region. This capability is largely independent of normal road transportation routes in and out of a city and casualties would remain on treatment during this process. Alternately, the Train can deploy its

Force Provider Kit in the form of a staffed, functional, Alternate Care Site for hospital bed overflow situations or as a specialized treatment center.

5. The use of standardized supplies, stores, and personnel yields a simplified on-site logistics plan coordinated by DoD military-civil support authorities already structured for such tasks in an emergency.

6. Existing Federal disaster organizations could easily be merged with this tangible asset.

7. The ability to use modified existing rolling railroad stock combined with advances in technology in the form of low-cost, modified life-support stretchers make this concept practical. Provisions for adding special-built rail cars for highly-infectious patients, rail cars for the storage of components of the National Pharmaceutical Stockpile, for mass mortuary capability, and for a multiple prepackaged rapidly deployable Alternate Care Sites, will all act to decrease the response time and increase the overall flexibility of this system.

8. The Disaster Train is designed to comprehensively interface with the active duty military, National Guard, Federal, State, and the local authorities involved in a pandemic response. It can quickly be positioned where or near it is most needed.

There are two major prerequisites for a successful "Disaster Train" system. The first is the availability of on-call *surge* medical personnel assigned to respond to a national disaster. With a mass trauma event, this would include general surgeons and anesthesiologists, internal medicine specialists, nurses, medical assistants, paramedics, pharmacists, lab technicians, and mortuary personnel.

In the case of a pandemic, this would involve pandemic-trained social workers, public health personnel, trained" pandemic responders", an augmentation of general medical and intensive care personnel, and an increased mortuary capability.

As mentioned, the CBRNE Response Enterprise encompasses approximately 18,000 DoD members assigned to respond to a catastrophic domestic incident with NORTHCOM in overall command and control. A "Disaster: Train would give this organization a powerful response tool to work with. Another approach would be to assign an Army Reserve MASH unit to NORTHCOM, give them infectious disease training, and use them to staff the train.

The second prerequisite for the Train is an effective Command and Control system than can integrate it into other on-going Federal, state and local emergency management efforts.Sponsored by the Defence Threat Reduction Agency, the DoD *Resource Augmentation for Civilian Consequence Management* (DRACCM) *Tool* is a relatively new software set that is capable of assessing the effect of CBRN exposures on civilian populations and medical infrastructures in order to inform DoD planners at the NORTHCOM / Joint Task Force for Civil Support level what additional resources might be required to support civilian authorities.[4]

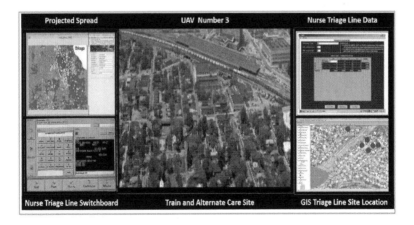

Figure 55. *Projected Real-time Fusion Display of Nurse-Triage Line Data for Use by the Disaster Train Outreach Teams.* Authors' Collection

The DRACCM package is envisioned to allow planners to calculate time-dependent casualties, and to assess beneficial the effects of medical countermeasures including the effects of non-ideal, late medical treatment. Models include chemical agent releases and Influenza with predictive resource shortfalls for civilian populations.

The tool can make predictive requirements for beds, ventilators, doctors, and other critical medical material, allowing a phase-in of needed medical resource augmentation packages from state, non-DoD Federal, and DoD sources. This would help direct the "Disaster" Train to effectively fill civilian gaps in medical staffing, materiel, and other personnel resources (Figure 51).[13]

Additional routing algorithms could help manage patient transport by the "Disaster" Train from high-density to low-density areas to evenly distribute casualties. Alternately, special routing algorithms could direct the *surge discharge* of existing stable hospital patients to Alternate Care Sites to free up hospital beds for newly arriving casualties.

The DRACCM software is also able to provide a quantitative analysis of a particular course of action while accurately predicting the flow of casualties to treatment centers over time and the amount of resources required to treat each patient. It is possible that with rigid contractor supervision, a Disaster Train could be economically assembled to serve as a significant asset for NORTHCOM and its CBRN Response Enterprise (CRE). The political and bureaucratic ramifications of this concept are extensive and outside the scope of this discussion. However, in a pandemic, a Disaster train(s) of this type would be a significant tool to minimize the critical problems caused by the vaccine gap, the lack of effective antiviral drugs, the lack of national medical surge capability, and the neglect in local planning for the largest poor low-resource communities in the United States.

As a final note, the first assembled "Disaster Train" would be an established piece of hardware rather than just a nebulous paper-response plan. As such, it could be used in practical field exercises to fully explore the potential of this type of response, establish its limitations, and delineate corrections for the inevitable deficiencies that are inherent in any new concept. This includes both the Train and its hypothesized NORTHCOM Fusion Center-based Command and Control System.

One annual exercise could involve the deployment of a fully staffed "Disaster Train" to perform a one-week NORTHCOM-sponsored MEDCAP full-service mission to areas of West Virginia, Ohio, or other poor *Gallup-Healthway's State of American Well-Being* populations that have a shocking current lack of health care for their communities. The Public Affairs advantages of this are self-explanatory.

It must be emphasized that there are worse things lurking in nature than another 1918-type pandemic. One acknowledged concern is a natural (or intentionally engineered) outbreak involving a recombinant strain of H5N1 or H7N9 Influenza that features a 40-60% mortality and an R_0 number higher than the 1918 H1N1 pandemic strain. An outbreak of this type would completely overwhelm all preparedness efforts to date- if a vaccine and an *effective* oral antiviral drug could not be rapidly dispensed to a majority of the U.S. population.

The human species is now living under historical population densities with increasing new infectious disease threats. This requires a change in the emphasis that we as a nation, place on public health and pandemic mitigation. Based on numerous continuing GAO Reports and Testimony, as well as real world events, the current Federal planning for a mass casualty biological event is only minimally functional for the poor, high-density, low-resource communities of many major metropolitan regions. The question then to be asked then, is if the United States does not employ a "Disaster Train" System, then what other method can provide such an adaptable, centralized, fast-response capability at an affordable cost to communities with failed local planning during a severe 1918-type pandemic?

*One can consider the assistance that a Disaster Train would
have provided if one has been available to support the 1918*

*slum areas of Philadelphia where it would have operated under
a military chain-of-command within a National Incident
Management System.*

*A successful improved integrated Pandemic Fusion Center for
global infectious disease surveillance would represent a major
advance in Public Health, and it could be crucial for fostering
the early containment of the next lethal pandemic outbreak in
the United States.*

Notes for Chapter 29

1 *America's Forgotten Pandemic*: The Influenza of 1918, Alfred W. Crosby Paperback, Second Edition, 2003 by Cambridge University Press. (ISBN0-521-54175-1).

2 Plumridge, John H., *Hospital Ships and Ambulance Trains*, Seeley; First edition (1975) ISBN-10: 0854220879, ISBN-13: 978-0854220878.

3 Starbuck ES, Koepsell J. *Are we prepared to help low-resource communities cope with a severe influenza pandemic?* Influenza Other Respiratory Viruses 2013; 7(6):909–913 (http://onlinelibrary.wiley.com/doi/10.1111/irv.12040/epdf).

4 Johnson, K., Pearce,F., et.al *Clinical evaluation of the Life Support for Trauma and Transport (LSTAT) platform*, Crit. Care. 2002; 6(5): 439–446. Jul 10. doi: 10.1186/cc1538 PMCID: PMC130145

5 Examining the Impact of Food Deserts on Public Health in Chicago. www.agr.state.il.us/marketing/ILOFFTaskForce/ChicagoFoodDesertReportFull.pdf

6 Pandemic Influenza: Community Planning and Response Curriculum for Community Responders, Volunteers, and Staff. Humanitarian Pandemic Preparedness (H2P) initiative, July 2009 https://www.cdc.gov/nonpharmaceutical-interventions/tools-resources/published-research.html).

7 Centers for Disease Control and Prevention. Interim pre-pandemic planning guidance: community strategy for pandemic influenza mitigation in the United States—early, targeted, layered use of nonpharmaceutical interventions. Atlanta, GA: US Department of Health and Human Services, CDC; 2007. https://stacks.cdc.gov/view/cdc/11425.

8 Qualls. N, Levitt A, Kanade N, et al. Community Mitigation Guidelines to Prevent Pandemic Influenza — United States, 2017. MMWR Recom Rep 2017; 66(No. RR-1):1–34. DOI: http://dx.doi.org/10.15585/mmwr.rr6601a1

9 The Flu: Caring for Someone Sick at Home, US CDC, Feb. 2013 (http://www.savethechildren.org/publications/technical-resources/avian-flu/).

10 "Section IV-Laboratory Biosafety Level Criteria". Biosafety in Microbiological and Biomedical Laboratories, 5th ed. (PDF). U.S. Health and Human Services. December 2009, pp. 30–59.

11 Mark R. Withers, George W. Christopher, Steven J. Hatfill, and Jose J. Gutierrez-Nunez, Chapter 11, "Aeromedical Evacuation of Patients with Contagious Infections" In Aeromedical Evacuation; Management of Acute and Stabilized Patients". Eds. William Hurd, John Jernigan. Springer Press.

12 Chui, P. Chong, B., Wagener, 2007, Applied Biosafety, Vol. 12, No. 4, pp 238-244

[13] DoD Resource Augmentation for Civilian Consequence Management (DRACCM) Tool Defense Threat reduction Agency DTRA-TR-15-17 July 2015 DTRA01-03-D-0014

30

THE CONCEPT OF PREDICTIVE VIRAL FORECASTING

AS OUTLINED IN THE BEGINNING CHAPTERS, the ability of an animal virus to infect man and acquire a capability for efficient person-to-person spread is not a straightforward proposition. It involves many factors. Some of these pertain to the environment and some of these involve human social structures and behavior (*the seed and the soil concept*).[1] Some of these factors remain ill-defined and poorly understood.

The ability to make a reasonable prediction of when a virus is getting ready for a species jump into humans would have large implications for preparedness. For human Influenza, we have already outlined how the WHO, CDC, and other international public health agencies participate in a *Global Influenza Surveillance and Response System* (GISRS). Each year, this early predictive warning system uses global Influenza virus isolates in an attempt to determine 6-months ahead of time, what actual Influenza strains will be dominant in the upcoming year. This is used to determine what type of a seasonal vaccine should be mass produced.

Because of the multiplicity of the various factors involved, these annual predictions for the north and south hemispheres may be only partially right or even completely wrong. However, the system does provide some degree of international surveillance for more lethal strains of this bird virus.

RNA "VIRAL TRAFFICKING"

Outside of Influenza, a small number of scientists and research groups are working to create a surveillance system for other animal RNA viruses.[2,3,4]

In Chapter Two we outlined the concepts of *Viral Spillover* and *Viral Trafficking* between different animal species as a basic biological mechanism for new human Emerging Infectious Disease (EID) outbreaks. The hypothesis is that if an RNA virus is naturally trafficking between two or more different non-human mammalian species, it may be prone for a species jump into humans with efficient human to human secondary transmission.[5,6,7]

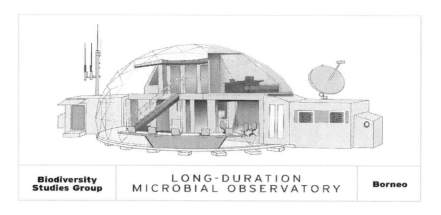

Figure 56. *Standardized Isolated "Microbial Observatory" For Predictive Global EID Surveillance.*

As a first step towards studying this concept for "predictive" EID surveillance, a small prototype laboratory should be set up in a region under high-risk for EID emergence under our current understanding. The purpose of this laboratory would be to test the equipment, techniques, and procedures for the possible real-time prediction of an actual human outbreak (Figure 56). The overall dynamics suggest that a surveillance system tailored to detect a wild-type virus in more than one species of host animal in the same environment, might be predictive for its impending jump into humans.[5,7]

To validate this hypothesis, the question becomes one of which viruses to look for, which animals to monitor for viral trafficking and in what area of the world should such a validating study be undertaken?

DEVELOPING A PROTOTYPE VIRAL FORECASTING SYSTEM

More than 20 virus families contain some strains that are pathogenic to humans, however, it is interesting that only 4 of these RNA virus families account for 65% of all the viruses that affect humans. These same 4 viral families also constitute more than half of all the currently known human viral EID.

This suggests a starting point for which viruses to examine. These families are the *Bunyaviruses, Flaviviruses, Togaviruses* and *Reoviruses*.[5,7] Because of the medically important members of the *Orthomyxoviruses, Rhabdoviruses, Coronaviruses* and *Filoviruses*, these should be examined as well. The *Hepeniviridae* and the *Paramyxoviridae* viral families should be examined as well.

The question as to which animal species should be examined for the presence of the trafficking of these viruses can also be answered. Out of the 4629-known species of mammals on Earth, rodents represent the largest Order with 2,277 different species. Bats represent the second largest Order of mammals with 1,240 species subdivided into the fruit-eating "flying foxes" and the smaller insectivorous bats.[5,7]

Together, the rodents and bats account for 75% of all the known mammalian species and both are known to transmit serious EID viral infections to humans. Their rich species diversity, social organization, and high population densities suggests that a predictive surveillance effort focused on rodents and bats would have high potential value.

Because arthropod vectors transmit some RNA viruses, a secondary project would be to collect and examine a region's insects to characterize these viruses in the region under study. As witnessed by the origin of the HIV/AIDS virus, the local non-human primate population in an area represents another important target for surveilling viral traffic.

Finally, there will need to be a method to screen the resident human population. This might be done by taking informed blood samples when the local inhabitants attend rural clinics for other health issues.

RT-PCR / DNA Microarray Technology

DNA Microarrays can provide an unprecedented enhancement for conducting on-site microbial surveys in harsh remote areas.[8,9] Until recently, performing such host-range surveys would have been a daunting task needing large teams of investigators and weeks of laboratory work to assess the viral background of the different species of mammals and insects in a region. However, advances in DNA Microarray technology now make such studies feasible. Collected biomedical samples may include animal blood and tissue, stool, saliva, crushed insect samples, soil, water, and vegetation. Hundreds of different pathogens can be scanned for simultaneously in these samples with results available within 23-hours from the start of analysis. DNA Microarray systems provide an unprecedented ability to conduct viral surveys in remote areas and in many cases, they allow identification to the strain and sequence level, yielding a possible genetic profile of all viruses in a sample.

The Affymetrix Axiom® Microbiome System is an example of how microarray technology can provide an unprecedented ability to conduct microbial surveys. This microbiome array is used by scientists to examine the normal human gut microflora and it allows identification to the species, strain and sequence level, yielding a genetic profile of all the microorganisms present in a stool sample. It has a comprehensive coverage of over 11,000 organisms across five microbial domains including the archaea, the bacteria, fungi, protozoa, and viruses. This type of technology promises to revolutionize field epidemiological studies.

Continuous small teams of multidisciplinary scientists would staff the proposed prototype jungle laboratory to initially characterize the normal host range of the endogenous animal viruses in its geographical area. When complete, this research will progress into a predictive "viral forecasting" program as the area is closely monitored for any changes of viral host range in the bat and rodent population of the region. To aid this process, a small number of captive laboratory animals would be housed in open but screened confinement in the jungle, to be used as "sentinel species."

To elucidate zoonotic viruses that are still unknown to science, pooled species samples can be subjected to random multiplex (RT)-PCR with 3'-locked random primers and the product sent to internationally designated reference laboratories for further analysis.[10] This data would then be used to add any new viruses to the Microarrays. When combined together, the use of these techniques will give the on-site laboratory the ability to act as a "microbial observatory" or "listening post."

THE USE OF FLOATING LABORATORIES

The tropical jungle represents a unique environment for scientific study, but it is one with numerous problems with respect to equipment maintenance, reagent and specimen cold chains, communication difficulties, heat with high humidity, tropical diseases, fast water crossings, multi-platform resupply requirements, and difficult overland movements.

One alternative would be a shallow draft, littoral/riverine research vessel. Such a floating, self-contained platform would have enough space for designated laboratories, liquid nitrogen generation for specimen archiving, and comfortable accommodation for up to 8 scientists with an administration office, library, and satellite internet access to the main scientific journals (Figure 57). The purpose of such a vessel would be to provide comfortable accommodation as well as the insertion, extraction, and logistical support of the inland research personnel involved with animal trapping and biomedical sample collection, and the molecular biologists involved in the study of viral host range and viral trafficking (including the Influenza viruses).

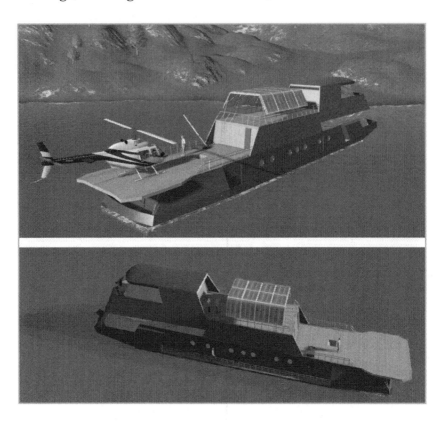

Figure 57. *Standardized Low-Latitude Research Vessel (LLRV) Designed as a Long-Duration Floating Microbial Observatory or "Listening Post" For New RNA Viral Emergence.* Credit: Asymmetrical Biodiversity Studies and Observation Group

The main advantage of using a littoral platform is the fact that by being mobile, it can relocate to study the range of micro-ecologies found in both native jungle and the encroached, fragmented, wildlife jungle reserves. Its disadvantages are that it is restricted to operating only in biodiversity hotspots that feature long navigable rivers. Because this vessel may be operated more remotely than a land-based facility, it carries a Medical Treatment Facility including a pharmacy and a small operating room for acute emergencies.

In addition, its Command Center has facilities for weather monitoring, precise electronic navigation, and an extensive communications suite. It can also support the rotary wing aeromedical evacuation of personnel suffering from a serious medical condition or trauma. The design of the vessel features safe waste management, water purification, interior climate control, and twin motor propulsion. Its cargo handling and storage system is designed to support continuous operations by up to 8 personnel for 3-months without any external resupply.

Long rivers such as the Amazon in South America or the Kinabatangan in Borneo, are characterized by scattered areas of high-density human habitation along the riverbanks.

One un-intentioned capability that emerges from the use of a littoral/riverine research vessel, is the fact that it could also be part of the response to a sudden outbreak of a new EID. During such an event, the research vessel would provide a high-technology focal point for disease characterization. Its on-board communication system would facilitate a unified incident command of the outbreak response by the host nation. In addition, it could provide contingency accommodation for host nation authorities.

If the concept is validated, a series of standardized land-based or floating "microbial observatories" could be deployed to other biodiversity hotspots using international scientific personnel and funding, with collected virus samples shared with collaborating laboratories specializing in whole viral genome sequencing for longitudinal genomic analyses. The goal is to conclusively demonstrate that a predictive "viral forecasting" system is possible. Shared collation of the resulting data over time may help elucidate the actual molecular mechanisms that drive viral cross-species jumps into man.

While this proactive approach to Global Public Health is still highly experimental, it rests on a body of peer-reviewed scientific research as well as several successful previous small efforts by other groups. The question now is where should the first prototype EID surveillance system be located?

THE KINABATANGAN FLOODPLAIN REPRESENTS A NATURAL LABORATORY FOR EID RESEARCH

To develop a predictive capability for detecting viral species jumps, it is important to consider where to look. Published research indicates that the ideal place to study "viral trafficking" would be in an equatorial "biodiversity hotspot" that still has a diverse number of animal species at a high density, together with an encroaching local human population.[5,11,12,13,14]

Under ecological threat since the 1950s, the Kinabatangan Floodplain is a "biodiversity hotspot" that is located on the east coast of the Malaysian State of Sabah in Borneo, surrounding the 560 kilometer Kinabatangan River.[15] This is the second longest river in Malaysian national territory and arguably the last forested alluvial floodplain in Asia. Much the native forested land in this area has been converted for agricultural development, mainly in the form of palm oil plantations.

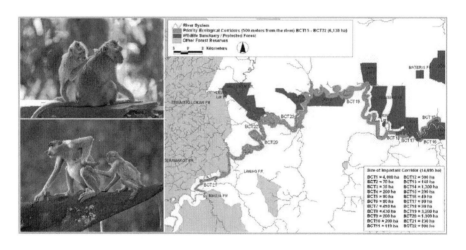

Figure 58. *The Kinabatangan Wildlife Sanctuary and Corridor of Life.*

However, in 2005, some 26,000 ha were set aside as the Kinabatangan Wildlife Sanctuary, crowding the resident endangered wildlife into a patchwork of primary and secondary forests with nearby encroaching human habitation.

The region currently fosters 1,056 species of plants, 300 different

species of birds, a variety of amphibians and reptiles and a diverse collection of mammalian species.[15] The largest cave system in Sabah is in
this region with an accompanying multi-species bat population. In addition, the Kinabatangan Rainforest is one of only two places on Earth
where 11 different primate species (including humans) can be found
together. This represents an almost perfect viral "mixing bowl."

A growing amount of data indicates that tropical areas that are subjected to ecological or demographic changes such as an expanding human population, deforestation, and changes in land use, can precipitate
enhanced viral trafficking between species and the possible outbreak of
an emerging zoonotic infectious disease. All these risk factors are occurring in the Kinabatangan floodplain in addition to an unnatural,
overcrowded, high multi-species primate density. This makes this region under high threat for EID emergence and a natural laboratory for
the study of viral trafficking of new emerging RNA viruses.

SUMMARY

Outbreaks of previously unknown or rare infectious diseases are occurring with an ever-increasing frequency as previously unknown viruses jump from their normal animal hosts into man. This is typically without warning and often with fatal dramatic results. It is essential to better understand how these new viruses emerge to cause human disease. The concept of "viral trafficking" suggests that a study of the normal viral diversity and host range in the rodents and bats living in a tropical biodiversity hotspot, may be able to detect regional alterations in the normal viral "ecology", and hence a predictive increased risk for a new infectious virus to enter a surrounding human population.

To validate this concept, a small, standardized prototype "Microbial Observatory" should be established on the Kinabatangan floodplain to detect viruses that are undergoing species trafficking as a prelude for a possible species jump into man.

If validated, such a predictive capability could be expanded to enhance the biological security of regional high-density areas in both the Americas and Asia, as well as help train the next generation of infectious disease researchers.

Notes for Chapter 30

[1] Morse, S.S. Factors in the emergence of infectious disease. Emerg Infect Dis. 1995; 1:7-15. [PMC free article] [PubMed]

[2] Wolfe ND, Daszak P, Kilpatrick AM, Burke DS. Bushmeat hunting, deforestation, and prediction of zoonosis emergence. Emerg Infect Dis. 2005; 11:1822–1827. [PMC free article] [PubMed]

[3] Sintasath DM, Wolfe ND, Zheng HQ, et.al. Genetic characterization of the complete genome of a highly divergent simian T-lymphotropic virus (STLV) type 3 from a wild Cercopithecus mona monkey. Retrovirology. 2009; 6:97. [PMC free article] [PubMed]

[4] Zheng H, Wolfe ND, Sintasath DM, et.al., Emergence of a novel and highly divergent HTLV-3 in a primate hunter in Cameroon. Virology.2010; 401:137–145. [PMC free] [PubMed]

[5] Parrish, C.R., Edward C. Holmes, E.C., David M. Morens, D.M., Park, E.C., Burke, S., et.al. Cross-Species Virus Transmission and the Emergence of New Epidemic Diseases, Micro and Mol Bio. Rev.2008.

[6] Morse, S., Mazet, J.A.K., Woolhouse, M., Parrish, C.R., Carroll, D., Karesh, W.B., Zambrana-Torrelio,C., Lipkin,W,I., Daszak, P., Prediction and prevention of the next pandemic zoonosis, Lancet. 2012 Dec 1; 380(9857): 1956–1965.

[7] Flanagan, M.L., C. R. Parrish, C., S. Cobey, S., Glass, G., R. M. Bush, R., and Leighton T. J. Anticipating the Species Jump: Surveillance for Emerging Viral Threats, Zoonosis Public Health, 2012 May; 59(3): 155–163. doi: 10.1111/j.1863-2378. 2011.01439.x

[8] Eunice C. Chen, Steve A. Miller, Joseph L. DeRisi, Charles Y. Chiu Using a Pan-Viral Microarray Assay (Virochip) to Screen Clinical Samples for Viral Pathogens J Vis Exp. 2011; (50): 2536. Published online 2011 Apr 27. doi: 10.3791/2536 PMCID: PMC3169278 PMID: 21559002
https://www.ncbi.nlm.nih.gov/pmc/articles/PMC3169278/

[9] Renois F, Talmud D, Huguenin A, Moutte L, Strady C, et.al. Rapid detection of respiratory tract viral infections and coinfections in patients with influenza-like illnesses by use of reverse transcription-PCR DNA microarray systems. J Clin Microbiol. 2010 Nov; 48(11):3836-42. doi:10.1128/JCM.00733-10. Epub 2010 Aug 25. https://www.ncbi.nlm.nih.gov/pubmed/20739481

[10] Clem, A.L., Sims, J., Telang, S., Eaton, JW., Chesney, J., Virus detection and identificationusing random multiplex (RT)-PCR with 3'-locked random primers, Virol Journal, 2007, 4:6

[11] Lederberg J. Infectious disease - an evolutionary paradigm. Emerg Infect Dis 1997; 3:417-23.

[12] Morse, S., Mazet, J.A.K., Woolhouse, M., Parrish,C.R., Carroll, D., Karesh, W.B., Zambrana-Torrelio,C., Lipkin,W,I., Daszak, P., Prediction and prevention of the next pandemic zoonosis, Lancet. 2012 Dec 1; 380(9857): 1956–1965.

[13] Myers, N., R. A. Mittermeier, C. G. Mittermeier, G. A. B. da Fonseca, and J. Kent. Biodiversity hotspots for conservation priorities. 2000, Nature, 403:853-858

[14] Woolhouse M, Scott F, Hudson Z, Howey R, Chase-Topping M (2012) Human viruses: discovery and emergence. Royal Society Philosophical Transactions Biological Sciences, 367: 2864–2871.

[15] Kinabatangan Corridor of Life Fact Sheet, 2007.

EPILOGUE

N **1918, A LETHAL STRAIN** of the Influenza Group A virus suddenly appeared in the United States. Over the following 12-months, it infected one-fourth of the total US population and globally it killed up to an estimated 100 million people. It was the third deadliest plague in recorded human history.

Each year as a public service, the Robert Wood Johnson Foundation (Johnson and Johnson) analyzes the overall individual health security in each state to prepare a *Health Security Preparedness Index* (NHSPI). Here, public health security is defined as the ability to minimize the threat and impact of a crisis that endangers the collective health of the U.S, population. The most likely cause of such an event is a pandemic RNA virus with no treatment or vaccine. In this respect, the NHSPI is the first national index that collectively measures the preparedness of each individual state and then gives a performance aggregate for national preparedness. The Index includes 129 measures that are grouped into six broad domains.

The 2019 release of the Index is the sixth in a series of annual data releases and it reveals that the U.S. readiness for a lethal pandemic remains far from optimal (6.7 out of a scale of 10). Large differences in state health security persist with clusters of states in the South-Central, Upper Mountain West, Pacific Coast, and Midwest regions lagging significantly behind the rest of the nation.

Some 39 percent of the U.S. population now reside in states with below-average health security levels. The number of States with a previous above-average health security Index fell from 34% in 2017, to just 19 percent in the latest Index release. This includes the states of North Carolina, Kentucky, Pennsylvania, Minnesota, and Iowa. The lowest index scores for all the states were in the areas of community planning and health care delivery, as well as environmental health and worker protection.[1] Although improvements have been made since 2013, the nation's weakest area of preparedness is developing the necessary supportive relationships between government agencies, community organizations, and individual residents, and in engaging these entities in emergency planning.

The study found that the hospitals in most states have a high degree of participation in the new DHHS concept of *Healthcare Coalitions*. These Coalitions bring hospitals and other healthcare facilities together with the inclusion of emergency management and public health officials. This is to respond to health events requiring extraordinary action.

However, over the past six years the above-average states in the Preparedness Index have become more geographically clustered and isolated from the below-average states. This clustering has created challenges by making it more difficult for the above-average states to offer mutual aid to neighboring below-average jurisdictions during a lethal pandemic.

The 2019 Index states that overall, health security in the United States is very slowly improving but it is at an uneven pace, leaving large segments of the American population under-protected. A number of states are losing health security and others are failing to keep pace with advances in policy and practice. The problems in Local Authority public health planning have already been discussed in Chapter 13.

During its layered top-down approach to national pandemic

planning, the U.S. government has seriously underestimated the ability of the State and Local Authorities to optimally manage a lethal Influenza outbreak in their communities. The current gaps and shortfalls in pandemic readiness are manifold, despite multiple iterations of organizational change and the formation of entirely new Federal Departments and Agencies since 2001. Over a decade of ever-changing "flip-flopping" of high-level federal guidance on even the simplest issues such as when to use a HEPA-filter mask, (now called a "respirator"), is indicative of a poorly functioning federal bureaucracy.

Senior Federal Agencies have failed to address critical issues in pandemic preparedness in a timely and coherent manner. Additionally, a combination of increasing global population numbers and the increasing level of American urbanization, as well as economic globalization and just-in-time inventories, have all combined to cause a serious set of new pandemic problems that were not a factor in 1918.

This places into question the effectiveness of the current National Pandemic Influenza Response Plan for anything except the care of the federal government, the military, some federal and state employees, senior state politicians and their staff, and a limited number of essential civilian personnel who will struggle to maintain medical and other essential services during a severe pandemic.

During such an event, the local/regional hospitals will become overwhelmed. Even worse, a minimum of some 123 million Americans will receive nothing in the way of antiviral medications or vaccines until the peak of the pandemic wave has almost passed.

Current planning continues to ignore the special needs of the economically poor, high-density, low resource communities in our 120 largest cities who will be affected the worst in a 1918-type event. As has been mentioned, the inhabitants of these areas will watch their neighbors, coworkers, or family members become ill and some will die around them, and all there will be is federal and state advice to stay away from others, to frequently wash their hands, and if sick, to stay home from work.

It is important to realize that another 1918-type pandemic event will happen again. It could be this time next year or 20-years from now, but it will happen, and it could conceivably involve an Influenza A strain that is much worse than in 1918. Conversely, it could involve a completely new, emerging, and even more lethal viral respiratory pathogen.

However, there is still hope for the basic U.S. Pandemic Influenza Response Plan. There is recent progress towards developing new and more effective Influenza vaccines and the ability to produce these based on cell culture technology. This is way past due. Progress is also being made in the development of new effective antiviral drugs that are much less likely to undergo viral resistance during a pandemic.

It is now time to concentrate on a strong, focused, bottom-up approach to pandemic preparedness. This should begin with the local neighborhoods, then up to communities, then to towns and cities, up to the counties, and States. This is what a Unified National Pandemic Influenza Response Plan should contain.

Planning is essential, but nothing ever goes according to plan. Therefore, flexibility and routes for alternate decision making are essential, as well preparing a catastrophic backup capability. We have suggested one of these in the form of establishing several regional multi-functional "Disaster Trains" operated by the US military as part of its NORTHCOM / Joint-Task Force for Civil Support mandate.

We now live under population densities that are a new phenomenon in human civilization and we have no precedent to indicate if we are nearing a threshold or not. As a consequence, every individual alive today is participating in an on-going global biological experiment. With no idea what will happen over the next 50-years. It would be prudent to prepare for the worst while we have the economy to do so.

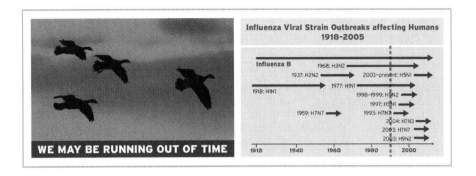

We must hope that our technology and social organization can advance further before the next severe lethal pandemic event occurs. Upon examining the increasing frequency of micro-outbreaks of new strains of the Influenza A virus, we may not have long to wait.

Steven Hatfill MD. MS. MS. M.Med
Robert Coullahan MS. CEM
John Walsh PhD

NOTES FOR THE EPILOGUE

[1] 2019 National Health Security Preparedness Index. https://nhspi.org/tools-resources/2019-key-findings/nhspi_2019_key_findings/

ABOUT THE AUTHORS

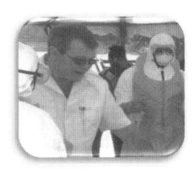

DR. STEVEN HATFILL is a specialist physician and a virologist with a military background and separate master's degrees in microbial genetics, radiation biochemistry, and experimental pathology. His medical fellowships include Oxford University, the NIH in Bethesda, and the NRC where he studied the Ebola Virus at the US Army Medical Research Institute for Infectious Diseases. His background includes training/certification as a UN Weapons Inspector and over a decade of teaching the emergency medical response to blast and ballistic injury. In 2015, he trained and helped to establish the Rapid Hemorrhagic Fever Response Teams for the National Disaster Medical Unit in Kenya, Africa. He has numerous peer-reviewed scientific publications. In 2018, he was awarded Honorary U.S. Army Parachute Wings with Bronze Star, in an exchange ceremony between the U.S. Army 1st Special Warfare Training Group (Airborne) and a former Regiment of an African Army. He is a National Fellow of the Explorers Club, a board member of several non-profit medical organizations and an Adjunct Assistant Professor in two departments at a leading US Medical School.

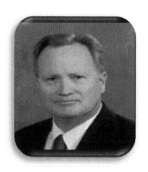

ROBERT J. COULLAHAN is the President of Readiness Resource Group Incorporated (RRG) which he founded in 2007. He has over 40-years of experience in U.S. preparedness, critical infrastructure protection, and technology development. In 9-years of military duty, he supported RDT&E at Redstone Arsenal and White Sands with active deployments to Southeast Asia. He holds an M.S. in Telecommunications, an MA in Security Management from the George Washington University and is a graduate of the Univ. of California. He is board certified in Emergency Management (CEM) and Security Management and served 20-years as a Senior Vice President at SAIC overseeing the Homeland Security Operations, NIMS, and Bioterrorism initiatives. He was Report Manager for the NG Bureau CBRN Enterprise Study, Co-Chair of the Infectious Diseases Working Group with AFMIC at Fort Detrick and leads programs supporting FEMA, the NG, DOE, National Laboratories, and critical infrastructure operator risk/resilience assessment /emergency management.

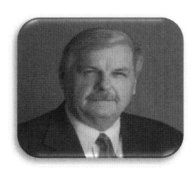

DR. JOHN J. WALSH, JR., PHD is Co-Director of the Vanderbilt University Medical Center Program in Disaster Research and Training. His specialty fields include disaster research in emergency management, preparedness policy, and human/organizational factors influencing disaster operations. He currently serves as the IAEM representative on the EMS Agenda 2050 Project. He is a founding member of the NESC on Medical Preparedness and is the current chair of IAEM's Credentials Committee.

He holds a MEP certification, is a Certified Healthcare Emergency Professional (CHEP), with a National Disaster Healthcare Certification in the specialty of Disaster Preparedness, Response, Mitigation and Recovery for the ANCC, and is listed on the ANCC Content Expert Registry. He is the former Assistant Director of the LSU Academy of Counter-Terrorist Education. Dr. Walsh is the recipient of the U.S. Department of Homeland Security, Under Secretary's Award for Program Support, Office of Weapons of Mass Destruction, Science & Technology Directorate.

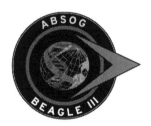

ASYMMETRIC BIODIVERSITY STUDIES AND OBSERVATION GROUP

threesecondsuntilmidnight.com
srjhatcoulwalsh@gmail.com

Printed in Great Britain
by Amazon

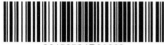